Progress in
Coronary Sinus Interventions

Clinics of CSI

Proceedings of the 2nd International
Symposium on Myocardial Protection
Via the Coronary Sinus
Vienna, February 2nd–5th, 1986

Edited by W. Mohl, D. Faxon, E. Wolner

Steinkopff Verlag Darmstadt
Springer-Verlag New York

W. Mohl, M.D. Ph. D.
2nd Surgical Clinic
University of Vienna
Spitalgasse 23
1090 Vienna, Austria

D. P. Faxon, M.D.
Department of Cardiology
University Hospital
75 East Newton Street
Boston, MA 02118 U.S.A.

E. Wolner, M.D.
2nd Surgical Clinic
University of Vienna
Spitalgasse 23
1090 Vienna, Austria

CIP-Kurztitelaufnahme der Deutschen Bibliothek

Clinics of CSI:

proceedings of the 2nd Internat. Symposium on Myocardial Protection via the Coronary Sinus, Vienna, February 2nd–5th, 1986 / ed. by W. Mohl ... – Darmstadt: Steinkopff; New York: Springer, 1986.
(Progress in coronary sinus interventions)
ISBN 3-7985-0695-7 (Steinkopff)
ISBN 0-387-91274-6 (Springer)
NE: Mohl, Werner [Hrsg.]; International Symposium on Myocardial Protection via the Coronary Sinus < 02, Wien >

Copyright © 1986 by Dr. Dietrich Steinkopff Verlag, GmbH & Co. KG, Darmstadt
Medical Editorial: Juliane K. Weller – Copy Editing: Cynthia Feast – Production: Heinz J. Schäfer

Printed in Germany

Type-Setting, printing and bookbinding: Vereinigte Buchdruckereien, Bad Buchau

Contents

Retrograde myocardial protection during surgery

ICSO and PICSO

Coronary sinus interventions and interventional therapy

Preface

This volume, the second in our series edited by the International Working Group on Coronary Sinus Interventions, presents the results of the 2nd International Symposium on Myocardial Protection via the Coronary Sinus held in Vienna, Austria, February 2–5, 1986.

Two years have passed since our first Symposium. The data and theories presented then demonstrated that the route via the coronary sinus is of great promise in the protection of ischemic myocardium. Nevertheless, when the meeting drew to a close, a significant number of questions remained unanswered. There was a general understanding that more thought and effort would be required to comprehend the basic mechanism and the underlying pathophysiologic and molecular processes, to clarify the intrinsic limitations and hazards of the techniques currently being investigated, and to realize in clinical settings the beneficial effects of more extensive applications of CSI already established in animal trials.

As a result of the first Symposium the interchange of ideas on both multidisciplinary and international levels has been enhanced. Many joint endeavours and independent research projects have been initiated. However, in order to provide safe and rational applications in humans, newly acquired data must be continously reassessed; this was our purpose in this second Symposium, a reassessment of the accomplishments of the previous two years, together with the identification of further areas for investigation, and the laying down of directives for future research. Furthermore, the meeting was intended to establish coronary sinus interventions as an accepted conventional therapy.

With the first volume serving as a basis for the series, Clinics of CSI discusses the clinical significance of a more complex understanding of the coronary sinus approach, with the aim of bringing together all the various aspects of the technique. To be as comprehensive as possible, the experience of anatomists, physiologists, bioengineers and technologists has been included.

This book could not have been produced without the aid of our many colleagues around the world whom we thank for their continuous support and untiring efforts.

We also gratefully acknowledge the help of Maria Fuchs, Juliane Weller, Irene Semlak, Monika Königswieser and Paul Simon in the organization of the Symposium and the publication of this book.

Vienna, June 1986   W. Mohl

1

Beck's Lectures 1986

To Beck and back

Dwight E. Harken
Clinical Professor of Surgery (Emeritus) Harvard Medical School,
Boston, Massachusetts (U.S.A.)

Summary: Dr. Claude S. Beck's arteriolization of the coronary sinus forms a basis for addressing the extensive laboratory work on myocardial protection via the coronary sinus. The paucity of clinical applications is stressed and some methods of overcoming these delays are mentioned. Future areas of clinical and laboratory work are suggested.

"He who would not learn the lessons of history is obliged to relive them".   Santayana

This Second International Symposium on Myocardial Protections via the Coronary Sinus has a firm broad basis in history, anatomy, physiology and brilliant multi-focal investigations. All of this has been magnificently put together and edited by Mohl, Wolner and Glogar in the published Proceedings of the First International Symposium in 1984 (8). These sources and personal conversations with key workers allow me to build on the primitive work of Doctors Beck (1) and Fauteux (4) several decades ago (Fig. 1).

My comments will address three areas:

   I. Dr. Beck recalled.
  II. Reference to the broad spectrum of solid laboratory work on myocardial protection via the coronary sinus.
 III. Human clinical obligations.

I. Dr. Beck recalled

First, reminiscences surrounding Dr. Beck, with whom I had the privilege of extensive personal acquaintance. I am commanded to open this volume with bases on Beck relating to his arterialization of the coronary sinus. I will return to that but it would be an injustice to narrow his gauge to *venous* arterialization. He is well known in three areas:
1. Mitral stenosis and valvulectomy with Drs. Eliot Cutler and Samuel A. Levine (3). These brave but disappointing adventures were abandoned after the one initial survival was followed by a series of deaths. Dr. Cutler gave me their valvulotome when may efforts at valvuloplasty were successful in 1948.
2. Cardiopulmonary resuscitation (CPR) (1). Here Dr. Beck's principles were important, his concept of thoracotomy frightening and the term "massage" unfortunate. It is not and never was *"massage"* (a bastard term). The correct term is *"manual systole"*. The emergency thoracotomy on the street wherever was too frequently tragic. It was dangerous to suffer simple syncope in Cleveland. If you awakened at all it was with a bloody shirt.

5

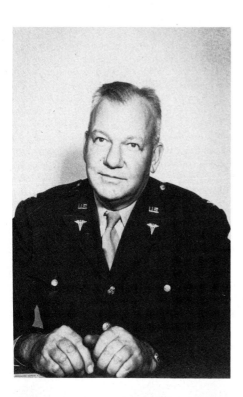

Fig. 1. Dr. Claude S. Beck, Colonel, World War II (courtesy of his daughter, Dr. Kathryn Kris), 1894–1971.

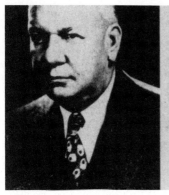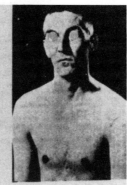

Fig. 2. Dr. Beck with a patient saved by open chest manual systole. Dr. Beck addressed this patient as "one from my Choir of the Dead".

That is an unfair and frivolous comment about a great man's honest belief. However, it was too easily applied and on balance, too often a lethal response to a less than lethal situation. The world awaited Kowenhoven, Knickerbocker and Jude who mercifully gave us *closed* chest manual systole and modern CPR (Figs. 2 and 3).

3. Myocardial revascularization. First, the Beck I operation on the arterial side by epicardial abrasion and stimulation of vascular adhesions. *Second,* on the venous side by partial closure of the coronary sinus and arterializing the venous system by a bypass graft from the aorta to the coronary sinus – the Beck II operation (Figs. 4 and 5).

6

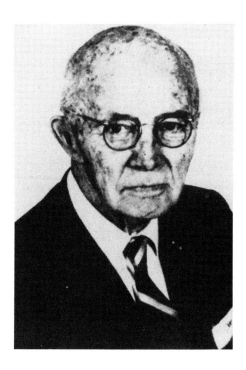

Fig. 3. Dr. Kowenhoven, proponent of closed chest manual systole (CPR).

In any discussion about coronary sinus operations or manipulation it is well to bear in mind the thin wall of the coronary sinus versus peripheral veins, e.g. saphenous vein. Figures 6 and 7 constitute a warning.

The Beck II operation was not widely accepted because of poor methods for patient selection, operative technique, high mortality and inadequate methods of evaluating patient operative results. Most of these factors have now been overcome. Dr. Beck's brilliant concept however, was to use this open highway to the heart via the open venous system to *save myocardium,* to prevent arrhythmias and to *salvage* lives. These goals are laudale

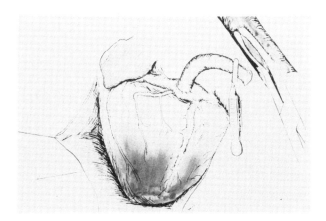

Fig. 4. Exposure of heart and anastamosis of saphenous vein to coronary sinus. Note non-arterialized sinus and veins. Courtesy of Dr. Charles P. Bailey.

7

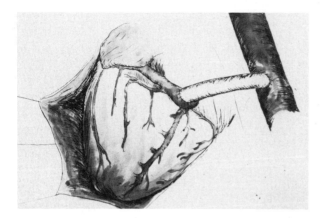

Fig. 5. Completed Beck II operation. Vein shunt aorta to coronary sinus. Note arterialization of venous system as artist's concept. Courtesy of Dr. Charles P. Bailey.

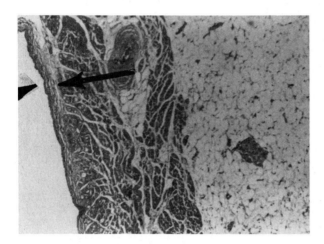

Fig. 6. Coronary sinus. Courtesy of Dr. Joel Umlar.

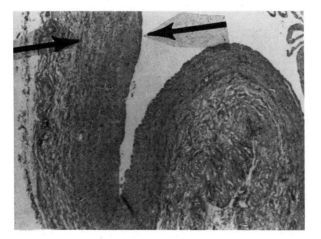

Fig. 7. Saphenous vein. Courtesy of Dr. Joel Umlar.

today and remain proper purposes for this Second International Symposium on Myocardial Protection via the Coronary Sinus. Save heart muscle and save lives.

Without thallium stress tests, angiography and metabolic studies, Dr. Beck had neither solid critical patient selection nor postoperative evaluation. Without modern vascular anastamotic technique on a heart stilled by cardiopulmonary bypass, there was a high surgical mortality and uncertain shunt size. It is little wonder that acceptance was low. Dr. Beck, with all his enthusiasm, energy, courage and enviable objectives was destined to fail before he began.

Even his 75% mortality of left anterior descending artery (LAD) ligation converted to 75% survival by various techniques has proved to be a false talisman. In fact, I have repeated LAD ligation after a variety of manipulations such as counterpulsation, epicardial abrasion, even myocardial trauma, and the salvage generally reaches that same 75%. I have even suspected that simple exsanguination short of death would a month later, enjoy a similar salvage. In short, it seems that many forms of trauma to animal hearts open enough inter-coronary communicators to be significantly protective against LAD ligation. Throughout our evaluation of any technique we must not overlook this simple factor. In short, Dr. Beck's arterialization of the venous system in humans had several reasons for failure. His methods of evaluating techniques in the laboratory were extensive but the salvage oif 75% after LAD ligation was and is not specific.

II. Laboratory studies on myocardial protection via the coronary sinus

The second area to be discussed is that of the multiple laboratory studies throughout the world to evaluate the coronary sinus and veins as pathways for myocardial protection. This relates directly to Dr. Beck's work.

It is not my purpose to review the spectrum of pressure controlled intermittent coronary sinus occlusion (PICSO) or coronary vein *retroperfusion*. We need not review the galaxy of patterns be they varying in time intervals, synchronized or other. We need not review the nearly endless repetition of excellent laboratory studies that do protect the ischemic myocardium. That was brilliantly documented at the First International Symposium last year and has scholarly documentation in the published Proceedings edited by Drs. Mohl, Wolner and Glogar. What I do feel compelled to address is the woeful lack of clinical application of these very promising concepts to relieve human suffering and death.

The evolution of break-throughs in many situations is in five stages:
  I) Concept.
 II) *Laboratory testing* of the concept and validation of the hypothesis.
III) *Selection of appropriate* patients based on knowledge of the life-cycle of their disease.
IV) *Successful clinical application* and appropriate documentation of the technique.
 V) Standardizing, simiplifying and *promulgating* the technique so that it can maximize patient service.

We have not progressed beyond Stage III. Many of the laboratory techniques have been well worked, many patient needs have been defined but we are spinning our wheels before patient service. We must not wait until all conceivable laboratory techniques have been exhausted before work in the laboratory can respond to human needs. We do not need to clarify all possible clinical needs or all conceivable laboratory problems before we start real service. We simply need to identify one or some areas where these techniques can help some specific patients. I am credited with the following definition of a safe device, i.e.:

> "A device is safe when it is safer than the disease it corrects and is the best available".

We can never be absolutely certain that the human response will be identical to that of the animal. This is to recognize the variables between laboratory animal and human pathologic processes. The endlessly pursue all conceivable animal variables, to avoid any possible errors of commission may cruelly expose humans to errors of omission.

The delays that we suffer from Regulatory Agencies may make the public suffer errors of omission. Commonly, satisfaction with the way things are prompts reluctance to deviate from the status quo even though change would constitute progress.

We must understand, even sympathize with the bureaucrat who says "no". "No" is safe for him. A "yes" may come back to haunt him if anything goes wrong with the device or technique. "No" is safe for the bureaucrat but possibly tragic for a particular patient. Remember that "the doubters" always will have an unfair advantage over "the doers". There are always niggling questions that can be asked. There are almost always more ways to be wrong than right with complex issues.

The manufacturers of essential devices may also delay because of their fear of litigation over a failed device. Or the manufacturer may delay samply because he sees no profit from the device. An enormous failure of application of a new technique may lie with the lack of courage or conviction on the part of the investigator or his clinical colleagues. In some parts of the world it has been known, as in the case of heart surgery, that the clinician's uncertainty has been bolstered by conscious or unconscious jealousy or even fear of patient loss. In short, apathy, antagonism, timidity or jealousy may block proper clinical application.

In any event, those who espouse the clinical service must be the prime movers. When the prime mover, be he investigator, clinician or both, has convincing evidence from the laboratory that fits a clear clinical need, he can expedite by taking his evidence *personally* to the regulatory agency be it Institutional Review Board, F.D.A., manufacturer or other for personal *hand processing*. Personal hand processing is the surest way to expedite and to avoid the desk top delay equivalent to a bureaucratic "no".

For the manufacturer who delays a clinician can serve by writing a letter defining a specific patient's need and indicating that the manufacturer must be responsible for any untoward patient effect for want of the device. This is not unwholesome blackmail – it is a helpful release for the manufacturer. That letter to the manufacturer was the precise technique which I used to obtain release of the first demand cardiac pacemaker in 1966.

In the case of the first caged-ball valve used successfully on March 10, 1960, I had less laboratory evidence but the *need* was established by following patients with aortic valve disease who suffered angina, syncope and left ventricular failure. I saw 87 such patients in the decade between 1950 and 1960. We followed these on the best medical care of those times. These people were unsuitable for anything but a prosthetic valve and no such valve existed. Of the 87, 77 were dead within 7 months. So, I did not need an absolutely safe device to be safer than the disease. Incidentally, those two successful patients of 1960 are still alive.

The first use of engineer Berkovits' direct current (DC) defibrillator was different and illustrates another method of expediting human service. We had found in our laboratory that we could use it for defibrillation 17 times before the animal's heart suffered as much coagulation necrosis as one shock caused with the alternating current (AC) defibrillator. So, in 1958, when a patient with ventricular fibrillation could not be reverted after 8 AC shocks, we rushed the DC defibrillator from the laboratory and restored normal rhythms with one shock. That was a simple introduction of a device in a "no choice situation". So it was also with the first "counterpulsation". We used it first in cardiogenic shock. It is often easy to identify "no choice emergency situations". It simply requires creativity and courage.

Now I have suggested methods for the clinical introduction of new devices and new techniques. Any of these may have application in your coronary sinus manipulation. The important point I make here is that we seem to be stuck on "dead center". I hope that this symposium will reveal many additional new clinical experiences of which I am unaware but there an be neither too many nor even enough.

III. Human clinical obligations

The third phase of this discussion is that of *"where now"* for coronary sinus manipulation? I have screened the recent cardiology and cardiac surgical programs and the paucity of human therapeutic programs is distressing. I find that Dr. Mark Hochberg is conducting a widespread survey to identify clinical uses. This should update his classical survey of laboratory work (6, 7). I find that Corday and colleagues (2) have worked with synchronized, antegrade and retrograde perfusion. Joel Gore (5) et al. In Dalen's Medical Department at the University of Massachusetts have used retroperfusion in perhaps a dozen patients with unstable angina instead of the intra-aortic balloon. He reports encouraging results. Mohl has had the most extensive experience, the latest of which is included in this volume. I too have tried further inquiry to find clinical activity and have come up woefully short.

So where do we go for clinical application now? Several places seem obvious and I apologize to any I should credit but do not. I claim no priority here. As Dr. Beck liked to say "Prophesy without experience is a dangerous philosophy".

First: patients unsuitable for coronary bypass surgery who have debilitating uncontrollable pain.

Second: malignant tachyarrhythmias as they are undergoing physiologic mapping.

Third: fresh myocardial infarcts that are being rushed to angiography for possible coronary artery bypass (CABG).

Whatever technique is to be tested clinically, *prior* planning for maximal appropriate documentation is mandatory. There are "gold standards" which are more objective than pain and less gross than deaths. These may be cardiac output, stroke volume, pulmonary wedge pressures, wall motion, ejection fractions and enzymes, etc. In any event, objectivity and specificity are real markers which render the clinical results credible.

Finally, in contrast let me add one more concept and challenge which justifies *more* laboratory investigation. *Cardioplegia* has been the greatest advance in open heart surgery in the last decade. Retroperfusion and antegrade perfusion for cardioplegia seem now to be finding some purpose in open heart operations. There is a potential area for great advance in cardiac transplantation. Our time limitation is now of of the order of four hours. If we could extend this by several additional hours by combined antegrade and retrograde perfusion utilizing various patterns, solutions and temperatures, we might extend organ harvesting in a field desperately short of organ supply.

The use of the mechanical heart helps the patient wait – perhaps you can bring the donor heart from a greater distance.

In conclusion, be it resolved that this Second International Symposium on Myocardial Protection via the Coronary Sinus celebrating the quantum jump from Beck to Mohl will launch equivalent clinical advances by the time of the third such symposium.

"We see so far because we stand on the shoulders of giants".

Sir Isaac Newton

References

1. Beck, CS (1970) Reminiscences of Cardiac Resuscitation: Review of Surgery, March–April
2. Corday, E.: Personal Communication
3. Cutler, E. C., Beck, C. S. (1927) Surgery of the Heart and Pericardium, Chapter IV: Nelsons's Loose Leaf Surgery. Thos Nelson and Son, New York
4. Fauteux M, Palmer JH (1941) The Treatment of Angina Pectoris of Atheromatous Origin by Ligation of the Great Cardiac Vein. Canadian Medical Assoc J, Vol 15: No 1
5. Gore, J.: Personal Communication
6. Hochberg MS, Austen WA (1980) Selective Retrograde Coronary Venous Perfusion Ann Thorac Surg Vol 24: No 6
7. ibid Personal Communication
8. Mohl W, Wolner E, Glogar D (eds) (1984) The Coronary Sinus, Proceedings of the First International Symposium on Myocardial Protection via the Coronary Sinus. Steinkopff Verlag, Darmstadt

Author's address:
Dwight E. Harken, M.D.
300 Mt. Auburn Street
Cambridge, Massachusetts 02138
U.S.A.

Nomenclature and distribution pattern of cardiac veins in man

M. v. Lüdinghausen

Anatomisches Institut der Universität München, Munich (West Germany)

Summary: Cardiac veins drain the myocardium of both ventricles and atria into the right atrium. Only the Thebesian veins empty additionally into other heart chambers.
The openings of the cardiac veins show different locations and sizes. They are arranged in a circle between the ostia of the caval veins. This circle-line is only partly identical with the area of embryonic venous sinus.
We distinguish the cardiac veins by their openings:
1. The coronary sinus and its tributaries (v. interventricularis anterior, v. cardiaca magna, v. interventricularis posterior, v. posterior ventriculi sinistri, v. obliqua atrii sinistri).
2. The sinus of the right atrium and its tributaries (vv. cardiacae anteriores, including the v. marginalis dextra, v. coni arteriosi, v. cardiaca parva – if existent).
3. The sinusoid openings of the interatrial septum, collecting the posterior left and right atrial veins (vv. atriales sinistrae et dextrae posteriores).
4. The sinusoid openings of the anterior wall of the sinus venosus, collecting the anterior left and right atrial veins (vv. atriales sinistrae et dextrae anteriores).
The atrial cardiac veins may play an important role for collateral circulation in the case of congenital or acquired obliteration of the coronary sinus and its tributaries.
In some cases compression of the cardiac veins by sclerotic arteries or intramural courses may interrupt the venous bloodstream. Obliteration of the coronary sinus, dilated inferolateral and inferomedial (subeustachian) fossae, as well as vestiges of cardiac venous sinus valves (Chiari network) are possible anatomic hindrances to successful catheterisation of the right atrium and its afferent vessels.

Introduction

In this unprecedented era of revolutionary development in clinical imaging, in no region of the body are breakthroughs better exemplified than imaging of the heart and circulation, especially of the morphology and physiology of cardiac vessels. In this field the cardiac venous system became more and more important.

However, a great deal of work remains to be done before the anatomy of great veins, long and short anastomic channels, small and large collecting veins, their differently formed and sized openings, and venous capillaries in the inner or outer myocardial layers of the cardiac chambers are fully understood. In connection with the progress of experimental and clinical investigations of coronary circulation, the nomenclature of some cardiac veins has changed for clinical use or ought to change to a more precise description.

This presentation is divided into two parts:

Part 1 consists of an updated delineation of nomenclature and classification of cardiac veins.

Part 2 deals with the morphologically caused hindrances to catheterisation and reperfusion of the right atrium, the coronary sinus and its tributaries.

Our study is based on 280 heart specimens from the gross anatomy dissection course.

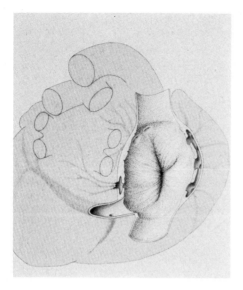

Fig. 1. The openings of the vv. cavae, coronary sinus, vv. atriales posteriores and anteriores (left) and of the right atrial coronary sinus (right) are arranged in a circle-line just above the tricuspid valve.

1. Nomenclature and classification

The cardiac veins drain the myocardium of both ventricles and atria into the right atrium. Only the Thebesian veins empty additionally into the other heart chambers. The openings of cardiac veins show different locations and sizes. They are arranged in a circle between the ostia of caval veins. This circle-line is only partly identical with the area of embryonic developed venous sinus (Fig. 1).

Because of the distribution patterns and locations of their ostia and orifices the cardiac veins may be classified as:

a) Coronary sinus and its tributaries,

b) vv. cardiacae anteriores and the subendocardial or intramural sinus coronarius atrii dextri,

c) vv. atriales sinistrae and dextrae posteriores and their sinusoid openings,

d) vv. atriales sinistrae and dextrae anteriores and their sinusoid openings, and

e) communications of the subepicardial collecting veins.

a) Coronary sinus and its tributaries

A variety of names have been used for the different cardiac veins, which tends to cause confusion. The distribution patterns and nomenclature of the cardiac veins are therefore partly reviewed here (Fig. 2).

It has become very common (1, 3, 4, 6) to use the terms "v. interventricularis anterior" instead of v. cardiaca magna and „v. interventricularis posterior" instead of v. cardiaca media (Fig. 3a, b). This happens in analogy with the names of the accompanying arteries in the anterior and posterior interventricular sulcus. The nomenclature commission of the International Society of Anatomists will accept these more logical terms at their next meeting.

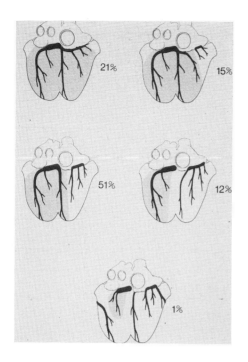

Fig. 2. Distribution pattern of the tributaries of the coronary sinus.

21%

15%

51%

12%

1%

Fig. 3a.

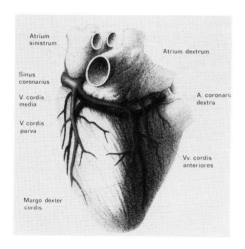

Atrium
sinistrum

Atrium dextrum

Sinus
coronarius

V. cordis
media

A. coronaria
dextra

V. cordis
parva

Vv. cordis
anteriores

Margo dexter
cordis

V. interventricularis anterior

Many investigators agree that this vessel takes its origin from the upper half of the ventral surface of the heart and from the anterior third of the interventricular septum. Therefore it is not as important as the v. interventricularis posterior, which drains not only the posterior walls of the ventricles, but additionally the apex cordis and the posterior two-thirds of the septal myocardium.

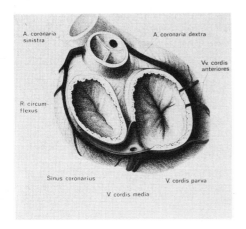

A. coronaria
sinistra

A. coronaria dextra

Vv. cordis
anteriores

R. circum-
flexus

Sinus coronarius

V. cordis parva

V. cordis media

Fig. 3b.

Fig. 3a, b. Anatomy of cardiac veins as shown in official textbooks; this occurrence of veins is found only in 30–35% of our cases.

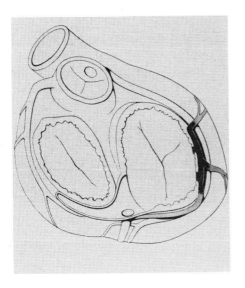

Fig. 4. A small cardiac vein runs extra- or intra-murally to the coronary sinus.

V. cardiaca magna

The v. cardiaca magna or great cardiac vein continues the anterior interventricular vein, runs parallel to the left circumflex coronary artery in the left atrioventricular sulcus, and enters via the coronary sinus the posterior aspect of the right atrium.

V. obliqua atrii sinistri (Marshall)

This vein is found in 56% of the cases; it lies over the posterior wall of the left atrium and represents a vestige of the left superior vena cava.

16

V. interventricularis posterior

This vessel has been regarded as a single stemmed cardiac vein. But in about 22% we found it splitting and forming islands. As mentioned previously it originates from the ventral surface of the apex (78% of the cases). Its main stem is developed, as a rule, in the distal part of the posterior interventricular sulcus, along which it runs, curving to the right towards to the terminal opening of the coronary sinus and emptying in it (72%). In 18% it may open directly into the right atrium. In 5% of our cases it had a significant communication to the venous system of the right heart and therefore may be called a branch of the anterior venous system.

b) Vv. cardiacae anteriores and the subendocardial or intramural sinus coronarius atrii dextri

The subepicardial veins of the right heart, the anterior cardiac veins including the small cardiac vein are some of the most confusingly described veins in the literature, probably due to the fact that variations occur most frequently in this region. In only one third of our specimens is there a well developed v. cardiaca parva. It begins over the lateral wall of the right ventricle, runs in the posterior atrioventricular sulcus well above the right coronary artery to terminate in the coronary sinus or the posterior interventricular vein (Fig. 3a, b).
In 10% of our cases the v. cardiaca parva runs extra- or intramurally from the inferolateral fossa or appendage to the coronary sinus or to the inferomedial fossa (subeustachian sinus) (Fig. 4).
In 60% a separate v. cardiaca parva does not exist. This means that the small cardiac vein is a tributary to the coronary sinus in exceptional and not in regular cases (5). But in most cases we find the root of the v. cardiaca parva, the right marginal vein, which is a tributary of the anterior cardiac system. The well developed anterior venous sys-

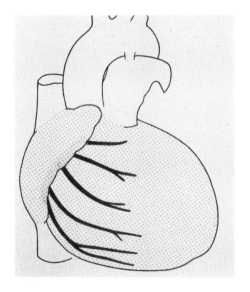

Fig. 5a.

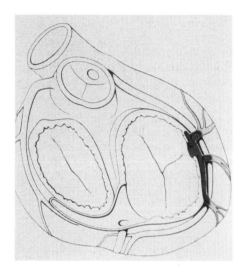

Fig. 5b.

Fig. 5a, b. Distribution pattern of anterior cardiac veins, which are emptying into an intramural right atrial coronary sinus.

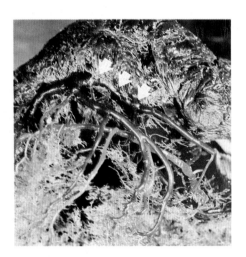

Fig. 5c. Corrosion cast with anterior cardiac veins and intramural tunnel (arrows).

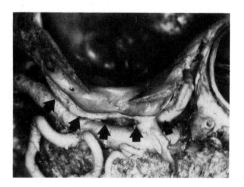

Fig. 5d. Intramural tunnel (arrows) in the lateral wall of the right atrium just above the supravalvular lamina.

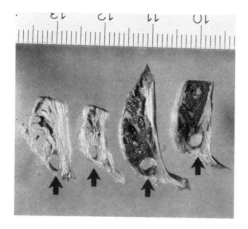

Fig. 5e. Section through the right atrial coronary sinus (arrows).

tem consists of three to six veins. It encloses all veins, which drain the right two-thirds of the anterior wall of the right ventricle. The anterior cardiac veins pass superficially or deeply to the right coronary artery, cross the anterior right atrioventricular sulcus and may empty by one or a few separate ostia into the right atrium. Generally they merge into the lower part of the anterior wall of the right atrium just above the supravalvular lamina (3).

In 60% the veins empty into an intramural tunnel or subendocardial venous lake which terminates in the anterior and posterior aspect of the atrium (Fig. 5a–e). A tunnel or lake like this was found in a length up to 12 cm with two or three openings to the right atrium (2) (Fig. 6a, b). It is called the sinus coronarius atrii dextri or right atrial coronary sinus. This sinus usually has a close connection to the inferolateral fossa or appendage above the acute margin of the right ventricle.

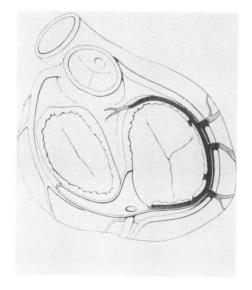

Fig. 6a.

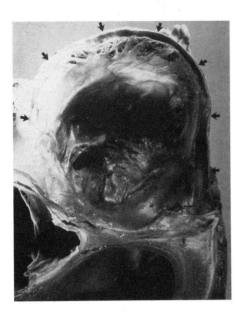

Fig. 6b.

Fig. 6a, b. Long intramural tunnel (up to 12 cm length) in the posterior, lateral and anterior wall of the right atrium (arrows).

Large conus vein

The presence of a large conus vein, which is a part of the anterior cardiac system, is of interest, because it may become a source of intersystemic collateral between the coronary sinus and anterior venous systems. A large conus vein receives most of the venous blood return from the anterior wall not only of the right ventricle, but also from the anterior part of the left ventricle (3%). It arises in the anterior interventricular sulcus, passes the arterial conus and empties, together with the other anterior cardiac veins, via the atrial sinus into the right atrium. In these cases the anterior interventricular vein or the great cardiac vein seems to be very small (Fig. 7a, b) (see p. 22 for Fig. 7b).

Septal veins

The venous drainage of the interventricular septum is not similar to the arterial supply by the anterior and posterior interventricular branch. Whereas the anterior interventricular branch of the left coronary artery supplies the anterior two-thirds of the septal myocardium, the corresponding vein only drains the one anterior third. On the contrary, the posterior interventricular branch supplies only the posterior third of septal myocardium, whereas the posterior interventricular vein drains the posterior two-thirds of the interventricular septum.

c) Vv. atriales sinistrae and dextrae posteriores and their sinusoid openings

Since in 60% of our cases the posterior veins of the left atrium empty into the coronary sinus (Fig. 8a, b), in 40% one, two or three small veins arise on the posterior wall

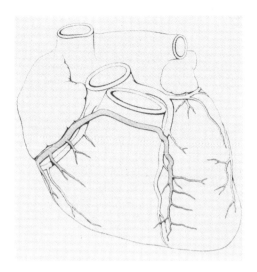

Fig. 7a.

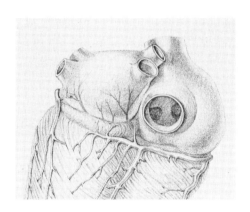

Fig. 8a.

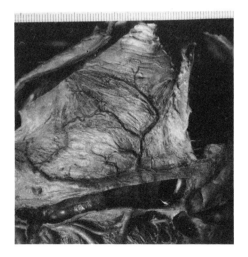

Fig. 8b.

Fig. 8a, b. Left posterior atrial veins empty into the coronary sinus.

21

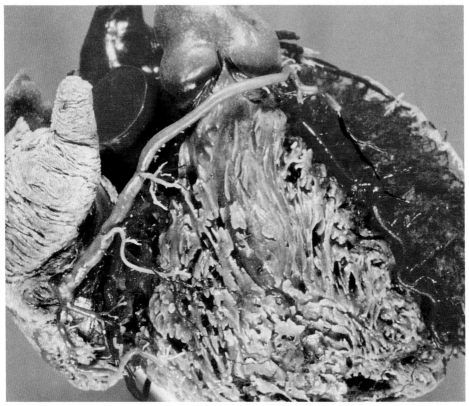

Fig. 7b.

Fig. 7a, b. Large conus vein arising in the anterior interventricular sulcus and emptying in the right atrium together with the anterior cardiac vein system.

of the left atrium (Fig. 9a, b). These veins run to the interatrial sulcus (Waterston) (3). Here the veins are collected in a thumbnail sized intramural lake or sinusoid in the wall of the interatrial septum, posterior of the fossa ovalis (Fig. 1). The lake empties via small or wide ostia into the right atrium.

d) Vv. atriales sinistrae and dextrae anteriores and their sinusoid openings

The anterior veins of both atria are inconstantly developed and distributed. Further studies will show the exact percentages. In approximately 40% of the cases we found single or a few venous lakes or collecting sinusoids in the anterior wall of the venous sinus near the ostium of the upper vena cava. These lakes drain the lateral left and right atrial wall and often show open communications to the right atrium. Formerly they were called crypts of Lannelongue (5). Sometimes we observed valve-like formations at the above mentioned openings. We believe that the anterior atrial veins additionally drain the myocardium of the sinus node area.

22

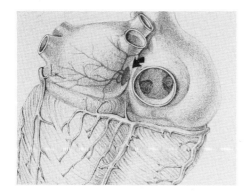

Fig. 9a.

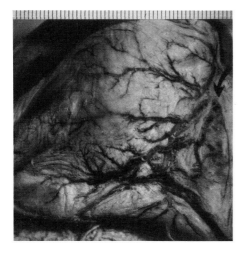

Fig. 9b.

Fig. 9a, b. Left posterior atrial veins collect into an intramural sinusoid of the interatrial septum (arrow).

e) Communications of the subepicardial collecting veins

The four cardiac venous systems (a–d) described above show some communications for collateral circulation. Venous collaterals are developed in axial or atrioventricular circles on the surface of the ventricles and atria of the heart:
– the venous network on the surface of the cardiac apex connects the large veins of the interventricular sulci and left and right cardiac margins. By this there are open communications of the tributaries of the coronary sinus and the anterior cardiac system.
– the venous network of both atria is composed of the anterior and posterior atrial veins and connects the coronary sinus and great cardiac vein with the anterior cardiac system.
The communicating veins are therefore called "intersystemic veins" (3).

2. Morphologically caused hindrances to catheterisation and retrograde perfusion of the right atrium, coronary sinus and its tributaries

a) Venous valves
b) Intramural courses of anterior interventricular vein
c) Compression of anterior ventricular or great cardiac veins
d) Occlusion of the coronary sinus
e) Atrial hindrances for catheterisation

a) Venous valves

To study the location, size and function of cardiac venous valves we removed the roofs of the coronary sinus and its afferent vessels. In 38% there was a wide open ostium of the coronary sinus without any vestiges of sinus septum, that means there was no remarkable Thebesian valve at the terminal of the coronary sinus (valvula sinus coronarii) (Fig. 10a).

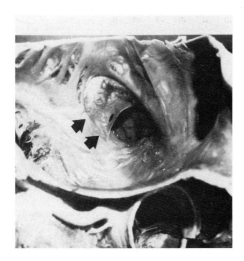

Fig. 10a. Remarkable translucent Thebesian valve (arrow) of the terminal opening of the coronary sinus.

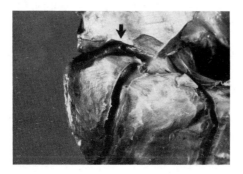

Fig. 10b. Valve of Vieussens (arrow) at the junction of the great cardiac vein and coronary sinus.

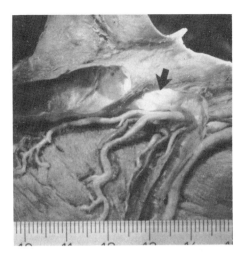

Fig. 10c. Ostial valve (arrow) of posterior interventricular vein directly emptying into the right atrium.

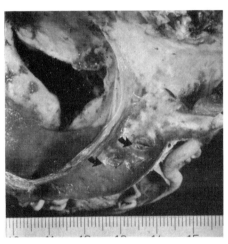

Fig. 10d. Ostial funnel valves (arrows) of posterior veins of the left ventricle, draining into the coronary sinus.

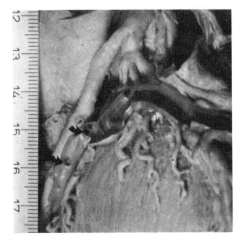

Fig. 10e. Atrophic ostial valves of the tributaries of the anterior interventricular vein (arrows).

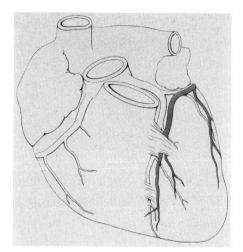

Fig. 11a.

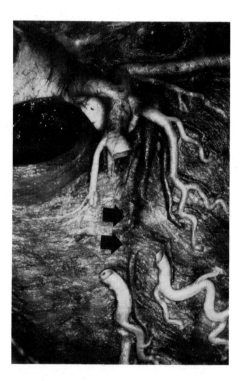

Fig. 11a, b. Intramural course of the anterior interventricular vein (arrow).

In 28% we noticed a crescent valve and in 24% a completely formed or net-shaped but thin and translucent valve (5). A valve of Vieussens at the junction of the great cardiac vein into the coronary sinus was macroscopically seen in about 62% of our cases. We found a complete occlusion by two cusps in 30%; whereas in 32% there was only one cusp or a rudimentary valve with incomplete occlusion (Fig. 10b).

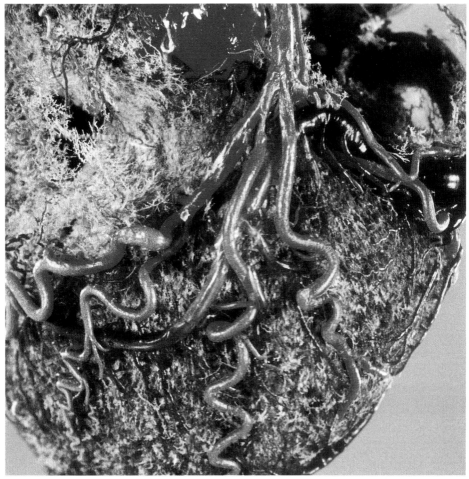

Fig. 12b.

Fig. 12a, b. Compression of the anterior interventricular vein by sclerotic branches of the left coronary artery.

All the other large cardiac veins, the tributaries of the coronary sinus as well as the branches of the anterior and posterior interventricular veins, and the posterior vein of the left ventricle characteristically show in about 30–48% of the cases fully developed or atrophic ostial valves immediately at the entry of a small vein into the larger vessel (Fig. 10c, d, e).

These ostial valves usually consist of a single fold, whose insertion occupies about two-thirds of the circumference of the entry. A special variety of the ostial valves is the funnel valve, especially found at the ostia of the tributaries of the coronary sinus itself (Fig. 10d).

b) Intramural courses of the anterior interventricular vein

In 5% of the cases the anterior interventricular vein dips into the myocardium of the interventricular sulcus and runs intramurally underneath a myocardial bridge for one or two centimeters. Here one can imagine that the vessel will be compressed in the systole and the bloodstream may be interrupted (Fig. 11a, b).

c) Compression of anterior interventricular or great cardiac veins

In about 49% of the cases we noticed significant compression of the anterior interventricular or great cardiac veins by sclerotic arteries of the main stem or branches of left cor-

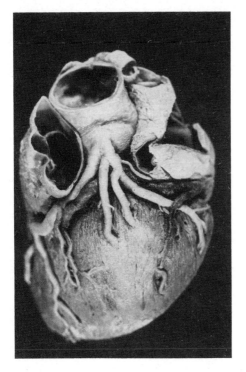

Fig. 12a.

onary artery (Fig. 12a, b) (see p. 27 for Fig. 12b). In a few cases the great cardiac vein seems to be ligated by a crossing small diagonal or left marginal branch of the left coronary artery (Fig. 13a, b).

d) Occlusion of the coronary sinus

Occlusion of the coronary sinus is a very rare malformation. Theoretically it may be congenital or acquired as well as asymptomatic or symptomatic. If of congenital nature, it can be combined with other cardiac malformations. We observed a congenital occlusion of the coronary sinus in a 70 year old man with cirrhosis of the liver and massive gastrointestinal bleedings. During dissection of the upper mediastinum we found a persistent left upper vena cava (v. vava superior sinistra), which emptied into an enlarged and terminal obliterated coronary sinus. The Thebesian valve was completely fixed in its surroundings. Besides this there was a remarkable collateral circulation of left atrial veins between coronary sinus and right atrium. If there is the possibility of occluded coronary sinus after endocarditis of the Thebesian valve is still unknown.

e) Atrial hindrances for catheterisation

Besides the occlusion of the coronary sinus itself we observed morphological hindrances to coronary sinus catheterisation and reperfusion in about 6% of the cases. Most of them

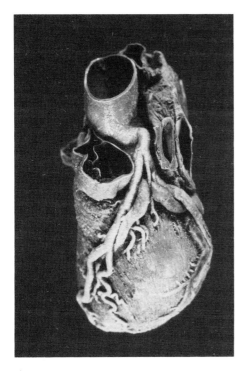

Fig. 13a.

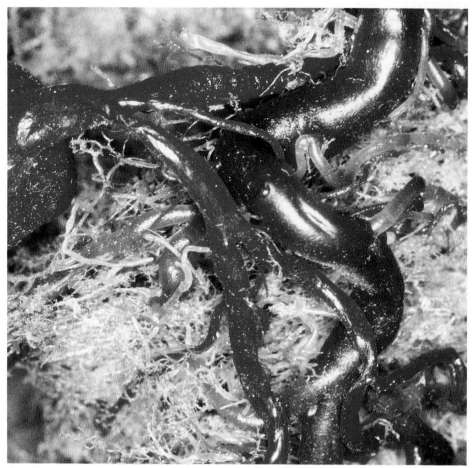

Fig. 13b.

Fig. 13a, b. Functional ligation of the anterior interventricular vein by a crossing small diagonal branch of the left coronary artery.

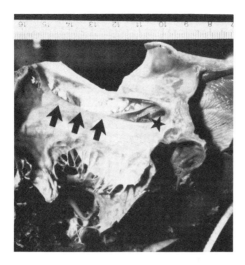

Fig. 14a.

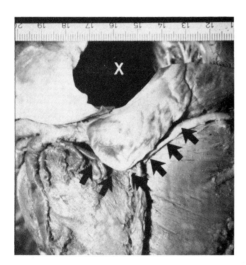

Fig. 14b.

Fig. 14. An enlarged inferomedial (subeusta-chian) fossa may be a possible hindrance for atrial catheterisation. a) The illuminated infero-medial fossa is marked with arrows, the ostium of the coronary sinus is marked with a star. b) The fossa looks like a diverticulum (arrows) of the right atrium; x = ostium of the inferior vena cava.

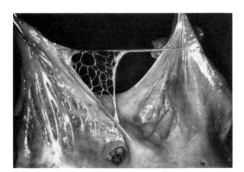

Fig. 15. Chiari-network with partial occlusion of the opening of the inferior vena cava. (Star: ostium of coronary sinus)

are diverticula or excavations of the medial or posterior walls of the right atrium described above: sinusoid openings of the posterior atrial veins dorsal the ovale fossa, the inferomedial (subeustachian) and inferolateral fossae (3), the first between the crista terminalis and the ostium of the v. cava inferior and the latter just above the right cardiac margin (Fig. 14a, b). In some cases these fossae and sinusoids may induce perforation during catheterisation.

In 2% of our specimens we found a well developed Chiari-network in the lumen of the ostium of the inferior vena cava (Fig. 15).

References

1. Aho A (1950) On the venous network of the human heart. Ann Med Exper et Biol Fenniae 28, Suppl I
2. v Lüdinghausen M (1984) Anatomy of coronary arteries and veins. In: Mohl W, Wolner E, Glogar D (eds) The Coronary Sinus. Steinkopff Verlag, Darmstadt, pp 5–7
3. McAlpin W (1975) Heart and coronary arteries. Springer Verlag, Berlin Heidelberg New York
4. Smith GT (1962) The anatomy of coronary circulation. Am J Cardiol 9: 327–342
5. Tschabitscher M (1984) Anatomy of coronary veins. In: Mohl W, Wolner E, Glogar D (eds) The Coronary Sinus. Steinkopff Verlag, Darmstadt, pp 8–25
6. Vlodaver Z, Amplatz K, Burchell HB, Edwards JE (1976) Coronary heart disease. Springer Verlag, New York Heidelberg Berlin

Address for correspondence:
Prof. Dr. M. v. Lüdinghausen
Anatomisches Institut der Universität
Koellikerstr. 6
D-8700 Würzburg
West Germany

The functional architecture and clinical significance of the cardiac venous system with special reference to the venous valves and Thebesian veins

A. Lechleuthner and M. v. Lüdinghausen

Anatomische Anstalt der Universität München, Munich (West Germany)

Introduction

At the 1st International Symposium on Myocardial Protection via the Coronary Sinus in Vienna (1984) we received intensive information on the anatomy and physiology of cardiac venous systems. Nevertheless, there were a few morphological questions left unanswered such as:

a) venous valves: where are they located, what do they look like and how do they work?

b) Thebesian veins: how do they appear and in what manner are they arranged?

c) cardiac venous architecture: what could be the clinical relevance?

Material and methods

This study is based on 150 mammalian heart specimens, which represent most classes including 50 human hearts.

Fresh heart specimens from the Institut für Tierpathologie der Universität München, were rinsed with physiological saline. The coronary arteries and veins were injected with Technovit (Kulzer, 6380 Bad Homburg, F.R.G.) and the specimens placed in a solution of 10% caustic potash. Further preparation, investigation and photography was done with a Tessovar-Zeiss stereoscope. Hearts of fresh cadavers of dogs (n = 5), rabbits (n = 3), and monkeys (macaca mulatta) (n = 3) were fixed in 2.5% glutaraldehyde and critical point dried, or were prepared by the method of Anderson et al. (2); aorta and coronary veins were injected with Mercox CL-2B (Jap.-Vilene Company Ltd., Tokyo, Japan). According to the method of Lametschwandtner and Mohl (3) the casts were frozen in distilled water and cut in slices 0.5 cm thick. After corrosion in 10% caustic potash the casts were prepared for SEM observation (Joul 35 CF Scanning Electron Microscope). Additionally, the vessels and chambers of a few hearts were injected with coloured Latexmilk (Unidispers-Color, Ciba Geigy, Basle, Switzerland and Semperit, Vienna, Austria). A few hearts were cleared according to the method of Spalteholz (4), to study the veins in the inner layer of the myocardium. The venous phase of the coronary angiography of 50 patients with coronary heart disease or cardiac valve failure was observed and documented with Kodak duplicating films.

Results

Undoubtedly, there are multiple venous valves; especially at the ostia of the tributaries of large collecting veins. Their quantity and quality depend on the size of the heart (Figs. 1 and 2). Small hearts exhibit only a few venous valves; most of them seem to be rudimentary (Fig. 3). In large animals, such as horses, elephants and giraffes, we found cardiac

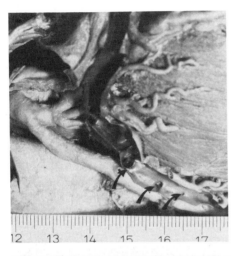

Fig. 1. Black arrows indicate orifices of ramification veins with valves.

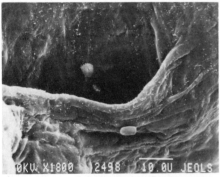

Fig. 2. Mouth of a small ramification vein (SEM; × 1800). The border functions like a valve.

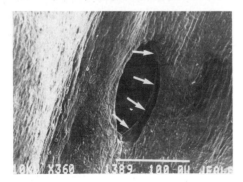

Fig. 3. Mouth of a small ramification vein (SEM; × 360). Arrows = rudimentary valve.

veins with more and stronger venous valves, which often prevent retrograde filling by contrast medium.

In most cases, the valves show one or two cusps, which preponderantly seem to be insufficient.

After injection only the atria and ventricles of fresh hearts in the classes investigated show Thebesian veins (Figs. 4–6). Thereafter they have their origin in the endocardial layer and sometimes bend in an approximate right angle, which makes them run parallel to the myocardial fibers. The distribution pattern of the subepicardial venous system is comparable to a venous network in which blood circulates in anastomosing vessels (Fig. 7). This renders flow direction unimportant, i.e. there are only a few openings available through which the blood can flow. This model of a venous ball is found in most mammalian hearts except the heart of Monotremata and Marsupialia.

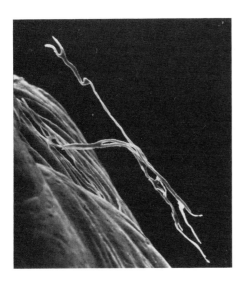

Fig. 4. Thebesian vein from the left ventricle of a rat (SEM; × 240), retrogradely filled with Mercox. The myocardium is corroded by caustic potash.

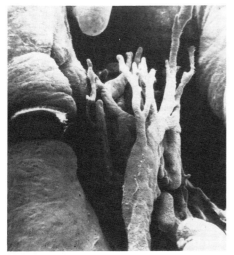

Fig. 5. Thebesian vein from the right ventricle of a dog (SEM; × 220). Preparation as in Fig. 4.

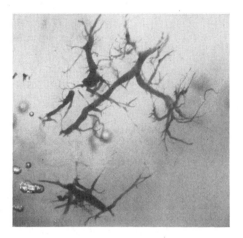

Fig. 6. Thebesianic veins from the right ventricle of a dog (stereoscope; × 80). Myocardium cleared according the method of Spalteholz.

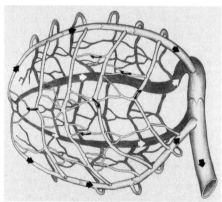

Fig. 7. Model of the subepicardial venous network, arrangement like a ball. Arrows indicate direction of flow.

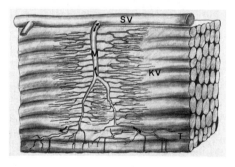

Fig. 8. Model of the myocardial venous network. KV = capillary veins; M = intramyocardial veins; T = Thebesian veins; SV = subepicardial vein.

Discussion

Myocardial venous drainage takes place during ventricular systole (5), in which phase the capillary blood is pressed by myocardial contraction to the subepicardial veins and in the deeper layers to the Thebesian veins (Fig. 8). They are – because of their capacity – soon able to collect large quantities of venous blood. This action is demonstrated angiographically after projection of both the systolic and diastolic phase together (Fig. 9).

36

The large venous stems of the interventricular and atrioventricular sulcus have a specific function as storage spaces, which collect the venous blood on its way from the capillary network (Fig. 10) to the right atrium.

This arrangement means that sufficient venous valves do not seem to be necessary because of the ostia are few and there is continuing massage by the elasticity of epicardium and myocardium.

Change in the resistance which appears at places where vessels differ in width is combined with a partially closing valve, which seems to be able to reduce or prevent venous reflux. Anderhuber (1) pointed out that valves in the venous system can develop during life at locations with special hydrostatic conditions. This would explain our observations that valves are found in the longer parts of a cardiac vein and on ramifications of them. Whether valves of the cardiac veins are sufficiently laid out during embryonic development, and only later become insufficient, is not known.

Thebesian veins in Placentalia are supposedly embryonic remains of the primitive sinusoidal network. Since the venous drainage takes place during systole, functional subepicardial venous drainage is more suitable than drainage by Thebesian veins. The presence of the latter is understood as venous drainage of parts of the myocardium which have no or only insufficient connections to the subepicardial venous system. Therefore, one may expect them in the chambers of the heart with lower systolic pressure (atria, right ventricle).

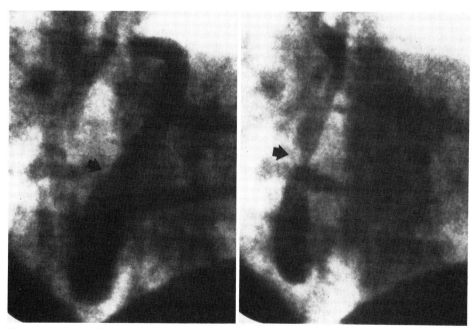

Fig. 9. Angiographic pictures of the coronary sinus and GCV. Left: ventricle diastole / atrium systole; arrow = incision by atrial myocardium crossing CS; Right: ventricle systole / atrial diastole; arrow = atrial myocardium relaxed. Venous drainage obtains highest value. Note the difference in the width of the CS.

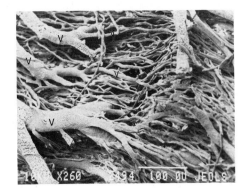

Fig. 10. Capillary venous network (SEM; × 260) of the subepicardial myocardial layer.

Conclusions

– Venous valves are especially found in the larger collecting veins of mammalian heart and on their ramifications. In human cadaver hearts they are normally found in insufficient conditions. Whether they are sufficient in the living individual and animal in any phase of cardiac action is unclear. An increase of the reflux resistance seems to be a probable conclusion.
– Thebesian veins are present: appearing with or without connections to the subepicardial venous network, especially in the myocardium of the atria, right ventricle, interventricular septum and papillary muscles.
– The success of retrograde arterialization anatomically depends on individual variable distribution patterns of the cardiac veins, the amount of veno-venous anastomoses, the efficacy of valves, and the connections to Thebesian veins.

Acknowledgments

We thank Prof. Dr. E. Struck (Clinical Hospital for Cardiovascular Surgery, Augsburg) for supporting our angiographic investigations, Fr. E. Mayer (Anatomische Anstalt der Universität München) and M. Spiess for excellent technical assistance.

References

1. Anderhuber F (1984) Venenklappen in den großen Wurzelstämmen der Vena cava superior. Acta Anat 119: 184–192
2. Anderson BG, Anderson WD (1980) Microvasculature of the Canine Heart Demonstrated by Scanning Electron Microscopy. Am J Anat 158: 217–227
3. Lametschwandtner A, Mohl W (1984) The Microcirculatory Vascular Bed of the Dog's Heart. A Scanning Electron Microscopy Study of Vascular Corrosion Casts. In: Mohl W, Wolner E, Glogar D (eds) The Coronary Sinus. Steinkopff Verlag, Darmstadt, pp 26–32
4. Spalteholz W (1914) Über das Durchsichtigmachen von tierischen und menschlichen Präparaten. Hirzel, Leipzig

5. Tsujioka K, Tomonaga G, Ogasawara Y, Nakai M, Tadaoka S, Goto M, Kajiya F (1984) Origin of Phasic Coronary Venous Flow and the Capacitance of Intramyocardial Coronary Vein. In: Mohl W, Wolner E, Glogar D (eds) The Coronary Sinus. Steinkopff Verlag, Darmstadt, pp 100–105

Authors' address:
Alex Lechleuthner
Anatomische Anstalt der Universität
Pettenkoferstraße 11
D-8000 Munich 2
West Germany

Enhanced cooperation – a challenge of cardiovascular research

W. Mohl

2nd Surgical Clinic, University of Vienna (Austria)

As early as 1880 Langer, a member of the first Medical Clinic at the University of Vienna, reported in the Academy of Sciences on the coronary venous system. Eight years later Pratt presented a theory according to which it should be possible to revascularize the heart via the coronary sinus. Both these memorable events led to a resurgence of interest in the 17th century research of Thebesius.

Today, much of our knowledge on the coronary venous vasculature, its anatomy and pathophysiology draws on hypotheses on the basic mechanisms of coronary sinus interventions (CSI), which have been advanced within the research activities focusing on the use of the coronary sinus as a means of protecting ischemic myocardium. Notwithstanding the major advances in this field, further enhancement of the basic understanding of the underlying pathophysiological and molecular mechanisms will, however, be indispensable if CSI are to become a viable approach in cardiac medicine.

In the early days famous scientists dedicating their research activities to the field of coronary sinus interventions failed, due to what when appeared to be irresolvable technological and methodological problems. This still held true for the Beck era, when lack of information on myocardial metabolism, function, measuring techniques as well as conceptual problems led to the temporary demise of the technique.

Since then, owing to enormous advances in science as a whole, a great deal of information has accumulated and is waiting to serve our needs. This puts us in an advantageous position.

Often, however, the problem is that we are somewhat at a loss when it comes to taking advantage of available information, simply because being an expert in one field does not mean that one is capable of exploiting information from another.

Thus, today, more so than ever, we are faced with the challenge of improving communication between experts from different fields, in order to ensure that the various researchers can make understood to each other what they want and what they need.

One major key to the ultimate success of our research will thus be enhanced communication and collaboration on a multidisciplinary basis.

Second, not only are we overwhelmed with information from fields other than the strictly medical domain but also with an enormous accumulation of data coming from our own areas. At this Symposium an enormous amount of information has been presented, including positive results in animal research and the first clinical trials on CSI; retroinfusion, for example, is on the threshold of leaving the trial stage and becoming a routine procedure in certain subsets of patients. But despite these promising prospects for the future it appears that coronary sinus research has not yet been taken to a point where it could be said that it has fully exploited its inherent potential.

To achieve this, greater standardization of the various methods and techniques currently applied in a great number of different research centers will be needed to avoid setbacks due to communication problems or translation and transcription errors. Furthermore, continuous reassessment of newly acquired data along multicenter lines will be needed if we are to ascertain that applications in human models will be safe and rational.

Moreover, further communication should encourage a climate more likely to enhance the free interchange between basic research concepts and the practical needs of clinicians. Such a scientific interchange, if carried out in appropriate forums and by other suitable means, would expedite the development and clinical applications of coronary sinus interventions and help establish them as a viable approach in cardiac medicine.

Author's address:
Werner Mohl, M.D. Ph. D.
2nd Surgical Clinic
University of Vienna
Spitalgasse 23
1090 Vienna
Austria

International Working Group on Coronary Sinus Interventions

W. Mohl, Secretary-General; D. Faxon, Chairman of the Organizing
Committee; J. Schaper, Chairwoman of the Scientific Advisory Board;
T. Ryan, Presiding Officer *pro tem.*

At a meeting of the Ad Hoc Committee on Coronary Sinus Interventions, held in Rust, Austria, December 2–5, 1984, it emerged as the general feeling of the attendees that the present state of coronary sinus research would legitimate, and indeed greatly benefit from, the establishment of a permanent panel for the free exchange of ideas between and within the various branches of coronary sinus research. Out of the conviction that such an organization would be very helpful in expediting knowledge in this rapidly growing and challenging field, the Ad Hoc Committee, presided over by Drs. Werner Mohl of Vienna and David Faxon of Boston, proposed that the necessary steps be taken for the establishment of a more formal organization that was to serve the purpose of fostering more direct and detailed discussions of current issues in the field of interventions via the coronary sinus.

Since then a great deal of thought has been given to this idea, and many scientists of outstanding renown in CS research were asked their opinion. Just before this Symposium there seemed to be a wide consensus that this international congress would provide and excellent setting for a formal meeting with the aim of establishing the International Working Group on Coronary Sinus Interventions as an official organization.

Minutes of the First Meeting
International Working Group on Coronary Sinus Interventions

Sunday, February 2, 1986: Mariott Hotel, Vienna, Austria, Prof. Thomas J. Ryan,
Presiding Officer, *pro tem.*

The meeting was called to order at 3.30 p.m. by Prof. Thomas J. Ryan, M.D. (Boston, U.S.A.), who agreed to serve as Presiding Officer, *pro tem.*

Dr. Werner Mohl (Vienna, Austria), as host and Chairman of the 2nd Symposium on Myocardial Protection Via the Coronary Sinus extended a welcome to the members attending from all parts of the globe.

In his introductory remarks Dr. Mohl pointed out that at the time of an informal meeting of scientists and clinicians interested in Coronary Sinus Interventions held in Rust, Austria, December 5th–8th, 1984 and Ad Hoc Committee called for the establishment of a more formal organization that would be identified as the International Working Group on Coronary Sinus Interventions. It was the purpose of the present meeting to identify the appropriate goals and suitable means of attaining the objectives of such an International Organization.

Professor Ryan opened the floor for general discussions and four basic topics emerged for primary considerations by those present:

1. A statement of the ultimate goal of the International Working Group on Coronary Sinus Interventions;
2. Development of a suitable organizational structure to achieve these goals;
3. Identification of specific individuals who will fulfil the necessary administrative and operational functions of this developing body whose composition will be international and whose expertise will be drawn the multiple disciplines of medicine and the natural sciences;
4. Membership dues, rights and privileges as well as other fiscal considerations.

After lengthy but hardly exhaustive discussions and using the Draft of Proposed By-Laws appearing in the Program and Abstracts of the 2nd International Symposium merely as a guideline, the following action items were Moved – Seconded – and Unanimously Approved:

1. The goal of the International Working Group will be to expedite the development and clinical applications of Coronary Sinus Interventions through scientific interchange carried out in the appropriate forums and other suitable means that are in keeping with the highest ideals of the medical/scientific community.
2. The International Working Group shall establish a *Secretariate* to be located in Vienna, Austria. The Secretariate will be headed by the Secretary-General of the Working Group, whose functions will be to execute and administrate the agenda developed by the Working Group and to perform such other functions as deemed appropriate by the General Assembly of the Working Group that shall convene at least biennially.
3. Dr. Werner Mohl of the Second Surgical Clinic, University of Vienna was unanimously elected to serve as the first Secretary-General, for a period no less than the convening of the General Assembly of the International Working Group on Coronary Sinus Interventions at the time of the 3rd International Symposium.
4. That a 3rd International Symposium on Coronary Sinus Interventions be held in Boston, U.S.A. two years hence.
5. That an **Organizing Committee** be appointed by the Secretary-General, consisting of a Chairman and at least 2 other individuals from the locale of the next scheduled International Symposium, whose function will be to develop, execute and fund the primary meeting of the Working Group that shall take place, at least biennially and be fittingly called an International Symposium.
6. That a nominating Committee comprised of Drs Mohl, Gore, Jacobs and Santoli develop from the general membership of the Working Group a suitable list of individuals drawn from the medical, surgical, basic and natural sciences communities, who could function as a **Scientific Advisory Committee** to the Working Group. It is recommended that the nominating Committee identify a suitable individual to serve as Chairman of the Committee, whose members shall include no less than 8, nor more than 12 individuals. It will be the function of the Scientific Advisory Committee to *identify* the best means of expediting research and the clinical applications – including but not limited to the dissemination of information, the potential development of common protocols, data registration and standardization of terms and methodologies.
7. Membership in the Working Group is considered to be open to individuals of the medical, scientific and industrial community who have demonstrated an interest in the development and application of new technologies relative to the Coronary Sinus Inter-

ventions. A member shall be considered in good standing with the right to vote and hold office by timely payment of dues that will be assessed to sustain the administrative expenses of the Secretariate and its standing Committees. It was moved, second and approved that current dues be $ 50 U.S. annually, or a sum of $ 90 U.S. be paid now for a period of 2 years.

8. It was agreed that a second Business Meeting be scheduled to take place at the close of the scientific session on Tuesday, February 4, 1986 at 6.15 p.m. to complete further organizational details.

The meeting was adjourned at 1700 hrs.

Minutes of the Second Meeting
International Working Group on Coronary Sinus Interventions

Tuesday, February 4, 1986: Mariott Hotel, Vienna, Austria
Prof. Thomas J. Ryan, Presiding Oficer, *pro tem.*
The meeting was called to order at 6.15 p.m. by Prof. Thomas J. Ryan, M.D. (Boston, U.S.A.), who served as Presiding Officer, *pro tem.*
After introductory discussions the following action items were Moved/Seconded and Approved:

1. An **Organizing Committee** was appointed by the Secretary-General, consisting of a chairman and vice-chairman, whose function shall be to develop, execute and fund the primary meeting of the Working Group that shall take place, at least, biennially and the fittingly called an International Symposium.

2. Dr. David Faxon of Boston University was unanimously elected Chairman of the Organizing Committee. Dr. Joel Gore of Worcester was unanimously elected Vice-Chairman of the Organizing Committee.
   The Chairman and Vice-Chairman shall be in charge of the planning, funding and implementation of the 3rd International Symposium on Coronary Sinus Interventions to be held in Boston, U.S.A. two years hence, on the occasion of which the General Assembly of the Working Group shall have the first of their biennial meetings. Both the Chairman and the Vice-Chairman shall serve for a period no less than the convening of the General Assembly of the International Working Group on Coronary Sinus Interventions at the time of the 3rd International Symposium.

3. That a **Scientific Advisory Committee** be created, which shall be headed by a Chairman, and which shall include no less than 8, or more than 12 individuals. It shall be the function of the Scientific Advisory Committee to identify the best means of expediting research and its clinical applications – including but not limited to the dissemination of information, the potential development of common protocols, data registration and standardization of terms and methodologies.

4. Commensurate with the list of individuals deemed most apt to serve on the Scientific Advisory Board, developed by the Nominating Committee comprised of Drs. Mohl, Gore, Jacobs and Santoli the following 12 scientists were, by unanimous vote, elected to serve on the Scientific Advisory Board: Dr. J. Dalen of Worcester, Dr. D. Glogar of Vienna, Dr. A. Jacobs of Boston, Dr. A. Juhasz-Nagy of Budapest, Dr. T. Kenner of Graz, Dr. M. von Lüdinghausen of Munich, Dr. S. Meerbaum of Los Angeles, Dr. P. Menasche of Paris, Dr. J. Schaper of Bad Nauheim, Dr. S. Vatner of Southboro, Dr. A. Wechsler of Durham, Dr. R. Weisel of Toronto.

5. It was unanimously carried that Dr. Jutta Schaper of Bad Nauheim be elected to serve as Chairwoman of the Scientific Advisory Board.
6. Members of the Scientific Advisory Board shall hold office at least until the convening of the General Assembly two years hence on the occasion of the 3rd International Symposium on Myocardial Protection Via the Coronary Sinus.
7. That the Secretariate be instructed to formally organize a not-for-profit, educational/scientific organization under the name of the International Working Group on Coronary Sinus Interventions that would be duly constituted under Austrian law and qualify as an International Organization that could serve as a repository for non-taxable funds from any of its constituent countries.
8. That the business of the Working Group be conducted by the General Assembly – comprised of members in good standing, convened at least biennially on the occasion of the International Symposium – or more often when deemed necessary. A majority vote of those attending shall prevail.
9. That between meetings of the General Assembly, the business of the Working Group – including its operational and fiscal policies – be conducted by an Operational Committee that will be composed of 1) The Secretary-General 2) The Chairman of the Organizing Committee and 3) The Chairman of the Scientific Advisory Committee.
10. That the agenda for the General Assembly of the Working Group to be held 2 years hence in Boston, U.S.A. shall include a re-evaluation of the structure and function of the Working Group on CSI as constituted.

The meeting was adjourned at 1900 hrs.

Addendum to the Minutes

It was also at this Symposium that the first honorary memberships of the newly founded International Working Group were conferred upon three scientists of the highest standing and international renown.

On the grounds of their outstanding contributions to coronary sinus interventions and the whole of cardiovascular research honoary membership was awarded to Drs. Eliot Corday and Samuel Meerbaum of Los Angeles, Ca., and Dr. Dwight E. Harken of Cambridge, Mass. (U.S.A.).

Pathophysiology of myocardial ischemia and reperfusion

The evolution of ischemic and reperfusion injury

D. H. Glogar

Kardiologische Universitätsklinik, Vienna, Austria

Introduction

This paper is based on an experimental model using a combination of in vivo and in vitro methods, to allow evaluation of the area at risk of infarction, infarct size and the periischemic borderzone as well as its changes over time. The purpose of this study was to characterize the topography and the time course of the developing infarction and the borderzone.

Following an ischemic insult a sequence of metabolic and cellular changes occur, of which the severity and extent appear to increase with the duration of ischemia, until changes which were initially reversible become irreversible (8, 9, 12). The definition of the borderzone and its clinical value remain particularly controversial. The concept of infarct size reduction by pharmacological and other interventions is based on the assumption that after coronary artery occlusion, there is a gradient of blood flow from the normally perfused myocardial tissue to the center of ischemia. this is accompanied by a comparable gradient of metabolic and cellular changes (1, 5, 6, 7, 11). While some interventions have only minimal cardioprotective effects on severely ischemic myocardial regions, more pronounced protective effects are observed using interventions on models with only moderate duration or severity of ischemia (9). It is uncertain, however, whether such regions with moderate ischemia may be protected only in the subepicardial region, or in the lateral and subendocardial borderzone as well. The present paper attempts to clarify the question of lateral and subendocardial distribution of the borderzone; to define its topographic location, considering differences between the apical and basal portions of the heart; and to investigate correlations between topographic boundaries and metabolic or blood flow data.

Methods and materials

Experimental preparation

Experiments were performed on anaesthetized mongrel dogs weighing between 15–25 kg. Anaesthesia was induced with sodium pentobarbital (30 mg/kg i.v.). The animals were intubated endotracheally and ventilated with a volume-regulated respirator using a mixture of O_2/N_2O. Anaesthesia was maintained with Piritramid (Dipidolor R., Janssen Pharmaceuticals, Beerse, Belgium; 8 mcg/kg/min.). Haemodynamic monitoring, recording of rectal temperature and maintaining a stable body temperature and continuous recording of the ECG were performed throughout the experiment.

Thoracotomy was performed in the 5th left intercostal space. The heart was prepared for temporary or permanent coronary artery occlusion of the left anterior descending coronary artery, distal to the first large diagonal branch, by permanent ligation or by a clip occluder.

Experimental protocol I (n = 14)

To determine the topography of the myocardium at risk and the borderzone, 5 minute sequential coronary artery occlusions were performed in 8 dogs. At the end of an initial 5 minute coronary artery occlusion, radioactive microspheres (for determination of regional myocardial blood flow) as well as microspheres of radiolabelled 99 m technetium human albumin macroaggregates, were administered into the left atrium. These would show the distribution of blood flow and a myocardium at risk of necrosis. After reperfusion of 45 minutes another 5 minute coronary artery occlusion was performed, at the end of which Thioflavin-S, a fluorescent dye, was injected, to indicate another myocardium at risk of necrosis. Following sacrifice, the heart was excised and perfused with coloured dyes administered into the ischemic coronary beds, to illustrate the extent of the ischemic and non-ischemic perfusion beds (2, 3). Infarct size was measured after incubation of heart slices in triphenyltetrazolium chloride. Regional myocardial blood flow was determined for these experiments in 4 distinct regions (Fig. 1), including the normal myocardium, the in vivo area at risk and the borderzone. The different regions were drawn on acetate paper for each heart slice, and the given regions were expressed as the percentage mass of an individual heart slice, or of the total left ventricular mass.

In another set of 6 experiments a similar protocoal was used, to assess metabolic changes during brief coronary artery occlusions of 5 minutes duration, followed by reperfusion.

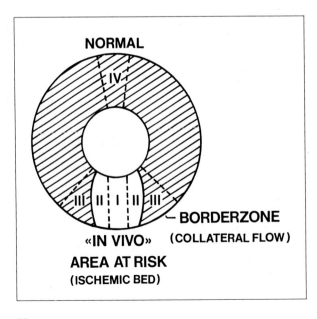

Fig. 1. Topographic regions for determinations of regional myocardial blood flow using radioactive microspheres.

Metabolic changes were measured by mass absorption spectrometry of myocardial PO_2, PCO_2 and pH (4). Changes in intramyocardial gas tensions were expressed (as described previously) as the maximum change of Pm CO_2 and the maximum trough (nadir) of Pm O_2.

Experimental protocol II (n = 8)

To investigate possible topographic changes in the area at risk, and in the periischemic borderzone, a similar protocol as before was used, but coronary artery occlusion was maintained permanently for 6 hours, after which the animals were sacrificed (5). Again an early myocardium at risk of necrosis was located, using radioactive labelled human albumin macroaggregates. This was compared to a late myocardium at risk, located by a fluorescent dye. The borderzone was defined as the myocardial region immediately adjacent to the myocardium at risk of necrosis (as indicated by either method) but still within the ischemic perfusion bed (Fig. 5). Changes in the extent of the borderzone over time were evaluated for the subendocardial, midmyocardial and subepicardial regions. In these animals, infarct size was determined, using triphenyltetrazolium chloride, and correlated with data of regional blood flow in the borderzone.

Experimental protocol III (n = 8)

To evaluate the effects of reperfusion on infarct size and on the topography of the borderzone, a model was used employing 4 hours of coronary artery occlusion, followed by 15 minutes of reperfusion. In eight experiments, infarct size was assessed by triphenyltetrazolium chloride, and the area at risk was determined, as described previously. In these experiments topographically defined biopsy specimens underwent post mortem analyses for tissue electrolytes, high energy phosphates, and tissue water content. Analysis by nuclear magnetic resonance spectroscopy was performed.

Experimental protocol IV

To evaluate the effect of therapy on infarct size and the distribution of the borderzone, animals were submitted to 6 hours of permanent coronary occlusion. The myocardium at risk of necrosis and the infarct size were determined, as described previously. Animals either underwent beta-blockade (propranolol 0,5 mg/kg i.v.) or combined alpha- and beta-blockade (labetalol 5 mg/kg i.v.). PICSO was started 15 minutes after coronary artery occlusion and compared with controls.

Statistical analysis

Data were expressed as mean values for each group and the standard error of estimate (SEM). Data were analyzed by student t-test for paired or unpaired observation, where applicable.

Results

Experimental protocol I

Eight animals were submitted to brief sequential 5 minute coronary artery occlusions. The myocardium at risk of necrosis was determined by "in vivo" methods and "post mortem" by infusion of a dye to distinguish perfusion beds. A representative heart slice of a midventricular section is shown in Fig. 2. Observe the decrease of the in vivo area at risk moving from the subendocardial region towards the subepicardium. In turn the peri-ischemic borderzone appears to increase in width at the lateral and midmyocardial regions. However, there was wide variability among individual experiments in the topographic extent of the borderzone. Particularly the subepicardial borderzone was variable, showing a continuous rim in some animals and only moderate increases towards the subepicardium in others.

In this series of experiments the myocardium at risk of infarction was $27,9 \pm 3\%$ of the left ventricular mass, as shown by radiolabelled human albumin macroaggregates; $30,2 \pm 2,9\%$ of the left ventricular mass by fluorescent dye. The ischemic perfusion bed, however, was significantly larger at $43 \pm 2,5\%$ of the left ventricular mass ($p < 0,001$).

The extent of the ischemic perfusion bed decreased from the apical transverse slabs towards the base of the heart (Fig. 3). Furthermore, apical slices appeared to be at a greater risk of severe ischemia, and displayed only a minimal degree of borderzone; while the extent of the borderzone appeared to increase towards the base of the heart, with decreasing size of the in vivo area at risk. Therefore, one would expect greater potential for salvage in the basal portions of the heart, with larger borderzones, while the apical portion of the heart may be unresponsive to various interventions.

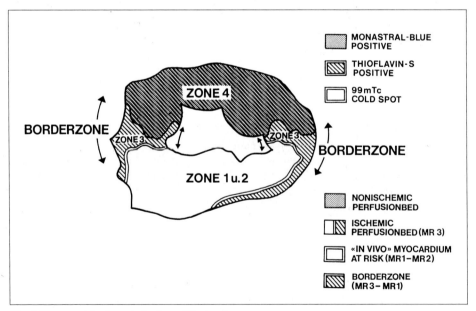

Fig. 2. Topographic characterization of the borderzone.

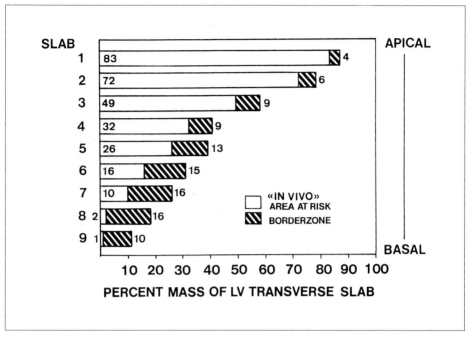

Fig. 3. Topographic distribution of area at risk and borderzone from base to apex of the heart after occlusion of the left ventricular anterior descending coronary artery.

A similar protocol of sequential 5 minute coronary artery occlusions, followed by reperfusion, was employed to study changes in myocardial metabolism using mass absorption spectrometry analysis. Results are shown in Fig. 4. Intramyocardial gas tensions changed rapidly, with intramyocardial $PmCO_2$ increasing as early as two to three minutes after coronary artery occlusion, reaching a peak briefly after reperfusion, and returning to baseline approximately 10 to 15 minutes after reperfusion. Thus, metabolic changes appear to be reversible after such brief ischemic insults. Similarly, intramyocardial PmO_2 shows rapid response with gradual decrease after coronary artery occlusion and quick recovery after reperfusion. While the centre of ischemia shows pronounced changes, the periischemic borderzone shows only minimal ones; particularly a mild decrease in intramyocardial PmO_2. This is probably caused by a moderate decrease in blood flow to the borderzone, compared to the non-ischemic region. The $PmCO_2$ remains basically unchanged, consistent with only a mild ischemia where there are no pronounced metabolic consequences.

Experimental protocol II (n = 8)
A model was utilized to determine possible topographic changes in the myocardium at risk of necrosis during the time course of an infarction, as well as changes in the borderzone. 6 hours of permanent coronary artery occlusions were administered to the proximal

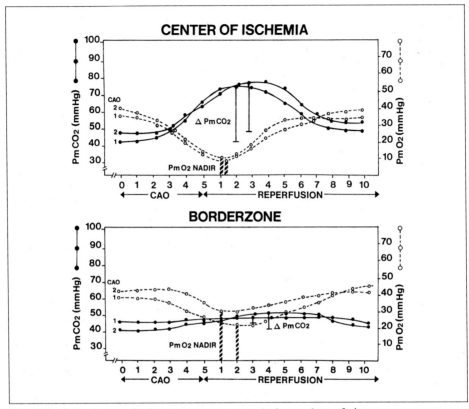

Fig. 4. Metabolic changes after brief coronary artery occlusions and reperfusion.

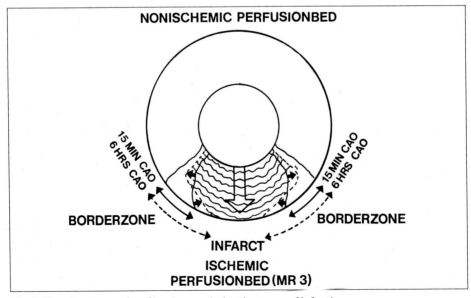

Fig. 5. Changing topography of borderzone during the course of infarction.

left anterior descending coronary artery. Results are shown in a schematic drawing (Fig. 5). As previously shown by Reimer et al. (10) the infarction develops like a wave-front phenomenon, progressing from the subendocardial region to the subepicardial portion of the left ventricular myocardium. After the first 15 minutes of occlusion the myocardium at risk of necrosis (determined by radioactive microspheres) was 24,8 ± 3,1% of the left ventricular mass; compared to 24,4 ± 2,2% of left ventricular mass after 6 hours of coronary artery occlusion. Infarct size correlated well with either myocardium at risk at 23,7 ± 2,0% of the left ventricular mass. As shown previously, the ischemic perfusion bed of the post occlusive LAD was significantly larger, at 40,7 ± 4,4% of left ventricular mass (p < 0,001). Similar to the model of sequential brief coronary artery occlusions, the borderzone, its location and topography, were evaluated and compared between 15 minutes and 6 hours of coronary artery occlusion. In the subendocardial region the initially small lateral borderzone, of 3,5 ± 1,6 mm on either side of the in vivo area at risk, decreased further after 6 hours of coronary artery occlusion, to 1,8 ± 1,1 mm (p < 0,05). There was, however, a significant, compensatory increase in the lateral borderzone in the midmyocardium from 3,3 ± 1,4 to 4,3 ± 1,6 mm after 6 hours of occlusion. The subepicardium increased from 9,6 ± 3,2 mm after 15 minutes of coronary artery occlusion to 14,3 ± 3,6 mm after 6 hours of occlusion (p < 0,05). These findings indicate dynamic changes in the borderzone and are consistent with the observation of Reimer and Jennings (8). While the time course of necrosis leads to a progression from the subendocardium to the subepicardium, there is a comparable wave front in the peri-ischemic borderzone, which displays increasing narrowing of the borderzone in the subendocardium, but significant expansion of it in the subepicardial region.

In the same set of experiments regional myocardial blood flow was determined by radio-labelled plastic microspheres illustrating distinct regions, as shown in Fig. 1. Fig. 6 shows

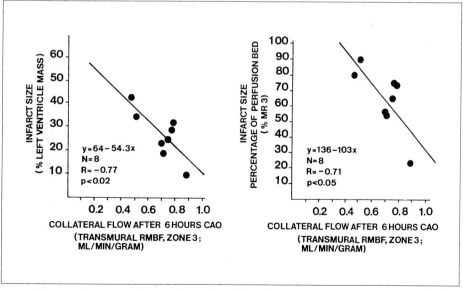

Fig. 6. Influence of collateral flow on infarct size and size of borderzone.

plots correlating infarct size with the extent of collateral flow in the borderzone. Animals with less impairment of collateral flow in the borderzone (and thus with a larger borderzone) are at a lesser risk of developing large infarctions. Animals with only minimal collateral flow develop large infarctions that may be as large as 90% of the ischemic perfusion bed.

Experimental protocol III

To investigate the effects of reperfusion, 8 dogs were submitted to 4 hours of coronary artery occlusion, followed by 30 minutes of reperfusion. Reperfusion led to significant myocardial salvage. The extent of the area at risk of necrosis (determined early after coronary artery occlusion) is a good indicator of the eventual infarct size (Fig. 7). An area at risk of necrosis which comprises less than 15% of left ventricular mass appears to be independently protected from infarction, probably because small regions at risk have larger borderzones and thus less ischemic flow impairment.

Furthermore, following these experiments of 4 hours of infarction and reperfusion, post mortem tests were performed, including analyses tissue characteristics by nuclear magnetic resonance, of tissue water content, of high energy phosphate metabolites and blood flow. The results of these studies show that nuclear magnetic resonance in particular, is an excellent discriminator of ischemic and non-ischemic regions. This may be of great clinical importance for the future. Fig. 8 shows a typical NMR spectrum from an infarct specimen and a non-ischemic specimen. The spin-lattice relaxation time T 1 is greater in the centre of ischemia, at $1{,}67 \pm 0{,}20$ sec, compared to the borderzone at $1{,}12 \pm 0{,}12$ sec ($p < 0{,}01$), and the non-ischemic myocardium at $0{,}91 \pm 0{,}32$

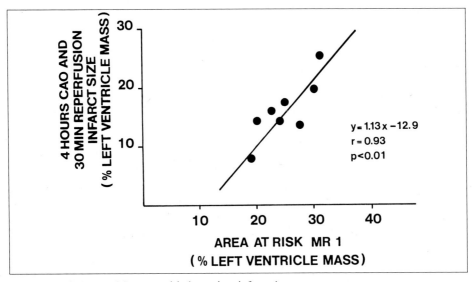

Fig. 7. Reperfusion model: area at risk determines infarct size.

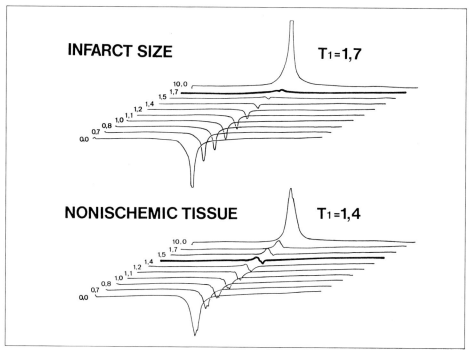

Fig. 8. Determination of relaxation time T 1 by nuclear magnetic resonance spectroscopy.

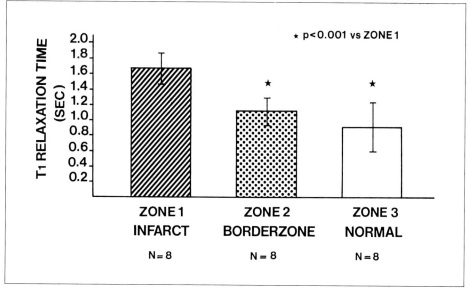

Fig. 9. Changes in relaxation time T 1 by ischemia.

(p < 0,01). There is, however, a wide overlap between measurements taken from the borderzone and the normal myocardium (Fig. 9).

Changes observed in T 1 relaxation times over topographic regions are probably due to changes in tissue water content occuring during the course of ischemia (Fig. 10). There is

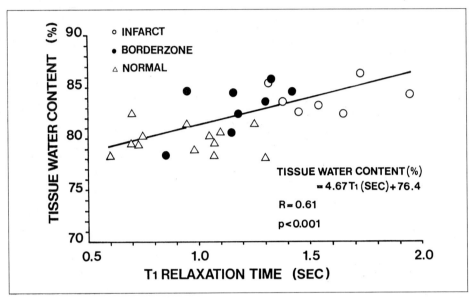

Fig. 10. Correlation between tissue relaxation time T 1 determinated by NMR spectroscopy and tissue water content.

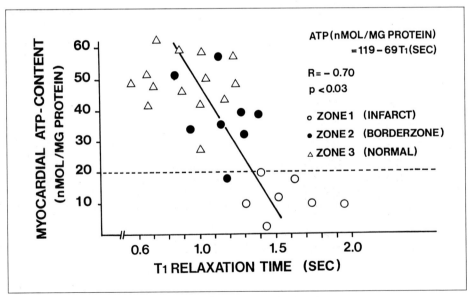

Fig. 11. Correlation between tissue relaxation time T 1 determined by NMR spectroscopy and myocardial ATP content.

58

also a good correlation between changes in tissue relaxation time and metabolic changes, measured as absolute concentrations of myocardial ATP content (Fig. 11). While there is an overlap of ATP content between normal and borderzone regions, the infarcted myocardium consistently shows ATP contents below 20 nmol/mg protein, after 4 hours of infarction.

Experimental protocol IV

The best discriminator, however, between mild ischemia of borderzone regions and infarction, is regional myocardial blood flow (Fig. 12). Betablockade has a tendency to decrease regional myocardial blood flow as well as collateral blood flow, particularly in the borderzone. Collateral blood flow, however, appears to increase after a combined alpha- and beta-blockade, particularly in the periischemic borderzone (Fig. 13). This may lead to pronounced changes, not only in the amount of collateral blood flow, but also in the topographical distribution of the periischemic borderzone. Similarly, PICSO induces pronounced changes in regional myocardial blood flow that appear to be of some importance in modifying the location and development of the borderzone (Fig. 14).

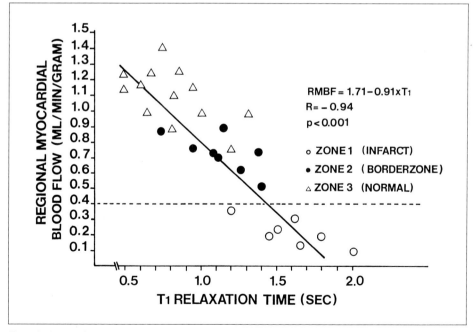

Fig. 12. Correlation between tissue relaxation time T 1 determinated by NMR spectroscopy and regional myocardial blood flow.

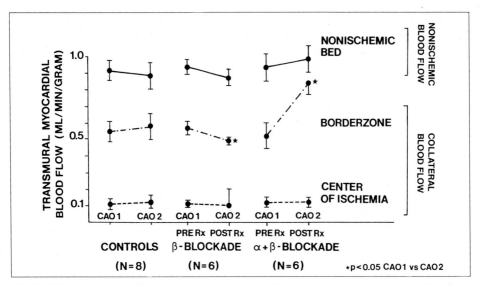

Fig. 13. Effect of alpha- and beta-blockade on collateral blood flow – model of sequential brief coronary artery occlusions.

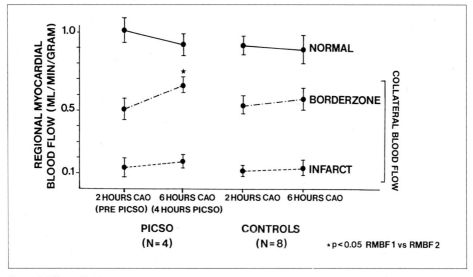

Fig. 14. Effect of PICSO on collateral blood flow.

Discussion

The purpose of the present paper was to define and to evaluate the time course of ischemia; particularly the changes in the periischemic borderzone. Several models were used for this purpose starting with brief, sequential coronary artery occlusion and progressing to permanent prolonged coronary artery occlusions, with and without reperfusion.

As shown previously, ischemia leading to infarction develops in a gradual fashion, from the subendocardial region progression towards the subepicardium. While 5 to 15 minutes of coronary occlusion appear to be associated with only temporary metabolic and functional changes, prolonged periods of ischemia lead to necrosis. Early reperfusion is likely to protect large portions of the ischemic myocardium from necrosis, although reperfusion as late as 4 hours after coronary occlusion also shows significant cardioprotective effects.

Among the parameters most significantly associated with the fate of the myocardium are blood flow data, and metabolic data, including high energy phosphates, tissue oxygen and carbon dioxide gas tension, etc. Measurements calculated using nuclear magnetic resonance spectroscopy are potentially of great use; for example, even proton relaxation measurement showed great discriminatory potential for the detection of ischemia.

The borderzone was defined as the myocardium immediately adjacent to the in vivo area at risk, but within the ischemic perfusion bed, thus receiving collateral blood flow to prevent infarction, during stable conditions. The borderzone was quite variable, in general of only minimal width along the subendocardium and increasing towards the subepicardium. Like the wave-front phenomenon of infarct expansion, the borderzone of the peri-ischemic regions also shows dynamic changes. The results from the present paper would suggest that the borderzone is increasing in width, starting from the apex of the heart towards the base of the heart. Prolonged duration of ischemia appears to modify the extent of the borderzone, by increasing its width along the subepicardium, producing a further increase in collateral blood flow to these regions. The subendocardial portion of the myocardium, however, appears to be at an increasing risk of infarction, probably due to the development of myocardial edema.

Acknowledgement

I greatly appreciate the secretarial assistance of Mrs. Gaby Bambasek in the preparation of this manuscript.

References

1. Braunwald E, Maroko PR (1974) The reduction of infarct size – an idea whose time for testing has come (Editorial). Circulation 60: 206
2. Glogar D, Ertl G, Kloner RA, Strauss HW, Davis M, Braunwald E (1980) The area at risk following coronary occlusion. Fed Proc 39: 398
3. Glogar D, Mayr H, Weber H, Mohl W, Sochor H (1982) Experimentelles Modell zur Erfassung eines in-vivo Infarktrisikogebietes unter Berücksichtigung des Kollateralflusses. Acta med Austriaca 9: 37
4. Hillis LD, Khuri SF, Braunwald E, Kloner RA, Tow D, Barsamian E, Maroko PR (1979) Assessment of the efficacy of interventions to limit ischemia injury by direct measurement of intramural carbon dioxide tension after coronary artery occlusion in the dog. J Clin Invest 63: 99
5. Hirzel HO, Nelson GR, Sonnenblick EH (1976) Redistribution of collateral blood flow from necrotic to surviving myocardium following coronary occlusion in the dog. Circ Res 39: 214
6. Kloner RA, Braunwald E (1980) Observations on experimental myocardial ischemia. Cardiovascular Research 14: 371

7. Maroko PR, Kjekshus JK, Sobel BE, Watanabe T, Ross JW jr, Braunwald E (1971) Factors influencing infarct size following experimental coronary artery occlusion. Circulation 43: 67
8. Reimer KA, Jennings RB (1979) The "wave front phenomenon" of myocardial ischemic cell death. II. Transmural progression of necrosis within the framework of ischemic bed size (myocardium at risk) and collateral flow. Lab Invest 40: 633
9. Reimer KA, Jennings RB (1981) Energy metabolism in the reversible and irreversible phases of severe myocardial ischemia. Acta Med Scand Suppl 651: 19
10. Reimer KA, Lowe JE, Rasmussen MM, Jennings RB (1977) The wavefront phenomenon of ischemic cell death. I. Myocardial size vs duration of coronary occlusion in the dog. Circulation 56: 786
11. Sobel BE (1984) Early intervention in acute myocardial infarction: one center's perspective. Am J Cardiol 54: 2E
12. Trump BF, Mergner, WJ, Kahng MW, Saladino AJ (1976) Studies on the subcellular pathophysiology of ischemia. Circulation 53: 1–17

Author's address:
D. H. Glogar, MD
Kardiologische Univ. Klinik Vienna
Garnisongasse 13
A-1090 Vienna
Austria

Reperfusion injury

A. D. Guerci

Coronary Care Unit, The Johns Hopkins Medical Institutions Baltimore, Maryland (U.S.A.)

The recent observations that coronary thrombosis is the proximate pathogenetic event in the overwhelming majority of acute myocardial infarctions (7) and that these thrombi can be dissolved with thrombolytic agents (6, 26) has ushered in an exciting era in cardiology. For the first time there is a clear understanding of the immediate cause of myocardial infarction, and effective therapies are already being developed (10, 23, 28). Unfortunately, reperfusion of ischemic myocardium is characterized by functional and morphologic changes which suggest that reperfusion itself may be deleterious.

Reperfusion after brief periods of ischemia (less than 20 minutes) is associated with prolonged mechanical dysfunction which is not adequately explained by the depletion of high energy phosphates (2, 12, 24). Reperfusion after longer periods of ischemia produces explosive myocellular injury, with sarcolemmal disruption, enzyme leakage, loss of volume regulation, mitochondrial swelling, and contracture of myofibrils. This histologic pattern, termed contraction band necrosis, is quite different from the histologic features of necrosis due to uninterrupted ischemia (13–15) and has stimulated the idea that reperfusion may actually contribute to the necrosis of reversibly injured myocardium.

Several hypotheses have been formulated to explain reperfusion injury; those which best account for the available facts are exaggerated sodium-calcium exchange and injury from oxygen derived free radicals. Other mechanisms, including cell swelling, the no-reflow phenomenon, and tissue hemorrhage, are more likely the consequences than the causes of reperfusion injury. Cell swelling is most prominent in myocytes which are already irreversibly damaged (14), and the no-reflow phenomenon and tissue hemorrhage appear to be confined to regions of myocardium which are already necrotic (17, 18).

Sodium-calcium exchange

The idea that exaggerated sodium-calcium exchange might be responsible for reflow injury originated in what has been called the calcium paradox: exposure to physiologic calcium concentrations after as little as two to three minutes of perfusion with calcium free media produces contracture and explosive cell death. First noted more than two decades ago (32), the calcium paradox is associated with morphologic features similar to those of post-ischemic reperfusion. These include profound mitochondrial disarray at an ultrastructural level, and cell swelling and contracture which are readily apparent under light microscopy. Although the histology of the calcium paradox may be viewed as a nonspecific response to altered membrane permeability and contracture, some data suggest that sodium-calcium exchange plays a primary role in reperfusion injury.

63

In isolated perfused hearts, 30 minutes of calcium free perfusion is associated with a 25% increase in intracellular sodium content. This sodium accumulation is the result of continued operation of a sarcolemmal sodium-calcium pump. The sodium-calcium pump can work in either direction, that is, it can exchange intracellular calcium for extracellular sodium, or intracellular sodium for extracellular calcium. In the absence of extracellular calcium, intracellular calcium is exchanged for extracellular sodium.

When calcium was added to the perfusate in these experiments, intracellular sodium concentrations quickly returned to normal. During this same time period, intracellular calcium more than doubled, with disastrous mechanical consequences. The hearts went into contracture for several minutes and ultimately regained only about 30% of baseline contractile function (27). Pharmacologic manipulation of intracellular sodium concentration during the period of calcium-free perfusion provided additional evidence of the importance of sodium-calcium exchange in the calcium paradox. When the accumulation of intracellular sodium during the period of calcium-free perfusion was prevented, restoration of normal perfusate calcium was not associated with calcium overload, and developed tension quickly returned to normal. Alternatively, hearts with massive sodium overload experienced a five-fold increase in intracellular calcium when they were again exposed to perfusate with normal calcium concentration. These hearts developed contracture, from which they did not recover. Thus, calcium influx is related to intracellular sodium concentration at the time of calcium reperfusion and the calcium influx seems to determine the resulting contractile abnormalities.

What is the relevance of the calcium paradox and sodium-calcium exchange to reperfusion injury? First, sodium accumulates in cardiac myocytes during ischemia as well as during calcium-free perfusion. In ischemia, the sodium overload is probably the result of passive inward leak of sodium as the activity of the sodium-potassium pump declines due to inadequate ATP supplies. Ordinarily, an increase in intracellular sodium would also stimulate the sodium-calcium exchange pump. During ischemia, however, declining levels of ATP permit the movement of calcium from mitochondria into the cytoplasm. Intracellular acidosis also reduces the binding of calcium to myofibrils. As a consequence of these effects, cytoplasmic calcium levels also rise during ischemia. This further inhibits the extrusion of sodium, because the elevated intracellular free calcium reduces the balance which would ordinarily favor sodium export via the sodium-calcium exchange mechanism.

These events set the stage for massive calcium influx at the time of reperfusion. With reperfusion, ATP and pH rise abruptly (25). Increased pH promotes the binding of cytoplasmic calcium to myofibrils, and increased ATP levels fuel the mitochondrial uptake of calcium, where calcium entry competes with ADP transport and ATP synthesis for the respiration dependent membrane potential. Intracellular calcium levels are in this way restored to normal, while intracellular sodium remains elevated. It is at this point that sodium-calcium exchange proceeds and the second feature common to reperfusion and the calcium paradox is established: massive calcium overload.

The clinical relevance of this sequence is suggested by another set of experiments with low sodium perfusate. In this study hearts were exposed to low or normal sodium during an hour of ischemia (perfusion less than 1% of control flow). In both the normal perfusate group and the low sodium group, the heart stopped beating, pH fell to 6.15, and ATP and phosphocreatine declined to approximately 30% and 10% of control values, respectively, by the end of the hour of ischemia. At the end of an hour of reperfusion with standard Krebs-Henseleit perfusate, control hearts had recovered only about 80% of phos-phocreatine and 50% of developed pressure. In contrast, hearts perfused with a low so-lium solution during the ischemic period had normal phosphocreatine levels and 95% re-covery of contractility (25). These results suggest that exaggerated sodium-calcium ex-change may indeed play an important role in reperfusion injury. In this regard it is worth noting that the failure of verapamil, administered at the time of reperfusion, to prevent reflow injury is not relevant to the hypothesis that excessive sodium-calcium exchange contributes to reperfusion injury. Verapamil does not affect the sodium-calcium exchange mechanism.

Oxygen derived free radicals

In recent years attention has focused on oxygen derived free radicals as mediators of re-perfusion injury. Free radicals are molecules with an unpaired electron, which is repre-sented in chemical formulas as a dot. The impaired electron makes free radicals highly reactive. Moreover, when a free radical reacts with a non-radical, another free radical must be formed. A typical reaction is outlined below:

$$R \cdot + XH \rightarrow RH + X \cdot$$

With regard to biological systems, and the heart in particular, free radicals may inactivate proteins by cross-linking and alter membrane permeability by the peroxidation of poly-unsaturated fatty acids (PUFAH). The general reactions are as follows (8):

Protein $- SH - HS + 2 R \cdot \rightarrow 2 RH + Protein - S - S$

PUFAH $+ R \cdot \rightarrow PUFA \cdot + RH$
PUFA $\cdot + O_2 \rightarrow PUFAOO \cdot$
PUFAOO $\cdot + PUFAH \rightarrow PUFAOOH + PUFA \cdot$

Two characteristics of the lipid-free radical interactions are noteworthy. First, the inter-action of a free radical with a polyunsaturated fatty acid can initiate a long chain reac-tion. Thus, a single free radical can alter hundreds of lipid molecules. Second, the poly-unsaturated side chains of cell membranes are important determinants of membrane permeability and the function of specific transport channels. Extensive lipid peroxidation may therefore eliminate any chance of recovery of otherwise reversibly injured cells.

Two systems have been identified which could, in theory, generate large numbers of free radicals during ischemia and reperfusion. In order to understand the first of these sys-tems, it must be recognized that cytochrome oxidase, the terminal enzyme in the electron transport chain, reduces most but not all of the oxygen consumed during oxidative phos-phorylation directly to water. A small amount, perhaps 5%, proceeds by a series of univ-alent reductions, during which the superoxide anion (O_2^-), hydrogen peroxide, and the hydroxyl radical (OH), are produced (9). Intramitochondrial superoxide dismutase and glutathione peroxidase ordinarily catalyze the reduction of these free radicals to oxygen, hydrogen peroxide, and ultimately, water. The highly reduced state which prevails at the time of reperfusion favors an increase in the univalent reduction of oxygen, and could overwhelm cell defenses against free radicals.

The second mechanism for free radical generation involves the enxyme xanthine oxidase (20). Normally an NAD+ dependent dehydrogenase, this enzyme is rapidly converted to an oxygen dependent, free radical generating oxidase during ischemia. Ischemia provides one of xanthine oxidase's substrates, xanthine, as ATP is degraded sequentially to ADP, AMP, adenosine, inosine, hypoxanthine, and finally, xanthine. Reperfusion provides the second substrate, oxygen. The reaction proceeds as follows:

$$\text{xanthine} + H_2O + O_2 \xrightarrow[\text{oxidase}]{\text{xanthine}} \text{uric acid} + 2 \cdot O_2^- + 2\,H^+$$

The oxygen paradox

The hypothesis that reperfusion actually causes necrosis rather than just hastening the death of cells which have already been irreversibly injured originated with the observation that reperfusion with oxygen containing solutions produced a unique set of abnormalities. In isolated hearts, a slow but steady leak of myocardial enzymes occurs during prolonged ischemia. Reperfusion with oxygen free media does little to change this pattern, producing only a small additional leak at the time of reflow. In contrast reperfusion with oxygen containing media is associated with massive enzyme release (11). While not specific of necrosis, enzyme leak is a marker for cell damage, and these studies focused attention on the potential toxicity of oxygen itself. More recently, the generation of oxygen derived free radicals has been demonstrated during post-ischemic reperfusion of isolated hearts (33). Consistent with expectations, this process reaches a maximum within seconds after reperfusion.

Free radical scavengers

Much of the evidence in support of the role of free radicals as mediators of reperfusion injury is indirect, derived from studies of the effects of free radical scavengers on reperfused hearts. These studies were conducted before the demonstration of free radical production at the time of reperfusion and, in general, have shown dramatic benefit.
In studies of transient global left ventricular ischemia in dogs, the addition of superoxide dismutase and mannitol to a standard cardioplegia solution was associated with 85% recovery of developed pressure 30 minutes after one hour of total ischemia. In contrast, hypothermia and conventional cardioplegia applied just before and during the ischemic period were associated with just 26% to 65% recovery (29). Similar results have been reported with superoxide dismutase and catalase in isolated rabbit hearts subjected to 210 minutes of global ischemia at 20 °C (4) and with superoxide dismutase alone in rabbit hearts subjected to 30 minutes of normothermic ischemia followed by 45 minutes of reperfusion (2). In the latter of these two studies, treated hearts regained 71% of contractile function and 93% of pre-ischemic levels of phosphocreatine, compared to 27% and 69% recovery, respectively, in control hearts.
Free radical scavengers have also been found to diminish the duration of myocardial stunning in models of regional ischemia. Dimethylthiourea and mercaptopropionylglycine, scavengers of the hydroxyl radical, and the combination of superoxide dismutase and catalase have been shown to be highly effective in this setting (3, 22). Typically in these studies the anterior walls of control hearts remain akinetic 60 to 90 minutes after a 15 minute occlusion of the left anterior descending coronary artery, whereas the anterior

66

walls of hearts treated with the free radical scavenger have by this time recovered 50% or more of baseline systolic shortening.

Perhaps the most exciting application of free radical scavengers has been in the reduction of infarct size. In a porcine model of 30 minutes of regional ischemia and one hour of reperfusion; superoxide dismutase reduced infarct size from 13.5% to 0.5% of the ischemic region. In canine models of 60 to 90 minutes of ischemia followed by one to 24 hours of reperfusion, superoxide dismutase, alone or in combination with catalase, has reduced infarct size by 35% to 78% (16, 31).

Two aspects of these studies are noteworthy. First, none of the free radical scavengers which have been shown to reduce infarct size is known to affect any of the determinants of infarct size: heart rate, collateral flow, preload, or afterload. Thus, explanation of the mechanism of action of free radical scavengers requires an alternative hyothesis (e.g. that oxygen derived free radicals do indeed mediate reperfusion injury). Second, in order to be effective, free radical scavengers must be present only at the time of reperfusion. Thus, pretreatment is not necessary.

Pretreatment with the xanthine oxidase inhibitor allopurinol 16 to 24 hours before and again just prior to experimental coronary ligation has also been shown to reduce infarct size. In a canine model of one hour of anterior descending occlusion followed by four hours of reperfusion, 23% of the ischemic region was infarcted in control hearts, compared to only 9% in allopurinol treated hearts (5). With 90 minutes of circumflex occlusion and six hours of reflow, allopurinol pretreatment reduced infarct size from 40% of the ischemic region to 22% (30). While the necessity of prolonged pretreatment renders this form of therapy somewhat impractical, the mechanistic implication of these studies is extremely important. As in the case of free radical scavengers, allopurinol has no effect on the known determinants of infarct size. Thus, reduction of infarct size by allopurinol in these canine models of ischemia and reperfusion is consistent with the free radical hypothesis and, more specifically, the xanthine oxidase system as a generator of oxygen derived free radicals.

Polymorphonuclear leukocytes

Leukocytes activated by inflammatory and immune processes release a wide variety of cytotoxic products including oxygen free radicals. Polymorphonuclear leukocytes begin to migrate into ischemic myocardium within hours of the onset of infarction. These phenomena raise the possibility that polymorphonuclear leukocytes contribute to necrosis in reperfused hearts. Available data indicate that this is so. Treatment with anti-polymorphonuclear leukocyte globulin has been reported to reduce infarct size by 30 to 40% into a canine model of 90 minutes of circumflex occlusion followed by six hours of reperfusion (21). The addition of a free radical scavenger to the animals treated with anti-neutrophil serum further reduced infarct size in these studies.

Summary

Reperfusion of ischemic myocardium is associated with a distinctive set of metabolic, functional, and morphologic abnormalities which suggest that reperfusion itself is deleterious. The reperfusion injury hypothesis began with the observation that reperfusion of isolated hearts with oxygen containing media produced massive enzyme leak and contracture, events not seen at a similar time in the course of uninterrupted ischemia or with reperfusion with oxygen-free media. The reperfusion injury hypothesis has received additional support from the realization that oxygen derived free radicals are generated by a variety of normal and pathologic processes (8, 20) that reperfusion of ischemic myocardium with oxygen containing media is indeed associated with a burst of free radical production, and that oxygen derived free radicals are highly toxic to the heart (19, 33). Exaggerated sodium-calcium exchange has also been implicated in reperfusion injury, and may be the means by which the free-radical generating xanthine oxidase system is activated (20, 25).

From a clinical perspective, the most gratifying aspect of studies of the role of oxygen derived free radicals in ischemic injury has been the dramatic reduction of infarct size observed when free radical scavengers are administered at the time of reperfusion. In particular, the administration of the free radical scavenger superoxide dismutase has reduced infarct size by 35 to 78% in canine models of 60 to 90 minutes of regional ischemia followed by four to six hours of reperfusion. These results are especially important in view of the emerging role of reperfusion as an effective means of limiting infarct size in humans. Reperfusion injury, a cruel paradox of modern therapy, appears to be a very real and very treatable pathophysiologic entity.

References

1. Ambrosio G, Becker LC, Hutchins GM, Weisfeld ML (1985) Reduction in Experimental Infarct Size by Recombinant Human Superoxide Dismutase Administration During Reperfusion (abstr). Circulation 72 (Suppl III): III-351
2. Ambrosio G, Jacobus WJ, Becker LC (1985) Evidence for Functional and Metabolic Reserve in Stunned Hearts (abstract). Clin Res 33: 165A
3. Braunwald E, Kloner RA (1985) Myocardial Reperfusion: A Double-Edged Sword? J Clin Invest 76: 1713–1719
4. Casale AS, Bulkley GB, Bulkley BH, Flaherty JT, Gott VL, Gardner TJ (1983) Oxygen Free Radical Scavengers Protect the Arrested, Globally Ischemic Heart upon Reperfusion. Surg Forum 34: 313–316
5. Chambers DE, Parks DA, Patterson G, Joy R, McCord JM, Yoshida S, Parmley LF, Downey JM (1985) Xanthine Oxidase as a Source of Free Radical Damage in Myocardial Ischemia. J Mol Cell Cardiol 17: 145–152
6. Collen D, Topol EJ, Tiefenbrunn AJ, Gold HK, Weisfeldt ML, Sobel BE, Leinbach RC, Brinker JA, Ludbrook PA, Yasuda I, Bulkley BH, Robison AK, Hutter AM, Bell WR, Spadaro JJ, Khaw BA, Grossbard EB (1984) Coronary Thrombolysis with Recombinant Human Tissue Type Plasminogen Activator: A Prospective, Randomized, Placebo Controlled Trial. Circulation 70: 1012–1017
7. Dewood MA, Spores J, Notske MD, Mouser LT, Burroughs R, Golden MS, Lang HT (1980) Prevalence of Total Coronary Occlusion During the Early Hours of Transmural Myocardial Infarction. N Engl J Med 303: 897–902
8. Freeman BA, Crapo JD (1982) Biology of Disease: Free Radicals and Tissue Injury. Lab Invest 47: 412–427
9. Fridovich I (1978) The Biology of Oxygen Radicals. Science 201: 875–880
10. Grupo Italiano per lo Studio dello Streptochinasi nell' Infarcto Miocardico (GISSI) (1986) Effectiveness of Intravenous Thrombolytic Treatment in Acute Myocardial Infarction. Lancet i: 397–401

11. Hearse DJ, Humprey SM, Bullock GR (1978) The Oxygen Paradox and the Calcium Paradox. Two Facets of the Same Problem? J Mol Cell Cardiol 10: 641–668
12. Hoffmeister HM, Mauser M, Schaper W (1984) Failure of Postischemic ATP Repletion by Adenosine to Improve Regional Myocardial Function. In: Mohl W, Wolner E, Glogar D (eds) The Coronary Sinus. Steinkopff Darmstadt, Springer Verlag, New York, pp 148–152
13. Jennings RB, Ganote CE, Reimer K (1985) Ischemic Tissue Injury. Am J Pathol 81: 179–198
14. Jennings RB, Reimer KA (1981) Lethal Myocardial Ischemic Injury. Am J Pathol 102: 241–259
15. Jennings RB, Schaper J, Hill ML, Steenbergen C, Reimer KA (1985) Effect of Reperfusion Late in the Phase of Reversible Ischemic Injury. Circ Res 56: 262–278
16. Jolly SR, Kane WJ, Bailie WB, Abrams GD, Lucchesi BR (1984) Canine Myocardial Reperfusion Injury. Reduction by the Combined Administration of Superoxide Dismutase Catalase. Circ Res 54: 277
17. Kloner RA, Alker KJ (1984) The Effect of Streptokinase on Intramyocardial Hemorrhage, Infarct Size, and the No Reflow Phenomenon During Coronary Reperfusion. Circulation 70: 513–521
18. Kloner RA, Ganote CE, Jennings RB (1974) The No-Reflow Phenomenon after Temporary Coronary Occlusion in the Dog. J Clin Invest 54: 1496–1508
19. Manson NH, Deardorff MB, Eaton LR, Hess ML (1985) Depression of Rabbit Papillary Muscle Mechanics by Leukocyte Generated Reduced Oxygen Intermediates (abstract). Circulation 72 (Suppl III): III: 85
20. McCord JM (1985) Oxygen Derived Free Radicals in Postischemic Tissue Injury. N Engl J Med 312: 159–163
21. Mitsos SE, Askew TE, Fantone JC, Kunkel SL, Abrams GD, Schork A, Lucchesi BR (1986) Protective Effects of N-2-Mercaptopropionyl Glycine against Myocardial Reperfusion Injury after Neutrophil Depletion in the Dog. Evidence for the Role of Intracellular Derived Free Radicals. Circulation 73: 1077–1086
22. Myers ML, Bolli R, Lekich RF, Hartley CJ, Roberts R (1985) Enhancement of Recovery of Myocardial Function by Oxygen Free Radical Scavengers after Reversible Regional Ischemia. Circulation 72: 915–921
23. O'Neill W, Timmis G, Bourdillon PD, Lai P, Ganghadarhan V, Walton J, Ramos R, Laufer N, Gordon S, Schork MA, Pitt B (1986) A Prospective, Randomized Clinical Trial of Intracoronary Streptokinase versus Coronary Angioplasty for Acute Myocardial Infarction. N Engl J Med 314: 812–817
24. Przyklenk K, Kloner RA (1985) Free Radical Scavengers Improve Contractile Function but not Adenosine Triphosphate Content of the "Stunned Myocardium" (abstr). Circulation 72 (Suppl III): III-350
25. Renlund DG, Gerstenblith G, Lakatta EG, Jacobus WE, Kallman CH, Weisfeldt ML (1984) Perfusate Sodium Modified Post-Ischemic Functional and Metabolic Recovery in the Rabbit Heart. J Mol Cell Cardiol 16: 795–801
26. Rentrop P, DeVivie ER, Karsch KR, Kreuzer H (1979) Acute Myocardial Infarction: Intracoronary Application of Nitroglycerin and Streptokinase in Combination with Transluminal Recanalization. Clin Cardiol 5: 354–356
27. Ruano-Arroyo G, Gerstenblith G, Lakatta EG (1984) Calcium Paradox in the Heart is Modulated by Cell Sodium During the Calcium Free Period. J Mol Cell Cardiol 16: 783–793
28. Simoons ML, Brand MVD, DeZwann C, Verheugt FWA, Remme WJ, Serruys PW, Bar F, Res J, Krauss XH, Vermeer F, Lubsen J (1985) Improved Survival After Early Thrombolysis in Acute Myocardial Infarction. Lancet ii: 578–581
29. Stewart JR, Blackwell WH, Crute SL, Loughlin V, Greenfield LJ, Hess ML (1983) Inhibition of Surgically Induced Ischemia/Reperfusion Injury by Oxygen Free Radical Scavengers. J Thorac Cardiovasc Surg 86: 262–272
30. Werns SW, Michael SJ, Mitsos SE, Dysko RC, Fantone JC, Schork MA, Abrams GD, Pitt B, Lucchesi BR (1986) Reduction of Infarct Size by Allopurinol in the Ischemic-Reperfused Canine Heart. Circulation 73: 518–526
31. Werns SW, Shea WJ, Driscoll EM (1985) The Independent Effects of Oxygen Radical Scavengers on Canine Infarct Size: Reduction by Superoxide Dismutase but not Catalase. Circ Res 56: 895–899
32. Zimmerman ANE, Hulsmann WC (1966) Paradoxical Influence of Calcium Ions on the Permeability of the Cell Membranes of the Isolated Rat Heart. Nature 211: 646–647

33. Zweier JL, Flaherty JT, Weisfeldt ML (1985) Observation of Free Radical Generation in the Post-Ischemic Heart (abstract). Circulation 72: (Suppl III): III-350

Author's address:
Professor Alan D. Guerci, M.D.,
Director, Coronary Care Unit,
The Johns Hopkins Medical Institutions,
Baltimore, Maryland 21205,
U.S.A.

Comparison of the effects of coronary artery occlusion on regional myocardial blood flow distribution and necrosis in conscious primates and dogs

M. Lavallee and S. F. Vatner

Department of Medicine, Harvard Medical School and Brigham and Women's Hospital, Boston, Massachusetts, and New England Regional Primate Research Center, Southboro, Massachusetts

Summary: The effects of acute coronary artery occlusion on regional myocardial blood flow distribution in the remote non-ischemic zone, the central ischemic zone and the lateral border zone of the infarct were evaluated in conscious primates and contrasted to the pattern observed in dogs. Prior to coronary artery occlusion, blood flow was 1.51 ± 0.11 for endocardial (ENDO) and 1.36 ± 0.11 ml/min/g for epicardial (EPI) layers with an ENDO-EPI ratio of 1.17 ± 0.05 for the primate myocardium. In dogs, blood flow before coronary artery occlusion was 1.26 ± 0.10 for ENDO and 1.06 ± 0.09 ml/min/g for EPI with an ENDO-EPI ratio of 1.22 ± 0.06. In primates, regional blood flow in the remote non-ischemic zone increased by $28.0 \pm 4.7\%$ and $31.7 \pm 3.6\%$ for ENDO and EPI layers respectively following coronary occlusion and remained elevated during the subsequent 24 hrs. A similar pattern was observed in dogs for the non-ischemic tissue. At the center of infarct in primates, ENDO and EPI blood flow were depressed by $97.9 \pm 0.7\%$ and by $97.9 \pm 0.8\%$ respectively, at 5 min after coronary occlusion and remained severely depressed throughout the 24 hr observation period. In contrast, at the center of infarct in dogs, there was less severe ischemia ($p < 0.01$) in EPI ($-80.9 \pm 3.5\%$) than in ENDO ($-97.1 \pm 0.9\%$). During the subsequent 24 hrs, blood flow returned to pre-occlusion levels in EPI and improved to $-84.8 \pm 5.0\%$ in ENDO, presumably due to opening of collateral channels. In primates, blood flow at the ischemic lateral border of the infarct was severely depressed and similar to the flow in the center of the infarct, while the non-ischemic lateral border of the the infarct had blood flow levels similar to the remote, non-ischemic myocardium. "Microsphere loss" was observed in the canine infarct but not in the primate infarct.

Introduction

Most of the current knowledge regarding the distribution of myocardial blood flow following acute coronary occlusion is based on experiments conducted in dogs. Very little is known about the response of the coronary circulation to acute occlusion in primates. We have recently characterized the effects of coronary occlusions for 24 h on transmural blood flow distribution in relation to tissue necrosis in conscious primates (14). The goal of this report is to review the effects of permanent coronary artery occlusion for 24 hours on measurements of regional myocardial blood flow and development of infarct in conscious primates and compare those results with data from a group of conscious dogs treated in a similar fashion.

Supported in part by U.S. Public Health Service Grants HL 26215 and HL 33065

Methods

Seven adult Macaca mulatta (6–8 kg) and four Papio anubis (22 and 29 kg) as well as 7 mongrel dogs underwent acute coronary artery occlusion 2–3 weeks after instrumentation. Under general anesthesia with sodium pentobarbital (30 mg/kg) for dogs and halothane (0.5 to 1.0%) for primates, the chest was opened at the fifth intercostal space and Tygon catheters were implanted in the descending aorta and left atrium. A snare made of polyethylene tubing and 2 silk was placed around the left anterior descending coronary artery distally to the first diagonal branch. The chest was closed in layers and the catheters were exteriorized for dogs or buried in subcutaneous pouches for primates.

During the 2–3 weeks recovery period, primates were trained to sit in chairs in the laboratory and dogs were trained to lie quietly on their side. On the day of the experiment, the primates were sedated with 6 to 8 mg/kg of ketamine hydrochloride, and the animals were placed in chairs after the catheters were exteriorized using lidocaine for local anesthesia. With the animals fully awake and alert, aortic and left atrial pressures were recorded through the fluid filled catheters connected to Statham pressure transducers (Oxnard, CA) and lead II ECG were monitored continuously on a stripchart recorder. After control measurements, the left anterior descending coronary artery was occluded for 24 h. Two dogs and two primates showing signs of discomfort after the induction of ischemia were treated with 0.25 mg/kg of morphine sulfate. Arrhythmias were not treated.

Regional myocardial blood flow measurements were made using the radioactive microsphere technique described by Domenech et al., 1969 (7), and utilized in our laboratory (14, 15, 23). The microspheres (15 ± 1 μ, 3M Co.) labelled with Ce-141, Nb-95, Sr-85, and Sc-46 were obtained in dry form and suspended in 0.01% Tween 80 solution (10% in dextran) and agitated in an ultrasonic bath for 60 minutes. Immediately before injection, the microspheres were agitated ultrasonically for 5 minutes and vortexed for 1 minute. Absence of microsphere aggregation was confirmed by microscopic examination. Before injection of microspheres, each animal was tested for possible adverse reaction to the Tween 80 solution (18). Microspheres (2–3 × 10⁶) in 1 ml of solution were injected prior to coronary artery occlusion and at 3–5 min, 1 hr and 24 hrs after coronary artery occlusion and flushed over a 15 second period with 6 ml of saline. Simultaneously, reference arterial blood samples were drawn at rates of 3.38 ml/min for small primates and 7.75 ml/min for dogs and baboons, starting 15 seconds prior to microsphere injection and lasting for 150 secs. The completion of coronary artery occlusion was confirmed at necropsy. Six animals died of ventricular fibrillation prior to 25 hrs. One Rhesus died within 2 minutes after coronary artery occlusion. Three others died within 20 min after coronary artery occlusion and one more died at 16 hrs after coronary artery occlusion. One dog died within 5 min of coronary artery occlusion, while the other 6 survived for 25 hours. After sacrifice of the animals with an overdose of barbiturates, the hearts were excised, the occluded vessel examined for the presence of thrombus, and the left ventricle, including the septum, was divided from base to apex in either 4–5 rings for rhesus or 6–8 rings for baboons and dogs. In all animals surviving more than 6 hrs after coronary artery occlusion, the heart rings were incubated at 37 °C for 40 min in 1% triphenyl tetrazolium chloride (TTC) solution and then in 10% formalin for 10 min to reveal normal (stained in dark red) and necrotic (non-stained) tissue (8, 16). Transmural myocardial samples obtained from normally perfused zones as well as from the necrotic areas were divided into 3 layers (endocardium, midwall and epicardium) and counted for 10 minutes in a multichannel gamma counter (Searle Analytic, Inc.) with appropriately selected energy windows to obtain regional myocardial blood flow. In primates, samples were also obtained immediately adjacent to the lateral border of the infarct from both normal and necrotic zones. Samples obtained from the infarct border zone and central ischemic areas were stained with hematoxylin-eosin and examined under light microscopy to confirm necrosis. For animals dying early after coronary artery occlusion, myocardial samples were obtained by dividing each ventricular ring into 5–6 transmural samples which were further divided in three layers.

The data anaylzed statistically using two-way analysis of variance (1).

Results

The pattern of infarction differed in dogs and primates. In primates, the infarcts were transmural with a distinct lateral border zone (Fig. 1a). In dogs, the epicardium was generally spared and the lateral border of the infarct was not as clearly defined (Fig. 1b). For the primates, the samples for regional blood flow determinations were taken in the central ischemic zones, the remote normal zones, and at both sides adjacent to the lateral edge of the infarct. In dogs, only the remote normal zone and the central ischemic zones were sampled, since the lateral edges of the infarct were not clearly defined.

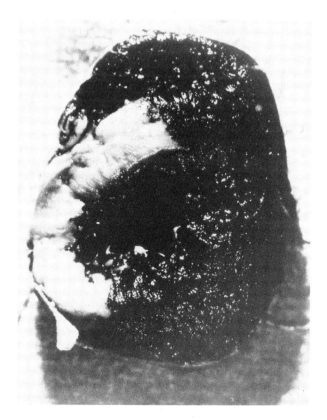

Fig. 1a. This photograph illustrates the pattern of infarct observed in a baboon, 24 h after coronary artery occlusion. The non-ischemic myocardium is stained in dark red by the TTC and the necrotic myocardium is TTC negative. Note the transmural distribution of necrotic tissue and the abrupt transition from normal to necrotic tissue at the lateral edge of the infarct.

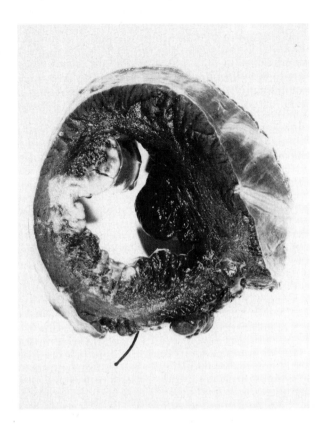

Fig. 1b. This photograph illustrates the typical pattern of infarct observed in a dog, 24 h after coronary artery occlusion. In contrast to the primate (Fig. 1a), the canine infarct occurred primarily in endocardial layers. Furthermore, the lateral edge of infarct was not as clearly demonstrated.

Hemodynamics

Prior to coronary artery occlusion baseline hemodynamics were similar in dogs and primates, except for heart rate, which was significantly higher ($p < 0.01$) in primates (155 ± 3.8 beats/min) than in dogs (96 ± 7.6 beats/min). With acute coronary artery occlusion, mean left atrial pressure rose similarly in both species, and remained elevated over the next 24 hrs. For both dogs and primates, mean arterial pressure was not changed from pre-occlusion baseline at 3–5 min and 1 hrs after coronary artery occlusion. A significant fall in mean arterial pressure (-18 ± 5.1 mmHg, $p < 0.05$) was observed in dogs at 24 hrs after coronary artery occlusion. In primates, the fall in mean arterial pressure was not statistically significant at that time.

Regional Myocardial Blood Flow

Non-Ischemic Zone:

In primates, at 3–5 min following coronary artery occlusion, blood flow rose in the non-ischemic myocardium both in ENDO ($28.0 \pm 4.7\%$) and EPI ($31.7 \pm 3.6\%$) layers. One hour after coronary artery occlusion, blood flow remained elevated by 24.2 ± 2.9% and 26.3 ± 3.8% in ENDO and EPI layers respectively and then rose further to 33.9 ± 7.2% (ENDO) and 42.4 ± 7.4% (EPI) at 24 hrs. The ENDO/EPI flow ratio was 1.17 ± 0.05 before occlusion and was not changed significantly following coronary artery occlusion. In dogs, acute coronary artery occlusion increased blood flow in ENDO (36.2 ± 5.3%) and EPI (38.0 ± 7.4%) layers. As in primates, blood flow in the non-ischemic myocardium remained elevated for the subsequent 24 hrs (Table 2). ENDO/EPI flow ratio was 1.22 ± 0.06 before occlusion and was not modified significantly by the induction of ischemia.

Central Ischemic Zone:

In primates, blood flow to the central ischemic zone fell similar in ENDO (97.9 ± 0.7%) and EPI (97.9 ± 0.8%) layers at 3–5 min after coronary artery occlusion and did not improve significantly over the subsequent 24 hrs (Fig. 2). No significant reversal of the ENDO/EPI flow ratio was observed at 3–5 min after coronary artery occlusion. At 1 hr and 24 hrs after occlusion, blood flow tended to be lower in ENDO layers. However, statistical significance was not observed, most likely due to the extremely low blood flow levels in both layers. In contrast, in dogs, blood flow in the central ischemic zone was depressed

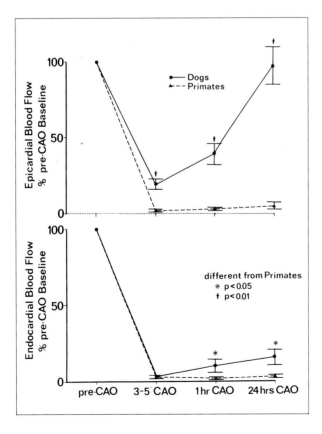

Fig. 2 (Top). The percent changes in epicardial blood flow in the central ischemic zone are compared for dogs and primates, at 5 min. 1 hr, and 24 hrs after coronary artery occlusion. Significant differences between the two species are noted by symbols.

Fig. 2 (Bottom). The percent reductions in endocardial blood flow in the central ischemic zone are compared for dogs and primates at 5 min. 1 hr, and 24 hrs after coronary artery occlusion. The symbols indicate significant differences between the species.

75

significantly more (p < 0.01) in ENDO (97.1 ± 0.9%) than in EPI (80.9 ± 3.5%) layers at 3–5 min after coronary artery occlusion, resulting in a reversal of the ENDO/EPI blood flow ratio. Blood flow rose in both layers over the subsequent 24 hr period. In ENDO layers, blood flow was still depressed by 84.8 ± 5.0% at 24 hrs, while in EPI layers, blood flow was no longer significantly depressed at 24 hrs after coronary artery occlusion (Fig. 2).

Lateral Non-Ischemic Border Zone:

In primates, regional blood flow in the normally stained tissue immediately adjacent to the necrotic myocardium was increased in ENDO (18.3 ± 10%) and EPI (21.8 ± 8.8%) layers respectively, at 3–5 min after coronary artery occlusion. These changes were similar to those observed in the remote, non-ischemic tissue. At 1 hour, regional blood flow remained elevated in both layers and then rose further at 24 hrs in ENDO (52.4 ± 18.4%) and EPI (57.6 ± 19.7%) layers (Fig. 3).

Lateral Ischemic Border Zone:

In primates, regional blood flow in the non-stained (ischemic) myocardium, immediately adjacent to the normally perfused tissue, fell both in ENDO (98.1 ± 1.1%) and EPI (96.5 ± 1.2%) layers at 3–5 min after coronary artery occlusion. These changes were

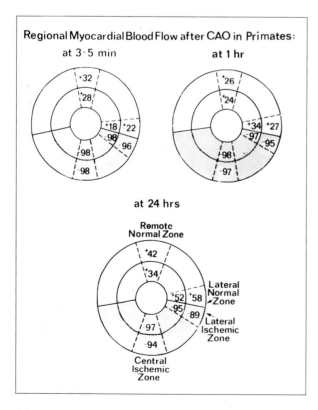

Fig. 3. The % changes from pre-occlusion baseline at 5 min. 1 hr, and 24 hrs in the remote non-ischemic zone (clear), the central ischemic zone (shaded), and adjacent samples from either the non-ischemic or ischemic tissue lateral to the edge of the infarct are indicated, for the primate myocardium. Similar reductions in blood flow for the tissue and the central ischemic zone or in the ischemic border of the infarct were found. The normal tissue immediately adjacent to that ischemic tissue, had blood flow levels similar to those found in the remote normal zone. (Reprinted with permission from American Journal of Physiology 246: H635–639, 1984.)

similar to those observed in the central ischemic zone (Fig. 3). At 1 hr after coronary artery occlusion, regional blood flow remained depressed in ENDO (97.4 ± 2.3%) and EPI (94.9 ± 3.3%) layers and did not improve significantly after 24 hrs of coronary artery occlusion in either ENDO (–95.0 ± 3.2%) or EPI (–88.9 ± 4.1%) layers. Thus, in terms of blood flow, the lateral ischemic edge of the infarct behaved similarly to the tissue located at the center of infarct.

"Microsphere loss"

In the necrotic tissue located at the center of the canine infarct, "microsphere loss" occurred as indicated by the reduced regional blood flow levels compared to the remote non-ischemic myocardium prior to coronary artery occlusion. In EPI layers, pre-coronary artery occlusion levels of regional myocardial blood flow in the central ischemic zone (0.82 ± 0.05 ml/min/g) were significantly less (p < 0.05) than in remote non-ischemic myocardial sites (1.06 ± 0.09 ml/min/g). In ENDO layers, regional myocardial blood flow was lower in the central ischemic zone (1.08 ± 0.06 ml/min/g) compared with the remote normal zone (1.26 ± 0.10 ml/min/g), but this difference was not statistically significant (p = 0.13). In primates, regional myocardial blood flow levels prior to coronary artery occlusion in normal (1.51 ± 0.11) and ischemic (1.54 ± 0.11) ENDO, as well as in normal (1.36 ± 0.11) and ischemic (1.37 ± 0.13) EPI were essentially similar, indicating that "microsphere loss" was minimal.

Discussion

There are major differences in regional myocardial blood flow distribution following acute coronary artery occlusion in primates as compared to those observed in dogs (11, 12, 14). First, in primates, coronary artery occlusion did not result in a reversal of ENDO-EPI blood flow ratio, which is consistently observed in dogs [2, 22, 25]. In primates, the reductions in EPI blood flow are essentially as severe as the reductions in ENDO flow. There was virtually no flow to ENDO and EPI layers following coronary artery occlusion. Lubbe et al., 1974 (17), as well as Weisse et al., 1976 (26) reported less severe reductions of transmural blood flow following coronary artery occlusion in anesthetized baboons with an open chest. Whereas in the present study, the ischemic area was identified precisely using the TTC technique, the approaches used previously by others did not allow an accurate delineation of the infarct for the determination of regional blood flow measurements. Any slight error would increase the blood flow levels significantly due to inclusion of normally perfused myocardium in the analysis. Moreover the study of Lubbe et al., 1974 (17), failed to indicate the existence of a transmural gradient in blood flow distribution prior to coronary artery occlusion. In our conscious primates, we found that prior to coronary artery occlusion, regional myocardial blood flow as distributed preferentially to the endocardium. It is possible that the combined effects of anesthesia and of an open chest procedure could obscure the transmural gradient of blood flow across the ventricular wall.

Another major difference between the two species was the failure of blood flow in either ENDO or EPI layers to improve over the ensuing 24 hrs period in primates. In contrast, in dogs, ENDO flow rose significantly at 1 hr and then further at 24 hrs, while EPI flow almost returned to control level over the 24 hr period. These differences can most likely be attributed to the presence of preformed collateral vessels in dogs [2, 13, 21, 22) whereas these vessels are sparse in the primate myocardium (5, 9).

Because of these important differences in perfusion of the ischemic tissue, the resulting pattern of infarct differed in the two species. In dogs, EPI layers were generally spared and the pattern of necrosis was variable at the lateral ischemic border. In primates, necrosis was transmural with a sharp demarcation between normal and necrotic tissue at the lateral ischemic border. This is consistent with the findings of Harken et al., 1981 (10), indicating that at the lateral border of the infarct, the distance between normal and anoxic tissue is less than 50 μm. In some animals, a small epicardial rim < 2 mm of non-infarcted myocardium was observed. Crozatier, et al., 1978 (5), previously noted this pattern in anesthetized baboons.

In the present study, the use of TTC staining technique permitted a clear identification of the area of necrosis and the evaluation of blood flow distribution in normal and ischemic tissue at the lateral ischemic border in primates. The validity of this histochemical technique has been recently demonstrated by comparison with histological identification of infarcted tissue (8).

Even at the boundary between necrotic and normal tissue, myocardial perfusion of tissue in the ischemic lateral edge of the border zone, did not significantly improve over time. These findings are consistent with post-mortem quantitative evaluations of collateral vessels in baboons undergoing acute coronary occlusion and with the absence of significant precapillary anastomoses between perfusion beds in primates (5, 9). Thus, the existence of either a lateral or an epicardial border zone, indicated by the TTC staining technique and confirmed by measurements of regional blood flow, was not demonstrated. Moreover, the stability of regional blood flow values at the lateral and epicardial border of the infarct, suggests that the amount of myocardium at risk early after coronary artery occlusion remains constant over the subsequent 24 hours, with no evidence of either a lateral or epicardial border zone. For the tissue immediately adjacent to the necrotic area, regional blood flow levels were almost identical to those observed in the remote, non-ischemic myocardium of the circumflex bed. Thus, the lateral border of the primate infarct is characterized by a sharp distinction between normally perfused and severely ischemic tissue.

Limitations in the accuracy of the radioactive microsphere technique in the study of regional myocardial blood flow distribution, following acute coronary artery occlusion, have been previously demonstrated in dogs. These studies have attributed "microsphere loss" either to dislodgement from the necrotic tissue (3, 19) or to apparent loss seondary to tissue edema, hemorrhage and inflammation following coronary artery occlusion (19, 21). In the present study this phenomenon was observed in the infarcted canine myocardium, since blood flow measurements prior to coronary artery occlusion in necrotic tissue, were significantly less than control measurements prior to coronary artery occlusion in the remote normal zone. Prior investigations indicated that physical loss of 15 μ microspheres is minimal and that "microsphere loss" can be attributed to edema, hemorrhage and inflammation (4, 21). Since we utilized 15 μ microspheres, the reduced levels of blood flow measured prior to coronary artery occlusion in the canine ischemic tissue, was most likely due to apparent "microsphere loss". Moreover, the tissue swelling is probably secondary to edema, since gross hemorrhage was not observed in the canine infarct. In contrast, microsphere loss was not observed in primates in either EPI or ENDO layers. This could be related to the severe transmural reductions in regional myocardial blood flow in primates and possibly to the lack of opening of collateral channels after the induction of ischemia. It is conceivable that edema formation is dependent upon the availability of collateral blood flow after coronary artery occlusion. Previous studies conducted in canine models of myocardial infarction indicated that tissue edema can hasten necrosis of the ischemic myocardium (6). In fact, procedures designed to limit tissue swelling associated with myocardial ischemia will ultimately reduce the amount of cellular disruption (20). This problem may not be as important at 24 hrs after coronary artery occlusion in the primate model of ischemia used in the present investigation.

In summary, as opposed to the pattern of infarct observed in dogs, the primate ischemic myocardium is characterized by 1) transmural reductions in myocardial blood flow at the center of infarct; 2) sustained decreases in blood flow over the 24 h occlusion period in the ischemic tissue with no evidence of opening of collateral channels; 3) a sharp distinction between ischemic and non-ischemic myocardium at the lateral edge of the infarct, with no evidence of either epicardial or lateral border zones; 4) absence of "microsphere loss" from the necrotic myocardium suggesting that tissue edema is not a feature of the myocardial infarct in primates.

References

1. Armitage P (1973) Statistical methods in medical research. Oxford, Blackwell Scientific Publications.
2. Bishop SP, White FC, Bloor CM (1976) Regional myocardial blood flow during acute myocardial infarction in the conscious dog. Circ Res 38: 429–438.
3. Capurro NL, Goldstein RE, Aamodt R, Smith HJ, Epstein SE (1979) Losses of microspheres from ischemic canine cardiac tissue. An important technical limitation. Circ Res 44: 223–227.
4. Consigny PM, Verrier ED, Payne BD, Edelist G, Jester J, Baer RW, Vlahakes GJ, Hoffmann JIE (1982) Acute and chronic microsphere loss from canine left ventricular myocardium. Am J Physiol 242: H392–H404.
5. Crozatier F, Ross J, Jr, Franklin D, Bloor CM, White FC, Tomoike H, McKown DP (1978) Myocardial infarction in the baboon: regional function and the collateral circulation. Am J Physiol 235: H413–H421.
6. Di Bona DR, Powell WJ, Jr (1980) Quantitative correlation between cell swelling and necrosis in myocardial ischemia in dogs. Circ Res 47: 653–665.
7. Domenech RJ, Hoffman JIE, Nobel MIM, Saunders KB, Henson JR, Subijanto S (1969) Total and regional coronary blood flow measured by radioactive microspheres in conscious and anesthetized dogs. Circ Res 25: 581–596.
8. Fishbein MC, Meerbaum S, Rit J, Ando V, Kanmatsuse K, Mercier JC, Corday E, Ganz W (1981) Early phase acute myocardial infarct size quantification: Validation of the triphenyl tetrazolium chloride tissue enzyme staining technique. Am Heart J 101: 593–600.
9. Geary GG, Smith GT, McNamara JJ (1981) Defining the anatomic perfusion bed of an occluded coronary artery and the region at risk to infarction. A comparative study in the baboon, pig, and dog. Am J Cardiol 47: 1240–1247.
10. Harken AH, Simson MB, Haselgrove J, Wetstein L, Harden III WR, Barlow CH (1981) Early ischemia after complete coronary ligation in the rabbit, dog, pig, and monkey. Am J Physiol 241: H202–H210.

11. Heyndrickx GR, Amano J, Patrick TA, Manders WT, Rogers GG, Rosendorff C, Vatner SF (1985) Effects of coronary artery reperfusion on regional myocardial blood flow and function in conscious baboons. Circulation 71: 1029–1037.

12. Heyndrickx GR, Manao J, Kenna T, Fallon JT, Patrick TA, Manders WT, Rogers G, Rosendorff C, Vatner SF (1985) Creatine kinase release not associated with necrosis after short periods of coronary artery occlusion in conscious baboons. J Am College of Cardiol 6: 1299–1303.

13. Hirzel HO, Nelson GR, Sonnenblick EH, Kirk ES (1976) Redistribution of collateral blood flow from necrotic to surviving myocardium following coronary occlusion in the dog. Circ Res 39: 214–222.

14. Lavallee M, Vatner SF (1984) Regional myocardial blood flow and necrosis in conscious primates following coronary occlusion. Am J Physiol 246: H635–H639.

15. Lavallee M, Cox D, Patric TA, Vatner SF (1983) Salvage of myocardial function by coronary artery reperfusion 1, 2 and 3 hours after occlusion in conscious dogs. Circ Res 53: 235–247.

16. Lie JT, Pairolero PC, Holley KE, Titus JL (1975) Macroscopic enzyme-mapping verification of large, homogeneous, experimental myocardial infarcts of predictable size and location in dogs. J Thorac Cardiovasc Surg 69: 599–605.

17. Lubbe WF, Peisach M, Pretorius K, Bruyneel KJJ, Opie LH (1974) Distribution of myocardial blood flow before and after coronary artery ligation in the baboon. Relation to early ventricular fibrillation. Cardiovasc Res 8: 478–487.

18. Millard RW, Baig H, Vatner SF (1977) Cardiovascular effects of radioactive microsphere suspensions and Tween 80 solutions. Am J Physiol 232: H331–H334.

19. Murdock RH, Cobb FR (1980) Effects of infarcted myocardium on regional blood flow measurements to ischemic regions in canine heart. Circ Res 47: 701–709.

20. Powell WJ, Jr, Di Bona DR, Flores J, Leaf A (1976) The protective effect of hypertonic mannitol in myocardial ischemia and necrosis. Circulation 54: 603–615.

21. Reimer KA, Jennings RB (1979) The changing anatomic reference base of evolving myocardial infarction. Circulation 60: 866–876.

22. Rivas F, Cobb FR, Bach RJ, Greenfield JC, Jr (1976) Relationship between blood flow to ischemic regions and extent of myocardial infarction. Circ Res 38: 439–447.

23. Vatner SF (1980) Correlation between acute reductions in myocardial blood flow and function in conscious dogs. Circ Res 47: 201–207.

24. Weisse AB, Kearney K, Narang RM, Regan TJ (1976) Comparison of the coronary collateral circulation in dogs and baboons after coronary occlusion. Am Heart J 92: 193–200.

25. White FC, Sanders M, Bloor CM (1978) Regional redistribution of myocardial blood flow after coronary occlusion and reperfusion in the conscious dog. Am J Cardiol 42: 234–243.

Authors' address:
Stephen F. Vatner, M.D.
New England Regional Primate Research Center
One Pine Hill Drive
Southboro, MA 01772
U.S.A.

Metabolic consequences of myocardial ischemia and assessment of coronary sinus interventions

Noninvasive evaluation by positron emission tomography

H. R. Schelbert and M. Schwaiger

Division of Nuclear Medicine and Biophysics, Department of Radiological Sciences, UCLA School of Medicine, University of California, Los Angeles, and Laboratory of Nuclear Medicine, Laboratory of Biomedical and Environmental Sciences*, University of California, Los Angeles, California (U.S.A.)

Introduction

Reductions in regional myocardial blood flow and oxygen supply trigger a sequence of functional and metabolic events. Regional myocardial function ceases almost instantaneously as blood flow and oxygen supply decline. The latter induce a series of metabolic alterations that result in reduced production of high energy phosphate compounds. Conversely, if blood flow is restored before irreversible injury occurs, energy metabolism rapidly resumes and undergoes a sequence of metabolic changes while recovery of regional myocardial function follows only slowly.

Numerous techniques exist for evaluating regional changes in blood flow and function. These parameters are undoubtedly important for defining the extent and severity of ischemia. Yet, it would seem that these changes associated with ischemia, in particular, myocardial function, reflect events that occur largely at the cellular level and are expressions rather than causes within the context of the pathophysiology of myocardial ischemia. Such events include alterations in substrate oxidation, a decline in ATP production and a fall in cellular high energy phosphate content (Figure 1). Alterations in energy metabolism during myocardial ischemia appear to follow a distinct pattern. Residual tissue blood flow including oxygen delivery and removal of inhibitory metabolic intermediates on one hand and energy demand on the other, influence the rate of progression of these metabolic alterations. They may proceed until reaching a point of no return with disruption of the cell membranes and ensuing cell death or reach a "new steady state" where residual energy production suffices for maintaining cell membrane integrity. For both conditions, the degree of functional impairment is indistinguishable. The amount of residual tissue blood flow may differ between both states, yet these differences are often small and escape detection by available techniques. Therefore, it would appear that characterization of residual metabolic activity holds the key for determining the tissue state in myocardial ischemia.

---

* Operated for the U.S. Department of Energy by the University of California under Contract ⊣ DE-AC03-76-SF00012. This work was supported in part by the Director of the Office of Energy Research, Office of Health and Environmental Research, by NIH Grants ⊣ HL 29845 and ⊣ HL 33177 and by an Investigative Group Award by the Greater Los Angeles Affiliate of the American Heart Association

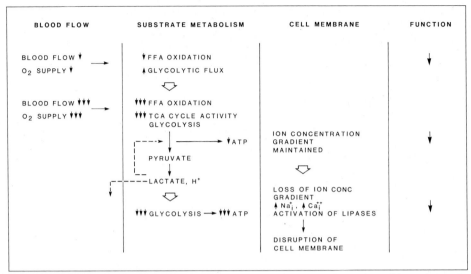

BLOOD FLOW	SUBSTRATE METABOLISM	CELL MEMBRANE	FUNCTION

Fig. 1. Schematic drawing of pathophysiologic events in myocardial ischemia. With moderate decreases in regional myocardial blood flow and oxygen supply, regional myocardial function declines or ceases completely. Metabolically, oxidation of fatty acid decreases in favor of increased glycolytic flux which may entail both enhanced anaerobic glycolysis and oxidation of glucose. More severe reductions in blood flow remain without further effect on segmental function but inhibit oxidative metabolism of free fatty acid and glucose. Anaerobic glycolysis with conversion of glucose to pyruvate and, further, to lactate, may persist as one of the few mechanisms remaining for production of ATP which then is used largely for maintaining basic cell functions, especially transmembraneous ion concentration gradients. Persistence of glycolysis depends upon removal of lactate and hydrogen ions from the cell via residual blood flow. If blood flow is too low and cytosolic concentrations of lactate and hydrogen ions increase, they inhibit glycolysis as one of the last resorts of ATP production. Transmembraneous ion concentration gradients can therefore no longer be maintained. An influx of sodium and consequently, calcium ions follows with activation of lipases and disruption of cell membranes leading to irreversible cell injury.

PET for the study of regional myocardial metabolism

The noninvasive study and measurement of regional myocardial metabolism of the human heart has long remained elusive but has now become possible with positron emission tomography (PET). This new imaging modality owes its unique capability to several features (5). The high contrast tomographic images are quantitative, that is, they reflect quantitatively regional tissue concentrations of tracers of biological processes. Regional radioactivity concentrations are measured from the cross-sectional images in counts per minute per gram myocardium. Secondly, a family of tracers of regional myocardial physiology is available. Positron emitting isotopes of oxygen, carbon, nitrogen and fluorine are labeled to physiologically active compounds without modifying their intrinsic biologic properties. They are administered in true tracer quantities which remain without effect on the biologic process under study. External imaging of uptake and turnover of radiotracers in myocardial tissue in response to an arterial tracer input function applied with tracer kinetic principles permits the in vivo measurement of regional physiologic pro-

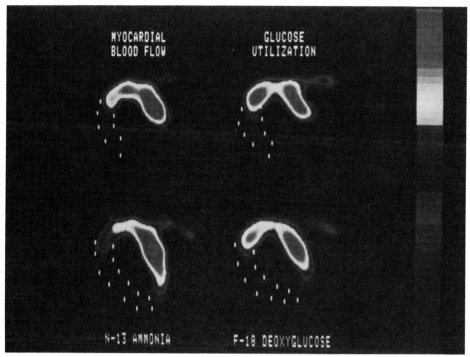

Fig. 2. Regional myocardial blood flow and glucose utilization in acute human myocardial infarction. Two contiguous cross-sectional PET images of blood flow (left panel), recorded after intravenous N-13 ammonia, and of exogenous glucose utilization (right panel), recorded after intravenous administration of F-18 deoxyglucose in a patient studied 52 hours after onset of acute symptoms and with documented acute myocardial infarction. The cross sections are seen from the patient's head. Note the absence of blood flow in the lateral and postero-lateral walls (dotted lines) associated with a proportionate decrease in glucose utilization in the same left ventricular segments.

cesses that are expressed in milliliters of blood or millimoles of substrate per minute per gram myocardium.

Myocardial ischemia and infarction by PET

When patients with acute myocardial infarction are studied within 72 hours of onset of symptoms, PET frequently reveals persistent metabolic activity in infarcted myocardial segments (13). In more than half of "infarcted" segments, that exhibit on electrocardiography evidence for acute myocardial infarction and in which blood flow and function are reduced or absent, glucose utilization as demonstrated with a tracer of exogenous glucose uptake, F-18 2-deoxyglucose (6, 7) is augmented either relative to blood flow (as determined with N-13 ammonia (8, 9)) or in absolute terms, that is, the "infarcted segment" utilizes more exogenous glucose than non-infarcted myocardium (Figures 2 and 3). Conversely, regional fatty acid metabolism is abnormal. Less C-11 palmitate, a tracer of myocardial fatty acid metabolism (10) accumulates in ischemic myocardium because of

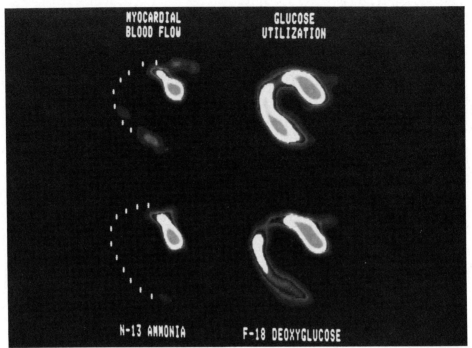

Fig. 3. Regional myocardial blood flow and glucose utilization in acute human myocardial infarction. Again, two contiguous cross-sectional images of blood flow are shown on the left, the corresponding cross-sectional images of exogenous glucose utilization are shown on the right. Note the decrease in blood flow in the anterior, lateral and posterior walls. In contrast to the patient shown in Figure 2, glucose utilization in the antero-lateral and posterior segments is preserved, indicating tissue viability.

reduced delivery of tracer, impaired metabolic sequestration and, consequently, enhanced back diffusion of tracer from tissue into blood. The characteristic biexponential tracer tissue clearance curve is markedly distorted. C-11 palmitate clears only slowly from "infarcted" myocardium, often associated with complete loss of the early rapid tissue clearance curve component as a reflection of impaired or absent oxidation of free fatty acid (Figures 3 and 4). In contrast, in the other half of "infarcted segments", both exogenous glucose utilization and fatty acid metabolism are reduced in proportion to the decreased blood flow or even entirely absent.

The abnormalities as observed in the human heart with PET are consistent with metabolic alterations described in myocardial ischemia from invasive animal experiments or as derived in in vitro experimental systems (2, 3). Substrate metabolism is geared towards production of energy which is stored in the high energy phosphate bonds of ATP. As shown schematically in Figure 5, the normal heart at rest spends about two thirds of the high energy phosphate for generating contractile force and about 15% for diastolic relaxation. About 3 to 5% are needed for maintaining transmembraneous ion concentration gradients and the remainder for "wear and tear", that is, for repair processes and cell upkeep. As production of high energy phosphate declines with myocardial ischemia, expenditures of ATP for generation of contractile force and for diastolic relaxation are mini-

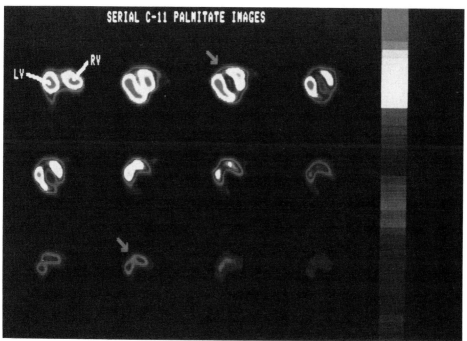

Fig. 4. Serial cross-sectional images through the mid-left ventricle obtained in a patient four days after an acute myocardial infarction with intravenous C-11 palmitate. The first five images were each recorded 3 minutes after tracer injection. Intermediate images recorded from 15 to 30 minutes are deleted from the figure. The late serial images each recorded for 5 minutes begin at 30 minutes (with the second image from the left in the second row, asterisk). The very early images depict the C-11 activity in the right and left ventricles (RV and LV). The tracer subsequently clears from blood into myocardium. Note the segmental reduction in C-11 palmitate uptake in the infarcted anterior wall (arrow). As indicated by the color code, the tracer rapidly clears from normal myocardium but is retained in the infarcted segment (arrow, third line).

mized and, mechanical function ceases as a consequence. Whatever energy is available, it is now spent for maintaining transmembraneous electrolyte gradients and for supporting basic cell functions, which are critical for survival and repair. Hence, it is the amount of ATP that still can be produced through either anaerobic or aerobic metabolism that may guarantee cell survival and thus account for tissue viability. From this point of view it would seem important to identify and measure residual metabolic activity in order to accurately identify remaining viable myocardium.

Ischemia initiates a now well defined sequence of alterations in substrate metabolism (Figure 7). Its rate of progression is largely determined by the magnitude of reduction in blood flow and oxygen availability. The amount of residual tissue blood flow may determine at what level the sequence of metabolic alterations stops and whether residual metabolic activity is maintained or whether ischemia rapidly proceeds to necrosis. There appears to be a consensus that β-oxidation of free fatty acid is the site most sensitive to oxygen deprivation (2). In other words, as blood flow, and with it, oxygen supply fall only moderately, flux of free fatty acid through the β-oxidative spiral declines and a disproportionately greater fraction of free fatty acid is diverted into the endogenous lipid pool.

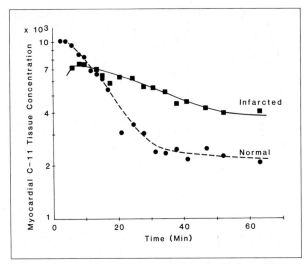

Fig. 5. Uptake and clearance of C-11 palmitate in normal and "infarcted" human myocardium. The two time activity curves were derived from the serial PET images obtained in the patient shown in Figure 4. In normal myocardium (solid circles), C-11 palmitate clears in a typical biexponential fashion with an early rapid and a slow clearance curve component. The early rapid phase reflects oxidation of C-11 palmitate. The relative size of the clearance curve component represents the fraction of tracer that is oxidized and the slope of the curve the rate of tracer turnover or flux of C-11 palmitate through β-oxidation and the TCA cycle. The "infarcted" segment (solid rectangles), reveals reduced tracer uptake. Importantly, the typical biexponential clearance curve morphology is no longer preserved with a loss of the early rapid clearance phase. This indicates a marked reduction in the fraction of tracer that is oxidized and its turnover rate or flux through the oxidative pathway consistent with impaired oxidation of free fatty acid in ischemic myocardium.

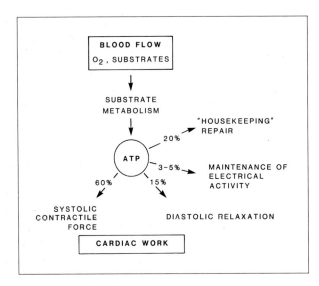

Fig. 6. Schematic representation of energy expenditure in myocardium for various tasks. Regional myocardial ischemia is conventionally assessed by techniques that evaluate regional myocardial blood flow and regional myocardial function or cardiac work. Both aspects of regional myocardial physiology are linked by substrate metabolism which generates high energy phosphate (ATP). In the heart at rest, approximately 75% of the energy is expended into mechanical function. The remainder is used for housekeeping (wear and tear, as well as repair) and maintenance of electrical activity (i.e., transmembraneous ion concentration gradients).

PET studies accurately reflect these changes as a decline in regional myocardial blood flow and regional myocardial C-11 palmitate uptake. The fractional distribution of C-11 palmitate as evidenced on the tissue clearance time activity curve shifts towards the large, slow turnover endogenous lipid pool as the relative size of the early rapid clearance

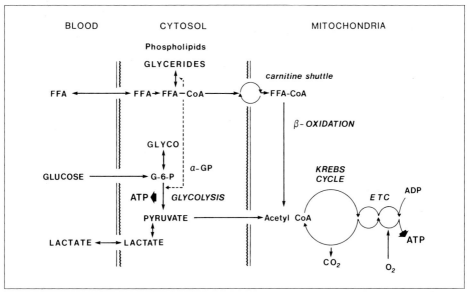

Fig. 7. Schematic representation of myocardial substrate metabolism. Free fatty acid (FFA) is considered the primary substrate of oxidative metabolism. Upon entering the cell, FFA is activated to FFA CoA which then is either deposited in the endogenous lipid pool in form of glycerides and phospholipids or transported via the carnitine shuttle into mitochondria for β-oxidation to acetyl-CoA and subsequent oxidation through the Krebs cycle (TCA cycle) to CO_2. Glucose is phosphorylated via the hexokinase reaction to glucose-6-phosphate (G-6-P), the transmembraneous uptake and phosphorylation step of glucose is traced by F-18 deoxyglucose. Glucose-6-phosphate is then either synthesized to glycogen (GLYCO) or catabolized through glycolysis to pyruvate which is transferred into mitochondria and enters the TCA cycle in form of acetyl-CoA. During glycolysis, α-glycerolphosphate (α-GP) is liberated and used for formation of triglycerides. Myocardial ischemia leads to any impairment of β-oxidation and an increase in glycolytic flux. Accordingly, more FFA-CoA enters the endogenous lipid cool. Oxidation of glucose with transfer of pyruvate into the TCA cycle may persist for some time. However, as oxidative metabolism becomes impaired, pyruvate is converted to lactate and, depending upon residual blood flow, either removed from the cell or if blood flow is absent, accumulates in cytosol and inhibits glycolysis.

phase and its clearance halftime decline (Figures 5, 8, 9, 10). A shift from free fatty acid to glucose utilization occurs (Figure 8). Glycolytic flux may initially remain largely aerobic with transfer of pyruvate (as the end product of glycolysis) into mitochondria and the TCA cycle for complete oxidation (4). However, with further decreases in oxygen supply, oxidation of glucose progressively declines and ATP production via anaerobic glycolysis remains one of the few residual sources of energy. The rate of glycolysis appears to depend largely upon the rate of removal of inhibitory metabolic intermediates as for example lactic acid and hydrogen ions. If tissue blood flow is maintained to some extent, self-contamination of the cell with these inhibitory metabolic intermediates can be avoided and cell membrane integrity be preserved. If on the other hand these metabolites cannot be removed, glycolysis decreases and ATP production no longer suffices to maintain a transmembraneous electrolyte concentration gradient. A massive influx of sodium and,

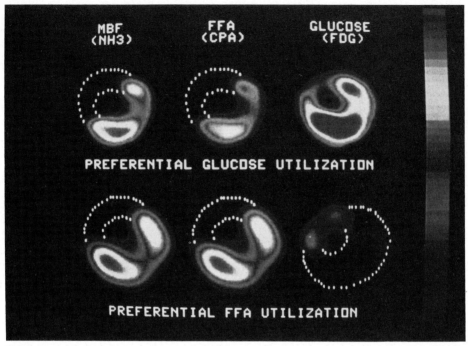

Fig. 8. Comparison between regional myocardial blood flow (MBF; evaluated with N-13 ammonia, NH₃) and uptake of C-11 palmitate (CPA) and F-18 2-deoxyglucose (FDG) in acutely ischemic myocardium in dog experiments. Myocardial ischemia was induced after partially stenosing the left anterior descending coronary artery and rapid atrial pacing. The upper panel shows a study in a dog after normal feeding, the lower panel a study in a dog after a 48 hours fast when free fatty acid plasma levels were high and glucose levels low. In this condition, free fatty acid becomes the primary substrate with little or no glucose utilization. Note the segmental reduction in blood flow in the anterior wall as shown on the cross-sectional images obtained after intravenous N-13 ammonia. Uptake of C-11 palmitate is reduced in the same segment in proportion to blood flow as shown in the upper and lower panels. Utilization of exogenous glucose is however augmented relative to blood flow (as shown in the upper panel) where tracer uptake in the ischemic segment is reduced when compared to normal myocardium, yet disproportionately less when compared to the reduction of blood flow. By contrast, in the dog fasted for 48 hours, no FDG uptake is noted in normal myocardium, whereas tracer uptake in the acutely ischemic segment is increased in absolute terms.

consequently, of calcium ensues, followed by activation of lipases and destruction of cell membranes, leading to irreversible tissue injury (1).

Conversely, if blood flow is restored either spontaneously or through therapeutic interventions, the sequence of functional and metabolic changes reverses. This information stems less from in vitro animal experimental systems but rather from studies with PET and tracers of blood flow and metabolism in acute and chronic dog experiments (11, 12). Reperfusion after only short coronary occlusions restores oxidation of FFA only slowly while improvement of function trails behind recovery of metabolism. Reperfusion after longer time periods of coronary occlusion, for example of 3 hours duration, does not result in an immediate improvement in segmental function. In fact, it often deteriorates even further or fails to change during the initial several days of reperfusion. This observa-

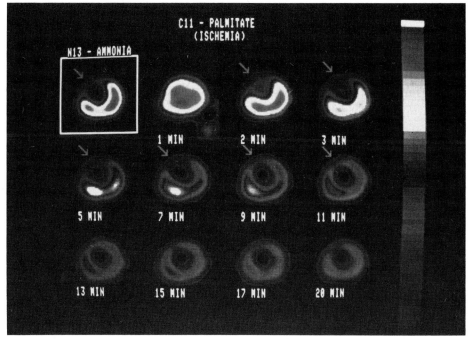

Fig. 9. Acute myocardial ischemia and tissue kinetics of C-11 palmitate in experimentally induced acute myocardial ischemia. Serial PET images were obtained through the mid-left ventricle beginning with the injection of tracer and continued for approximately 40 minutes. The initial images reveal most of the tracer activity in the ventricular cavity. After clearance of C-11 palmitate from blood into myocardium, the left ventricular wall is well visualized. Note reduced tracer uptake in the acutely ischemic segment which is proportional to the segmental decrease in blood flow (inset, left upper corner, N-13 ammonia). The subsequent images reveal the clearance of tracer from normal and from ischemic myocardium.

tion emphasizes the limited value of changes in regional function in response to reconstitution of blood flow as an accurate predictor of tissue outcome. As blood flow recovers, glucose utilization is markedly augmented during the early reperfusion period (Figure 11). C-11 palmitate turnover remains initially depressed but subsequently improves as glucose utilization returns to control levels (Figure 12). Thus, a reversal in metabolic events appears to occur during reperfusion. These observations suggest an initial resumption of glycolysis, that is largely anaerobic, while mitochondrial function may remain depressed for some time. As the latter recovers, fatty acid oxidation normalizes and glucose utilization returns to control values. These observations further indicate the limitations of regional wall motion abnormalities or their changes early after reperfusion as accurate predictors of late functional outcome and stress the importance of metabolic studies in myocardial ischemia.

Returning to the observations with PET in patients with acute myocardial infarction, at least two mechanisms may account for the metabolic findings. In about half of the segments that revealed persistence of metabolic activity on PET early after the acute event, function improved spontaneously over the following four to six weeks. This was associat-

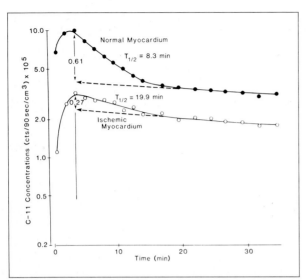

Fig. 10. Uptake and clearance of C-11 palmitate in normal and acutely ischemic myocardium in a dog experiment. The time activity curves were derived from the serial PET images shown in Fig. 9. Note the typical biexpotential clearance pattern of C-11 palmitate in normal myocardium. The fractional distribution of tracer between the two metabolic pools can be estimated by extrapolating the late slow clearance phase back to the time of peak activity. In this dog experiment, approximately 60% of tracer entered the early rapid clearance phase (oxidation) and cleared from myocardium with a halftime of 8.3 minutes. In acutely ischemic myocardium, tracer uptake is markedly reduced as compared to normal myocardium. Moreover, a significantly smaller fraction enters oxidative pathways with markedly prolonged clearance halftimes (about 20 min). The time activity curve is consistent with impaired oxidation of free fatty acid in acutely ischemic myocardium. (Reproduced with permission)

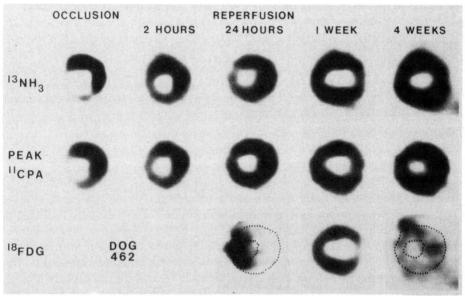

Fig. 11. Serial changes in blood flow, regional C-11 palmitate and FDG uptake in a dog during coronary occlusion and subsequent reperfusion. Note the similarity in segmental reductions of blood flow ($^{13}NH_3$) and C-11 palmitate (peak ^{11}CPA) uptake during occlusion and at two hours of reperfusion. Blood flow and C-11 palmitate subsequently return to normal. The F-18 2-deoxyglucose (^{18}FDG) image at 24 hours reveals enhanced glucose utilization, consistent with increased glycolytic flux. Augmented glucose utilization accurately predicted subsequent functional recovery in all dog experiments; absence of glucose utilization at 24 hours by contrast indicated tissue necrosis. As blood flow and C-11 palmitate uptake normalize, FDG uptake in the reperfused segment declines and no longer differs from control myocardium.

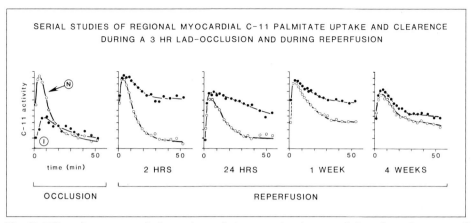

SERIAL STUDIES OF REGIONAL MYOCARDIAL C-11 PALMITATE UPTAKE AND CLEARENCE
DURING A 3 HR LAD-OCCLUSION AND DURING REPERFUSION

C-11 activity

time (min)   2 HRS   24 HRS   1 WEEK   4 WEEKS

OCCLUSION   REPERFUSION

Fig. 12. Effect of coronary occlusion and reperfusion on regional myocardial uptake and turnover of C-11 palmitate. Serial time activity curves in normal (N) and ischemic/reperfused (I) myocardium are compared in the same dog during a 3 hour coronary occlusion followed by 4 weeks of reperfusion. Note the decrease in relative size and clearance rate of the early clearance curve component during coronary occlusion and early after reperfusion. Subsequently, the time activity curve normalizes with a return of the early rapid clearance curve component (oxidation of C-11 palmitate). At 4 weeks, C-11 palmitate uptake and clearance are similar in both segments, indicating a recovery of FFA metabolism.

ed on PET with normalization of metabolism. In the other half of segments which failed to improve function, metabolism deteriorated further. Functionally, these segments behaved similar to those that were without metabolic activity early after the acute myocardial infarction.

Indeed, these segments with preserved metabolic activity and spontaneous functional recovery may represent "stunned myocardium", whereas in segments with no functional recovery or even further deterioration over time, low grade tissue perfusion may have initially allowed persistence of largely anaerobic glycolysis. Because of marginal blood flows, variations in energy demand and failure of spontaneous restoration of blood flow, metabolic activity may have slowly declined until ATP production fell to levels that were inadequate to maintain transmembraneous electrolyte gradients and prompted cell membrane disruption and cell necrosis.

It is the latter group which deserves careful therapeutic attention. Therefore, quantitative criteria are required for predicting which segments will regain function spontaneously and which ones will not. These criteria are likely to include the amount of residual tissue blood flow and mass of viable tissue. It will be the latter group of segments which will require aggressive interventions to enhance or enable removal of inhibitory metabolic intermediates and/or improved delivery of blood flow and oxygen. It is possible that the first objective can be accomplished initially by improving plasma flow so that tissue viability can be maintained until more aggressive treatment modalities can be implemented to ensure adequate oxygen and substrate delivery and with it, salvage of critically injured myocardium. Such improvements have indeed been observed in patients with chronic ischemic heart disease which revealed a similar metabolic pattern in functionally impaired segments. Surgical bypass grafts to these segments and, thus, restoration of blood flow, did indeed result in a slow improvement in segmental myocardial function (14).

Implication of PET studies for assessing effects of coronary sinus interventions

In the absence of any tangible experience with PET, effects of coronary sinus interventions on regional metabolism and their appearance on PET images are difficult to predict and remain therefore mostly speculative. Further confounding is the fact that the mechanism underlying tissue preservation through coronary sinus interventions remains largely unknown. Current hypotheses range from improved tissue plasma flow to improved delivery of oxygen. The first would primarily prevent self-contamination of tissue by inhibitory metabolites or, at least, lower the rate of rising levels of lactate and hydrogen ions in tissue. In terms of PET studies, this might result in improved levels of blood flow in underperfused segments using diffusible tracers and a possible increase in the rate of exogenous glucose utilization as an expression of accelerated glycolysis. If retroperfusion however improved tissue oxygenation in addition to improved plasma blood flow, then the augmented glycolytic flux may be followed by a recovery of fatty acid metabolism or, specifically the return of the initial rapid clearance curve component as a sign of restored fatty acid oxidation followed by an improvement in regional myocardial function.

Acknowledgements

The authors wish to thank M. Lee Griswold for preparing the illustrations and Kerry Engber for her skillful secretarial assistance in preparing this manuscript.

References

1. Hochachka PW (1986) Defense strategies against hypoxia and hypothermia. Science 231: 234–241
2. Liedtke AJ (1981) Alterations of carbohydrate and lipid metabolism in the acutely ischemic heart. Progr Cardiovasc Dis 23: 321–336
3. Neely JR, Rovetto MJ, Oram JF (1972) Myocardial utilization of carbohydrate and lipids. Prog Cardiovasc Dis 15: 289–329
4. Opie LH (1976) Effects of regional ischemia on metabolism of glucose and fatty acids. Circ Res 38 (Suppl I): 152–174
5. Phelps ME (1977) Emission computed tomography. Sem Nucl Med 7: 337–365
6. Phelps ME, Hoffman EJ, Selin CE, Huang SC, Robinson G, MacDonald N, Schelbert H, Kuhl DE (1978) Investigation of [^{18}F] 2-fluoro 2-deoxyglucose for the measure of myocardial glucose metabolism. J Nucl Med 19: 1311–1319
7. Ratib O, Phelps ME, Huang SC, Henze E, Selin CE, Schelbert HR (1982) Positron tomography with deoxyglucose for estimating local myocardial glucose metabolism. J Nucl Med 23: 577–586
8. Schelbert HR, Phelps ME, Hoffman EJ, Huang SC, Selin CE, Kuhl DE (1979) Regional myocardial perfusion assessed with N-13 labeled ammonia and positron emission computerized axial tomography. Am J Cardiol 43: 209–218
9. Schelbert HR, Phelps ME, Huang SC, MacDonald NS, Hansen H, Selin C, Kuhl DE (1981) N-13 ammonia as an indicator of myocardial blood flow. Circulation 63: 1259–1272
10. Schelbert HR, Schwaiger M (1986) PET studies of the heart. In: Phelps M, Mazziotta J, Schelbert H (eds) Positron Emission Tomography and Autoradiography: Principles and Applications for the Brain and Heart (Chapter 12). Raven Press, New York, pp 581–661
11. Schwaiger M, Schelbert HR, Ellison D, Hansen H, Yeatman L, Vinten-Johansen J, Selin C, Barrio J, Phelps ME (1985) Sustained regional abnormalities in cardiac metabolism after transient ischemia in the chronic dog model. J Am Coll Cardiol 6: 336–347

12. Schwaiger M, Schelbert HR, Keen R, Vinten-Johansen J, Hansen H, Selin C, Barrio J, Huang SC, Phelps ME (1985) Retention and clearance of C-11 palmitic acid in ischemic and reperfused canine myocardium. J Am Coll Cardiol 6: 311–320
13. Schwaiger M, Brunken R, Grover-McKay M, Krivokapich J, Child J, Tillisch JH, Phelps ME, Schelbert HR. Detection of tissue viability in patients with acute myocardial infarction by positron emission tomography. J Am Coll Cardiol (in press)
14. Tillisch J, Brunken R, Marshall R, Schwaiger M, Mandelkern M, Phelps M, Schelbert H., Prediction of reversibility of cardiac wall motion abnormality using positron tomography, ^{18}fluorodeoxy-glucose and ^{13}NH$_3$. N Engl J Med (in press)

Authors' address:
Heinrich R. Schelbert, M.D.
Division of Nuclear Medicine and Biophysics
UCLA School of Medicine
Los Angeles, CA 90024
U.S.A.

Panel Discussion
Marker of Ischemia, Marker of Reperfusion Injury

Chairmen: S. F. Vatner, H. R. Schelbert

Spotnitz:

I was very interested in some of your comments on the differences between dogs and humans and the amount of edema that we see with global ischemia and reperfusion. From our own observations we thought that there may be a species-related reason for that.

Vatner:

Our information related to some indirect observations on edema. In the studies where we did a permanent coronary occlusion without reperfusion we sacrificed the dogs and the primates 24 hours later. We looked at the values of regional myocardial blood flow using radioactive microspheres. Basically, the observation was that if you give an injection of microspheres before coronary occlusion, and then measure the control levels 24 hours or sometimes later, you find that the blood flow in the nonischemic zone prior to occlusion is about 1 ml/min/mg. And if you look at the precoronary occlusion blood flow in the ischemic tissue, it is about 20% lower than that. The early studies suggested that there was some microsphere loss to the ischemic process. But then later studies by Hoffman's group and Jennings and Reimer suggested that most of that microsphere loss could be accounted for by edema. In other words, if the ischemic tissue had swelled by 20%, the same number of microspheres would be in there, but you measure only 80% of the orginal value. We observed that in the dogs as well but we did not observe that in the primates. And from the inability to demonstrate that microsphere loss, which is thought to be due to cell-swelling and edema, we theorize that perhaps the baboon infarcts were not as edematous as the canine ones. But we never went further than that to define the mechanisms.

Spotnitz:

According to some of our own observations in humans with acute myocardial infarction, in the operating room we can actually feel an area of edema that does correspond to the endocardial area of the infarction. Do your studies suggest that there had been some increased thickness of the reperfused myocardium in the area of myocardial infarction, and whether there was a difference in that type of observation between species?

95

Vatner:

I think the wall thickness measure is affected by many factors. During ischemia you get reduced diastolic wall thickening, partly due to the lack of blood flow in the wall. During reperfusion you get a rebound effect with a small increase in wall thickening. And then over a period of weeks, again wall thickening decreases below control levels as scar formation occurs. Both of these phenomena are seen in dogs and primates. The data this morning were presented mainly for the changes of wall thickening from control levels. I think that the systolic shortening or thickening pretty much reflects the contractile state, rather than the extent to which there is edema or other changes.

Spotnitz:

A common methodological problem, at least in some of the surgical studies that I have looked at, had been the use of epicardially placed sonomicrometers to measure ventricular dimensions and ventricular functions, under circumstances when investigators knew or might infer that myocardial edema would occur during the experiment. One example that I remember very well is a study on hemorrhagic shock in which the authors were looking at a variety of things with epicardially placed crystals, and I think that in this setting mass may be increasing as much as 25%, and wall thickness may be increasing in the order of 10%. I do not think anyone really understands exactly how data measured under those circumstances could be interpreted. But there are related problems. People have been unable to report changes in mass or wall thickness systematically. And I think there are basic problems about edema formation that worry me. Firstly, I do not know the true measure of preload, and secondly, there is the use of elastance measurements following globular ischemia and reperfusion, the validity of which has not been unchallenged.
In an experiment we are doing in our lab. now, where we are looking at globular ischemia and reperfusion, we see the elastance being unchanged and the conventional hemodynamics changing markedly over the same time. So, I think there are a number of problems with those models that need to be worked out.

Meerbaum:

Dr. Spotnitz, what is your reproducibility of the measurements of the mass that you have made? Did you get your data from humans or from an animal?

Spotnitz:

Your are asking about the validation of our methods, Dr. Meerbaum, is that right? In dogs the standard error of estimate is about ± 7 g for those techniques. Actually, the method has some built-in problems with the dogs, one of which is that it is a preload dependent measurement of mass, so that if you measure mass at different endsystolic volumes, you either have to normalize to a standard volume or else you have to do all your measurements at the same endsystolic volume or a similar one. And what we do under circumstances where we cannot work at the same endsystolic volume in dogs, is to have each investigator write his particular preload dependence and then subsequently correct the data. We do not think that the method is accurate below mass changes of 10 g in dogs. Now, in humans the techniques is nowhere near as well worked out. And what we did was to basically run a study in which we correlated echodata with simultaneous or near simultaneous angiograms, so that we could do a regression correlating that ring area with the angiographic masses and thereby translate them. The correlation coefficient in that study was only 0.74 between the technique we used from mass and the angiographic values. The more important questions, how reproducible the measurement is, is the technique in serial measurements done under conditions of unchanged masses, and the related question, is the algorithm preload dependent, as the canine algorithm is. Until very recently we have been reluctant to talk about any data from conditions where endsystolic volume was changing in humans, until we had worked that out. We now feel that for endsystolic volume changes of the type we have seen in the operating room, the algorithm is not preload dependent. It is reasonable. We do not know about the reproducibility, but I would not believe in any mass changes of less than around 15 g in humans. And I think there is really a lot of scatter in the data and a lot of measurements are to be done. Well, in the transplants, things are a little different, because we use a multisectional algorithm and we feel, based on the observations we have made, that we can pretty reliably taken the mass change of 10 g and that it has physiologic meaning.

Vatner:

I would like to ask Dr. Guerci to tell us on what basis he believes there is reperfusion injury. In other words, almost all of the studies on reperfusion have shown more diminution of infarct size and salvage of regional function. With that in mind, why do you think that there is reperfusion injury?

Guerci:

I think there are two lines of evidence to support the idea that reperfusion under the proper conditions can actually cause necrosis of cells, that is, that there is truly an injury associated with reperfusion. I alluded to one of these briefly this morning and did not mention the other at all. The first line of evidence was established in the 1970's in studies of the oxygen paradox, done in Dr. Hearse's laboratory in England. Now this gets a little tricky because Dr. Hearse used the leak of creatine kinase as a marker for reperfusion injury, and subsequent studies have shown very clearly that necrosis is not required for CPK to leak from myocytes. Dr. Spieckerman and his colleagues in the Federal Republic of Germany showed two or three years ago that creatine kinase can leak from reversibly injured cardiac myocytes. They rendered these cells hypoxic for a sufficient period of time to produce morphologic changes. Reoxygenation was associated with a very large creatine kinase leak. Properly timed reoxygenation very clearly dissociated the creatine kinase leak from necrosis, so that when the cells were re-examined some period of time later, they were morphologically normal and contracting. Whole animal preparations and clinical observations also show very clearly that an ischemic insult of insufficient duration to cause necrosis may result in a large leak of creatine kinase. Dr. Vatner and his colleagues have been able to dissociate creatine kinase release from necrosis in a canine model of myocardial ischemia. In studies of coronary reperfusion in humans, Dr. Ganz's group in Los Angeles found that very early reperfusion with streptokinase was, in some cases, associated with high serum creatine kinase levels and complete recovery of regional function. Data such as these demonstrate that enzyme leak is not synonymous with necrosis.

Nervertheless, enzyme leak represents some form of injury. Getting back to Dr. Hearse's studies in England, in one group of isolated perfused hearts, a prolonged period of hypoxia was associated with a very small and steady release of creatine kinase. When these preparations were reoxygenated, there was a very large creatine kinase leak into the perfusate. Finally, when the same isolated, perfused hearts were reperfused with nitrogen instead of oxygen, there was only minimal creatine kinase leak. The same results were obtained with ischemia, that is the creatine kinase leak was exaggerated by reflow with an oxygen-containing solution but not with a nitrogen-containing solution. I think evidence of this sort indicates there is at least some form of damage associated with reoxygenation and that it is really reoxygenation more than reperfusion per se. I think the more important line of evidence that reperfusion may itself cause injury to myocytes which are not yet irreversibly damaged, is that free radical scavengers, which have no known haemodynamic effects, no effect on collateral blood flow, and no known direct effects on cell membranes, reduce infarct size in model of transient coronary occlusion and reperfusion. In other words, these drugs have no effects on any of the known determinants of infarct size, yet they reduce infarct size. Similarly, allopurinol appears to be a completely inactive compound with regard to the determinants of infarct size. Its only known activity is to inhibit xanthine oxidase activity. Nevertheless, it, too, has been associated with reduction in infarct size in experimental models of coronary occlusion and reperfusion. So, the oxygen paradox and myocardial salvage, due to the administration of free radical scavengers, are the best evidence that I can provide in support of the idea that reperfusion injury is not just a figment of my own or someone else's imagination.

Corday:

I think there is increasing evidence about the type of reperfusion, its condition, and whether it occurs with coronary bypass graft investigations or with angioplasty. There are many reports in the literature of a very successful reperfusion. The angiogram shows that vessels had been reopened and yet an infarct has occurred. There is functional evidence that something went wrong and an ischemic condition is taking place. I think the work done by Haendchen, working with Meerbaum in my lab., showed that this occurs within seconds after the establishment of the blood supply to an occluded area. The first evidence of this is a local swelling in the ischemic zone where the balloon had occluded the artery. And usually, when we identify it with 2D-echo, according to Haendchen and his publication in 1983, we can be sure that this is going to be followed by an infarct. However, Haendchen also showed that if he uses synchronized retroperfusion, he can often overcome these phenomena. He also shows that he can prevent reperfusion injury, as exhibited by a brightness to the ischemic area and also a swelling, by subjecting these animals to synchronized retroperfusion. Just what the mechanism is, I am not sure, but it involves a return of oxygen to the area. But – Meerbaum and I have discussed it in the past – why should the retroperfusion prevent the reperfusion injury? Is it replacing the oxygen more gradually? In our animal experiments we find that if we perfuse quickly we very often see this reperfusion injury, but if we do it gradually we do not run into this trouble. What the brightness in the echo during reperfusion means we do not know, but we think it is due to calcium deposition in the mitochondrias.

Guerci:

If I may just add two brief points, to bridge the gap between what is known to be possible and what actually happens in myocardial ischemia and, more specifically, reflow. First, there were data presented at the American Heart Association meetings by investigators who administered oxygen-derived free radicals to hearts in some kind of preparation. They were able to demonstrate a functional disturbance, that is, declining mechanical function. Thus, there is at least some evidence that free radicals are toxic when they are present. Secondly, in my own institution, Dr. Jay Zweier, using electron spin resonance, has demonstrated the generation of oxygen-derived free radicals in reperfused rabbit hearts. The peak formation of free radicals in this preparation occurred in the first 20 or 30 seconds after reperfusion. This is another important piece of evidence that free radicals are not only toxic to the heart but are produced under conditions of reperfusion.

Vatner:

I would like to remain a little sceptical. I would like to see a study where there is no intervention at the same time that reperfusion occurs and to determine, if one could, if there is a difference in the amount of infarction at that time. Having seen how research evolved over the past 15 years, I remember that the first studies suggested that reperfusion injury occurred on the basis of creatine kinase release and the appearance of haemorrhagic infarcts. Subsequently it had been demonstrated that neither one of these signs are evidence of reperfusion injury. Furthermore the initial effects that you see with reperfusion in the first few hours and up to 24 hours after reperfusion, are not necessarily seen 2 to 4 weeks later. There is a marked reduction in the inflammatory process, edema, and a recovery of function, as long as the occlusion has not been too long. So I would like to hold off on a final comment about whether there is substantial reperfusion injury, until several years from now when we will have more data.

Meerbaum:

I would like to say I agree with Dr. Guerci. I think this is about all the evidence than can be quoted. I think we can positively say that reperfusion per se creates this injury. We need more data but let us look at what we do know, and that is the stunning effect. We followed up some work done by Haendchen, where increased regional wall thickness was seen post reperfusion and appeared to predict ultimate necrosis, by studies done in patients who received intravenous streptokinase. Although we only have a small number of cases so far, and we do not have a pre-reperfusion control in some cases, it does appear that in humans one sees increased endsystolic wall thickness in the area that ultimately will have an infarct. We have seen it in two cases. So what does this mean? Is there just more blood flow? Possibly. But, in any case, it appears that this early increase in enddiastolic wall thickness is a predictor of infarction. At least in the dog, we did not see that increased wall thickness with reperfusion in areas where there was no infarct.

Vatner:

You mast have an increase in diastolic wall thickness with reperfusion. If you do not see it, you do not measure appropriately. Then is huge hyperemia, i.e. increase in blood flow, whether or not edema occurs, which would also make the diastolic wall thickness increase. Dr. Maurer, for how long does this swelling occur?

Maurer:

For hours, if not days; it takes time to absorb the edema. Wall thickness was associated with increased mortality in the dogs and with the eventual infarct.

Vatner:

I truly think that this is a transient increase in wall thickness, that goes away and is eventually replaced by wall thinning.
I guess it is important not to lose sight of the fact that with prolonged ischemia, of one, two, or three hours, with reperfusion intervening or not, you are going to have an infarct. And there is no way to salvage all the tissue when there is ischemia for that length of time. I do not want to be in the position to say that ischemia is good for you, and that if we can have ischemia and combine reperfusion and retroperfusion, you can maybe enhance the amount of normal tissue, and end up with more normal tissue that you started with.

Corday:

Dr. Vatner, what we are saying is, we are looking at this echo and watching it as soon as we perform reperfusion. And we know that we are reperfusing. The blood is getting in there with the angio in the animal. However, seconds later we see a thickening that persists for a period of a week. When the autopsy the animal after that, there is an infarct on that side and when we are using the whole series of animals, if reperfusion is going on when we do this, we do not see this sudden thickening. So it appears to us that a sudden

100

appearance of edema might be an explosive event, probably because the animals' tissue does not enjoy this sudden increase in oxygen concentration. If you see an abnormal mitochondrium you can feel pretty certain that the mitochondrial function is altered. But suppose the EM studies are normal, does that mean that you have intact mitochondrial function? I think these two are not correlated because you can have normal mitochondrial function, while at the same time function is still depressed. The mitochondrial function is perhaps of more importance than just about anything else, and the mitochondrial ability to generate ATP is more important to cellular electro-mechanical function than is the actual level of ATP, because we all know that the ATP level is markedly depressed following ischemia. But can the mitochondria generate ATP with what remains in the cell, because we all know that ATP nucleotide precursors tend to be washed out with reperfusion?

Vatner:

What type of marker is useful to determine ultimately if there is reperfusion injury or ischemic injury? What marker would you use to assess this? I think, my personal bias is that any marker, if done within the first 24 hours, probably is not very meaningful, because major changes will then occur over the next several weeks. Is there something other than the measurement of the infarct size versus the area at risk that can be used? It appears that the enzymes are not very accurate in predicting the amount of recovery. I believe all the functional techniques are flawed to the extent that lack to recovery of function does not mean lack of recovery of tissue, because even if there is a small infarct in the wall this still might inhibit wall motion considerably. Are there any metabolic changes?

Schelbert:

I think there are several ways of determining this, at least with radionuclear techniques or radioisotope techniques. One method is that one can measure, that one can make an image of what you actually see on cardiac tissue.
An old method – Dr. Corday already mentioned it – was the calcium phosphate deposit. One can hind ferrophosphate with technetium and get excellent images of the infarct. But a problem with that is that it takes some time and usually you can do those studies only about 10 to 12 hours after an infarct. But in reperfusion it occurs earlier. There is now a newer technique, which I think is more specific. It is using a labelled antimyocyte antibody and that seems to be fairly fast. In other words, one can apply this technology from very early on. It seems to me, however, that what we are interested in is not so much the data. I think the physician is interested in the sick patient, rather than the dead. So, for us it would be more interesting to study or demonstrate what tissue is sick and perhaps can be healed. And from our standpoint we looked at various tracers which had been used in the past such as sodium, to determine an agent which would tell us something about tissue viability. Studies in patients would indicate that if you use sodium and then look at

the image early after the injection and you see a detect, and if that defect disappears over time, then this, in general, is a fairly good indicator of tissue viability. On the other hand, recent clinical studies have shown that even in defects which did not resolve with time, function would return. And that carries some doubt about the validity and the sensitivity of sodium redistribution studies in assessing tissue viability.

While Dr. Sochor was with us, we did some studies in dogs after reperfusion, to determine the extent of the area at risk and to look at sodium as an indicator of tissue viability. Now, it turned out in this study that there was a direct relationship between the histological degree of tissue necrosis and ferrophosphate uptake. Sodium uptake by necrotic tissue, ischemic, and normal tissue essentially was unchanged. The extraction fraction, as such, was uneffected by necrosis. So it seemed to us that the sodium itself was not a good marker of tissue viability and we believe that the redistribution is simply a function of residual blood flow. What seemed in this study to be a very good marker of the tissue viability was the measurement of extractions such as glucose extractions uptake.

Corday:

For 14 years now I have been on the problem of trying to develop a technique that would be simple, that we could take to the bedside, that would tell us what is happening to the cardiac function. I took over Princemetall's lab. at that time and we started working on radionucleids and developed a technology that got us only so far. We developed the technique of radiocardiography. Which is now being brought back into clinical use. But the big nuclear machine is pretty clumsy, and you cannot get it into the bedside, and some of us hesitate each time we order it. Fortunately, when the two-dimensional echo came along about 10 years ago, I had feelings that it might be the tool. We get excellent images but it is not a case of having a quick look and saying, "It is ballooning", or "It is contracting", or "It is kinetic". I remember the days with Master and Dack: the three of us would go into a room and decide whether the patient had an acute coronary or not by watching the contraction. One person said, "It is contracting", and the other person said, "It is ballooning". But finally we were afraid that that we were getting too much radiation. That was the state of the art. Then when angiography became the most popular technique for imaging, we could see the tremendous error of how four experts were looking at the movement of this single frame and would come up with different opinions, one saying that it was kinetic, the other saying it was contracting. This is a classic example which shows that it is not a very accurate technology. The thing is, we have to be able to quantitate, we have to take it out of the guessing phase, and I think that 2D-echo is beginning to show some promise.

Schelbert:

You know, in a way I agree with your quantitative technique. I think that it is clearly needed. I would not be that negative about radionuclear techniques. I think that is the way to go. We can measure fairly simply, once the software is developed, glucose uptake rates in millimoles, and go down to very low utilization rates. There is no question, I think, that this is very important. On the other hand, our observations also found that often the decision has to be made of whether tissue is viable or not and we do not find that function helps us in discriminating between viable or irreversibly injured tissue. It makes sense because I think that as you cut down the oxygen supply and high energy phosphate production, the cell goes back and runs on a very low level of energy. It cuts down on function just to survive and I think metabolic indices may be more sensitive and tell us where the tissue is that can be salvaged. I think, coming back to retroperfusion, that it would make more sense to me if we could identify areas which could be salvaged, so that we could intervene where we would not otherwise know whether there is, in fact, any viable tissue left.

Effects of ischaemia on the canine myocardial β-receptor-effector mechanism

C. K. Spiss, M. Weindlmayr-Goettel, M. Zimpfer, H. Drobny,
and W. Freissmuth

Boltzmann-Institute of Experimental Anaesthesia and Research in Intensive
Care and Department of Pharmacology, University of Vienna, Vienna (Austria)

Introduction

Myocardial β-receptors are actively regulated by the neurotransmitter norepinephrine. Previous studies showed an ischaemia-induced increase in sympathetic tone, leading to a time-dependent alteration of cyclic AMP level, catecholamine content and β-adrenergic receptor density in ventricular myocardium. The aim of the study was to investigate possible changes of the myocardial β-receptor-effector mechanism under acute ischaemia.

Methods

Myocardial ischaemia was induced via hydraulic occlusion of the LAD in chronically instrumented dogs anaesthetized with 2% isoflurane. After 90 minutes of ischaemia portions of the ischaemic and non-ischaemic basal parts of the left ventricle were removed. Myocardium of each part was placed in liquid nitrogen for tissue norepinephrine determination by high performance liquid chromatography. Additional myocardium was minced in cold TRIS-sucrose buffer and homogenized. Particulate fractions were prepared by differential centrifugation. A crude 1000 g pellet was used for the adenylate cyclase assay. β-receptor density and affinity were determined in a microsomal pellet. Binding experiments were performed utilizing (– 125 J) jodocyanopindolol. Data obtained in isoproterenol competition experiments were subjected to computerized nonlinear least square curve fitting in order to quantify the relative amount of β-receptors in the high affinity state.

Results

The ischaemic myocardium showed a significant decrease of norepinephrine content (Table 1).
No significant increase in the β-adrenoceptor density and affinity could be observed (Fig. 1). However, isoproterenol-mediated adenylate cyclase stimulation was significantly reduced in the ischaemic myocardium (Fig. 2). These data were consistent with the findings obtained in the competition experiments (Fig. 3) where a rightward shift and an increase in the slope of isoproterenol competition curves could be observed.

105

Table 1. Tissue-norepinephrine (ng/g).

Normal ($\bar{x} \pm$ SEM)	Ischemic ($\bar{x} \pm$ SEM)
168 ± 67	16 ± 5.7*

$* p \leqq 0.05$

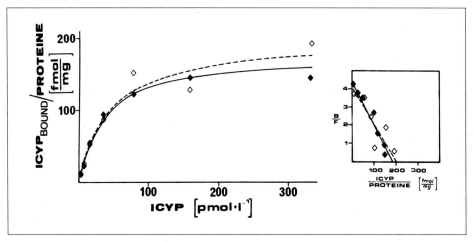

Fig. 1. Saturation isotherm of specific (–) [^{125}I]odocyanopindolol (ICYP) binding to membranes from ischemic (♦) and control (--- □) dog myocardium.

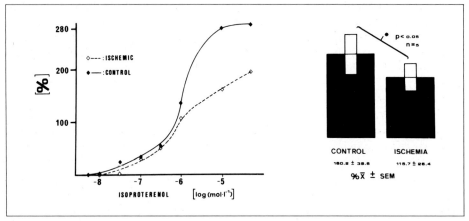

Fig. 2. Stimulation of adenylatecyclase activity by (–) isoproterenol in membranes from control and ischemic myocardium.

Discussion

During acute ischaemia the effects of circulating catecholamines can be extremely deleterious. The alterations in the cardiac action potential can lead to life-threatening arrhyth-

106

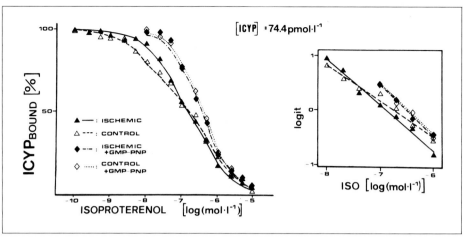

Fig. 3. Competition of (–)isoproterenol with (–)ICYP binding to cardiac membranes in the absence and presence of [100 μmol · l^{-1}] guanylimidodiphosphate (GMP-PNP).

mias, sinus tachycardia and increased contractility leads to increased myocardial oxygen consumption. The reduced oxygen supply may extent the zone of ischaemia or infarction. In our model 90 minutes of ischaemia produces no significant changes in β-adrenoceptor density. However, adenylate cyclase responsiveness to isoproterenol was significantly reduced, indicating an uncoupling of the β-adrenoceptor from the regulatory N_S-protein. This finding was verified in the competition experiments which show a paired formation of the agonist-specific, high affinity state of the β-adrenoceptor in the ischaemic myocardium.

Further work is needed to establish the mechanism of these changes and to define more precisely clinical consequences of these alterations.

References

1. Buja LM, Muntz KH, Rosenbaum P et al (1985) Characterization of a potentially reversible increase in β-adrenergic receptors in isolated, neonatal rat cardiac myosides with impaired energy metabolism. Circ Res 57: 640–645
2. Devos C, Robberecht P, Nokin P et al (1985) Uncoupling between β-adrenoceptor and adenylate cyclase in dog ischaemic myocardium. Naunyn-Schmiedeberg's Arch Pharmacol 331: 71–75
3. Maise AS, Motulsky HS, Insel PA (1985) Externalization of β-adrenergic receptors promoted by myocardial ischaemia. Science 230: 183–186
4. Mukherjee A, Wong TM, Buja LM, Lefkowicz RJ, Willerson JT (1979) β-adrenergic and muscarinic cholinergic receptors in canine myocardium, effects of ischaemia. J Clin Invest 64: 1423–1428

Authors' address:
C. K. Spiss
L. Boltzmann Institute of Experimental
Anaesthesia and Research in Intensive Care
University of Vienna
A-1090 Vienna, Austria

Myocardial metabolism during pacing-induced ischemia in man. Temporal relationship with changes in post-stenotic coronary flow

W. J. Remme, H. A. C. M. Kruyssen, X. H. Krauss, C. J. Storm, and D. C. A. van Hoogenhuyze

Department of Cardiology, Zuiderziekenhuis Rotterdam (The Netherlands)

Summary: Metabolic markers of myocardial ischemia may be useful to validate interventions during the early phase of infarction. The relative sensitivity of myocardial lactate (L) production and release of nucleosides (Hypoxanthine, H) as metabolic markers of ischemia and the temporal relationship of changes in these metabolites to alterations in regional coronary flow, assessed with a continuous intracoronary infusion of ^{81m}Kr, were studied in 16 patients (pts) with left coronary artery disease (CAD). During incremental atrial pacing, arterial L and H levels remained constant. L production and H release occurred early and simultaneously, before angina, but several minutes after a decrease in ^{81m}Kr perfusion in > 90% stenosis areas. During maximal pacing heart rates, ^{81m}Kr perfusion decreased to $67 \pm 8\%$ of control in > 90% CAD and to $78 \pm 4\%$ in 70–90% stenosis areas (both $p < 0.05$ vs control). Maximal increases in coronary venous L (0.8 ± 0.1 mmol/l vs. 0.58 ± 0.04 mmol/l (control), $p < 0.05$) occurred 15 seconds post-pacing (p-p) and in coronary venous H at 1 min p-p (5.8 ± 1.5 μM vs. 1.5 ± 0.14 μM (control), $p < 0.01$). After pacing, ^{81m}Kr perfusion was still significantly reduced ($79 \pm 6\%$ of control) 5 min p-p. Although angina had disappeared and L metabolism normalized at 2 min p-p, significant H release persisted at 5 min p-p, indicating ongoing silent ischemia.

Introduction

Metabolic markers of myocardial ischemia may be useful to validate interventions during the early phase of infarction. Although in humans myocardial lactate production and release of nucleosides occur already during short periods of ischemia (2, 4–7), it has been demonstrated in animals that during prolonged periods of ischemia the duration of lactate production is limited, whereas hypoxanthine release appears to persist (1, 12), indicating ongoing breakdown of high-energy phosphates. These data suggest that during prolonged ischemia, e.g. the early phase of myocardial infarction, nucleosides and oxypurines may be particularly useful to indicate the degree and duration of myocardial ischemia. It is the purpose of this study to investigate the temporal relationship between changes in lactate and nucleoside metabolism and regional alterations in coronary flow in patients with coronary artery disease.

Methods

Study population. Sixteen patients were studied (15 men and 1 woman) during cardiac catheterization. Studies were carried out without premedication after an overnight fast, using the Seldinger technique. A 7 Fr Amplatz or Judkins left coronary artery catheter was positioned in the left coronary artery ostium via an arterial Desilet system in the right femoral artery. The sidearm of this catheter was used to record arterial pressures and for sampling of arterial blood. Next, a 7 Fr Swan Ganz catheter was positioned with its tip in the pulmonary artery from a femoral vein and a 7 Fr Zucker catheter advanced from the right brachial vein into the midportion of the coronary sinus. Throughout the study a sterile Rubidium-81/Krypton-81m generator was continuously perfused with glucose 5% and the eluate passed directly into the left coronary artery.

Planar imaging of the myocardial distribution pattern of Krypton-81m was performed in the 45° LAO position during 15-second intervals with a General Electric Portacamera, connected on line to a Medical Data System A_2 computer (Fig. 1). Regions of interest were constructed with a light pen on a visual display unit over areas with > 70% coronary lesions, over normal regions, total heart, aorta and background areas. Calculations were made of total counts per area per timeframe divided by total counts over the heart during the same period. The methodology used to ensure stable baseline distribution patterns without streaming artefacts, has been described in detail elsewhere (9, 10).

Arterial (a) and coronary venous (v) blood (1 ml) was sampled simultaneously, at prefixed intervals during the study, quickly transferred into tubes with 1 cc icecold 8% HCLO4 and vigorously shaken. After centrifugation, the supernatant was stored at −20 °C. Lactate was determined enzymatically in triplicate as described before (10) (standard deviation 0.012 mmol/l) and Hypoxanthine by dual column HPLC (standard deviation 0.2 µmol/l). The study protocol consisted of a 10 minute baseline period, 30

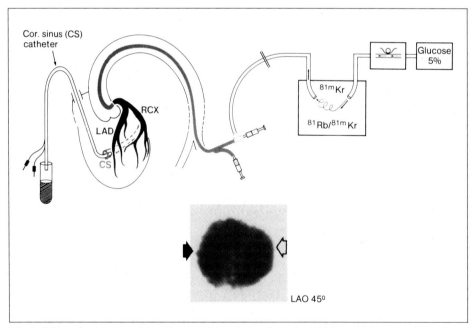

Fig. 1. Schematic representation of krypton-81m elution from the rubidium-81/krypton-81m generator and perfusion of the left anterior descending (LAD) and circumflex (RCX) area. Imaging is performed in the 45° LAO projection. Normal distribution of krypton-81m over both regions in a patient without coronary artery disease is shown at the bottom of the figure (reprinted with permission from (7)).

minutes after the last coronary angiogram, followed by atrial pacing with increments in heart rate of 10 beats/2 minutes, until angina or atrioventricular block occurred. Scintigraphic, hemodynamic and metabolic determinations were performed at fixed intervals during pacing, e.g. at 100 and 120 beats/min, during maximal pacing heart rates, followed by measurements 15 seconds, 1, 2 and 5 minutes after pacing.

Results

All patients had significant (> 70%) coronary artery diameter narrowing of at least one branch of the left coronary artery within the sampling area of the coronary sinus catheter. In all, there were 15 areas with > 90% CAD and 7 with 70–90% CAD. At rest, krypton-81m perfusion was reduced in 5 areas, 4 in infarct-related areas and 1 in a region without any sign of a previous infarct. Signs of ischemia were absent in all patients, except for significant hypoxanthine release in 2 patients with reduced krypton-81m distribution during the control period, indicating silent ischemia at rest.

During pacing, Krypton-81m distribution decreased at an early stage (100 B/min) in > 90% CAD areas, before any sign of ischemia, followed 4 minutes later by a significant reduction in 70–90% regions. During maximal pacing heart rates, krypton-81m perfusion had decreased to 67 ± 8% of control in > 90% CAD and to 78 ± 4% in 70–90% CAD areas (Fig. 2). Krypton-81m perfusion was still significantly reduced in > 90% CAD areas 5 minutes after pacing (79 ± 6%, p < 0.05 vs. control). Although in 70–90% areas Krypton-81m distribution was diminished as well, 5 minutes post-pacing, these changes were not significantly different from baseline values.

The arterial levels of lactate and hypoxanthine remained unchanged during pacing. Lactate production and hypoxanthine release occurred early and simultaneously, at 120 beats/min, before angina was present. A maximal increase in coronary venous lactate lev-

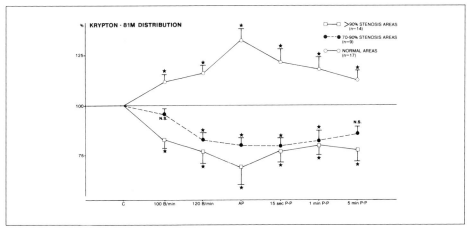

Fig. 2. Percentage changes in Krypton-81m distribution from control values in > 90% and 70–90% stenosis areas and in normal regions, during and after incremental atrial pacing.
AP = maximal pacing heart rates; B/min = beats/minute; C = control; n.s. = not significant; P-P = post-pacing; sec = seconds.

111

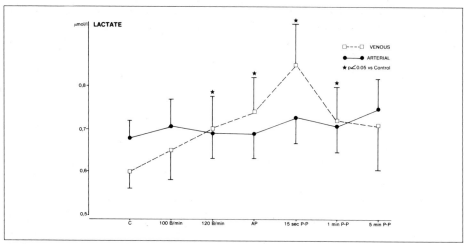

Fig. 3. Arterial and coronary venous lactate levels during and after incremental atrial pacing. Maximal efflux of myocardial lactate occurs 15 seconds post-pacing.
AP = maximal pacing heart rates; B/min = beats/minute; C = control; P-P = post-pacing; sec = seconds.

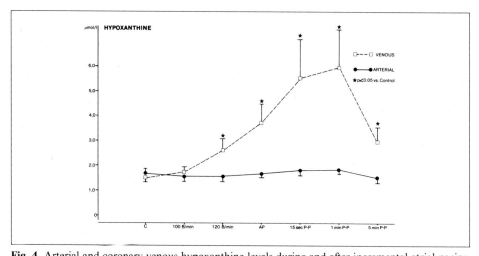

Fig. 4. Arterial and coronary venous hypoxanthine levels during and after incremental atrial pacing. Maximal increase in venous hypoxanthine levels is found at 1 minute post-pacing. Significant hypoxanthine release is still present 5 minutes after pacing.
AP = maximal pacing heart rates; B/min = beats/minute; C = control; P-P = post-pacing; sec = seconds.

els was observed 15 seconds p-p (0.83 ± 0.10 mmol/l vs. 0.58 ± 0.04 mmol/l during control, $p < 0.05$ (Fig. 3)), whereas the greatest elevations in coronary venous hypoxanthine levels occurred 1 min p-p (5.8 ± 1.5 μM vs. 1.5 ± 0.14 μM during control, $p < 0.01$ (Fig. 4)). Lactate production was short lasting with normal extraction values already at 2 min p-p. Hypoxanthine release, on the other hand, was still present 5 min p-p

112

(coronary venous hypoxanthine 2.8 ± 0.5 μM, p < 0.05 vs. control). Finally, whereas significant changes in ^{81m}Kr-distribution and hypoxanthine release occurred in all patients, angina and lactate production were only observed in 14 patients.

Discussion

In this study an impressive increase in coronary venous hypoxanthine levels was observed, starting early during pacing, only a few minutes after changes in coronary flow. This relatively early release of the oxypurine indicates that in humans during pacing-induced stress, ATP-breakdown is observed soon after changes in coronary perfusion, simultaneously with anaerobic glycolysis. This observation is rather unexpected, as in animal experiments nucleoside production appears to follow lactate production (12). It does not agree as well with the findings from an earlier study on hypoxanthine release during pacing-induced ischemia in humans, which indicated that hypoxanthine release occurred after lactate production (6). In the latter study, a different biochemical assay technique was used, however, which did not differentiate between hypoxanthine and xanthine, and as such is less sensitive than the HPLC method. The high levels of coronary venous hypoxanthine observed in the present study therefore may be explained in part by the improved assay technique. More importantly, however, in the present study repetitive sampling in the post-pacing period was carried out, which allowed us to assess the optimal time period during which peak hypoxanthine release occurred, e.g. at 1 minute post-pacing. Likewise, the assessment of lactate production values was improved by sampling in the direct post-pacing period, e.g. at 15 seconds after pacing (8).

The lactate production values are rather low in the present study compared to previous investigations in similar patient groups (10, 11), which indicates a low level of ischemia. In view of this, the impressive increase in coronary venous hypoxanthine levels and the fact that hypoxanthine release did occur in all patients with coronary flow changes suggest that hypoxanthine is more sensitive as a metabolic marker of ischemia than lactate.

After pacing, coronary flow changes persisted for some time after the disappearance of general signs of ischemia and normalization of lactate metabolism. This ongoing decrease in ^{81m}Kr perfusion has been described before (10). The present data suggest that silent myocardial ischemia persists as well after pacing, however only evidenced by hypoxanthine release. Whether this is because hypoxanthine is more sensitive as a metabolic marker of ischemia than lactate or whether it is due to inhibition of glycolysis during prolonged ischemia (3), is unknown. However, the observation does indicate that the assessment of hypoxanthine may be of value when longer periods of ischemia have to be identified, e.g. when validating the efficacy of therapeutic interventions during the early phase of ischemia.

References

1. De Jong JW, Verdouw PD, Remme WJ (1977) Myocardial nucleoside and carbohydrate metabolism and hemodynamics during partial occlusion and reperfusion of pig coronary artery. J Moll Cell Cardiol 9: 297–312
2. Fox AC, Reed GE, Glassman E, Kaltman AJ, Silk BB (1974) Release of adenosine from humans hearts during angina induced by rapid atrial pacing. J Clin Invest 53: 1447–1457

3. Gudbjarnason S (1971/1972) Acute alterations in energetics of ischemia heart muscle. Cardiology 56: 232–244
4. Kugler G (1979) Myocardial release of inosine, hypoxanthine and lactate during pacing-induced angina in humans with coronary artery disease. Eur J Cardiol 9: 227–240
5. Parker JO, Chiong MA, West RO, Case RB (1969) Sequential alterations in myocardial lactate metabolism, ST-segments, and left ventricular function during angina induced by atrial pacing. Circulation 40: 113–131
6. Remme WJ, De Jong JW, Verdouw PD (1977) Effects of pacing-induced myocardial ischemia on hypoxanthine efflux from the human heart. Am J Cardiol 40: 55–62
7. Remme WJ, De Jong JW, Verdouw PD (1978) Changes in purine nucleoside content in human myocardial efflux during pacing-induced ischemia. In: Kobayashi T, Ito Y, Rona G (eds), Recent advances in studies on cardiac structure and metabolism. Volume 12, Cardiac adaptation. University Park Press, Baltimore, pp 409–413
8. Remme WJ, Krauss XH, Storm CJ, Kruyssen HA, van Hoogenhuyze DCA (1981) Improved assessment of lactate production during pacing-induced ischemia. J Moll Cell Cardiol 13: 76 (abstr)
9. Remme WJ, Cox PH, Krauss XH, Kruyssen HACM, Storm CJ, van Hoogenhuyze DCA (1985) Visualization of myocardial blood flow changes with intracoronary [81m]Kr. In: Biersack HJ, Cox PH (eds) Radioisotope studies in cardiology. Martinus Nijhoff, Dordrecht, pp 263–281
10. Remme WJ, Krauss XH, van Hoogenhuyze DCA, Cox PH, Storm CJ, Kruyssen DA (1985) Continuous determination of regional myocardial blood flow with intracoronary krypton-81m in coronary artery disease. Am J Cardiol 56: 445–451
11. Remme WJ, van Hoogenhuyze DCA, Kruyssen D (1986) Acute hemodynamic and antiischemic effects of intravenous diltiazem in man (abstr). JACC (to be published)
12. Verdouw PD, De Jong JW, Remme WJ (1978) Hemodynamic and metabolic changes caused by regional ischemia in porcine heart. In: Kobayashi T, Ito Y, Rona G (eds) Recent advances in studies on cardiac structure and metabolism. Volume 12, Cardiac adaptation, University Park Press, Baltimore

Authors' address:
Willem J. Remme, M.D.
Department of Cardiology
Zuiderziekenhuis
Groene Hilledijk 315
3075 EA Rotterdam
The Netherlands

Functional transport properties of the arterial and venous coronary tree

A. Hoeft, H. Korb, J. Böck, H. G. Wolpers, and G. Hellige

Zentrum "Physiologie und Pathophysiologie" der Universität Göttingen
(West Germany)

Summary: Coronary sinus interventions are based on the possibility of accessing myocardial tissue via the coronary vascular system. Since synchronized retrograde perfusion techniques can theoretically only deliver blood to the capillary vessels if the volume injected per diastole exceeds the capacity of the venous vessels, an experimental study on mongrel dogs was carried out to determine the volume distribution within the coronary vascular tree under in vivo conditions. The total coronary blood volume, as determined by transcoronary dye dilution technique, was about 11 ml/100 g of myocardial tissue under resting coronary blood flow and about 15 ml/100 g during vasodilation by adenosine infusion. The relation between the arterial and the venous compartment of the coronary vascular tree was derived from kinetic measurements of myocardial oxygen uptake during transient hyperemia after adenosine bolus injections and amounted to 1 : 2. Based on these experimental results a model of the arterial and venous coronary tree was developed by the aid of Strahler's law for natural branching systems, which could be used to estimate the dimensions of a particular segment of the branching system. The venous capacity of a human heart (200 g left ventricular weight) would amount to 14–16 ml according to this model. The normally used perfusion flows would therefore only be sufficient to fill the epicardial veins down to a size of approximately 2 mm in diameter. If a more selective perfusion into smaller epicardial veins could be performed, a volume of more than 1 ml per diastole is required, to access the capillary vessels by a vein less than 2 mm in diameter with a draining area of less than 25 g in weight.

Due to these results, the synchronized retrograde perfusion of the coronary sinus is very unlikely to affect the myocardial tissue by capillary perfusion, a blood displacement by redistribution within the venous system due to back pressure effects is more conceivable as the reason for the reported positive effects of this methods.

Introduction

The intracoronary blood volume as well as the transmural distribution of coronary vascular space has been experimentally determined by several investigators (4). The estimates of coronary blood volume vary considerably, probably because of the different techniques used and whether blood in epicardial coronary arteries and veins is included in the measurements. In addition to this problem, in all studies, total coronary blood volume was determined and no distinction between the arterial and venous part of the coronary vascular tree was made. However, more detailed information about the functional structure of the venous coronary vessels seems to be desirable, since recently developed techniques for the treatment of myocardial ischemia try to access the myocardial tissue via the coronary sinus. The application of these methods, which in part use a synchronized retrograde perfusion, should only be possible if the volume delivered per diastole into the coronary venous vessels exceeds the volume capacity between the site of injection and the desired site of action, i.e. the capillary vessels. Since little is known about the blood volume within the coronary venous system and about total coronary blood volume including the epicardial vessels the present study has been designed to determine the necessary data of the coronary vascular tree under in vivo conditions.

115

Methods

All experiments were carried out on mongrel dogs in piritramide anaesthesia and artificial respiration with nitrous oxide and oxygen. Catheters were inserted via brachial and femoral vessels under X-ray control, the analog signals of the measuring devices were digitized online and processed by a microcomputer.

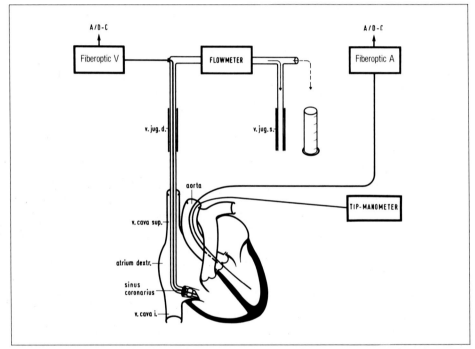

Fig. 1. Experimental design for the determination of total and venous coronary vascular volume. Total coronary volume was determined by simultaneous measurements of coronary sinus outflow and transcoronary mean transit time of an intravascular dye tracer (indocyanine green). Coronary sinus blood flow was measured by an extracorporeal electromagnetic flowprobe (Flowmeter) within a bypass system, which allowed volumetric calibration. For measurements of the transcoronary mean transit time a dye bolus was injected into the right atrium. The resulting arterial and coronary venous dye dilution curves were recorded by a fiberoptic device (Fiberoptic A and V) and digitized online by a microcomputer (A/D-C). The mean transit time was derived by deconvolution of the concentration time courses.
The determination of coronary venous volume is based on kinetic measurements of myocardial oxygen uptake and myocardial energy demand (for details see text). The myocardial oxygen uptake was calculated for each heart beat from arterial and coronary venous oxygen saturation (obtained by Fiberoptic A and V), coronary sinus blood flow and hemoglobin content. The energy demand per stroke was derived from hemodynamic parameters, which were measured by a left ventricular catheter tip manometer (Tip-Manometer).

Determination of total coronary blood volume by transcoronary dye dilution

Total coronary blood volume was determined by the product of the mean transit time of an intravascular tracer and coronary blood flow. For the measurements of mean intravasculuar transit time (mtt) a dye bolus was injected into the right atrium (indocyanine green, 12.5 mg) and the arterial and coronary venous dye dilution curves were recorded by means of a fiberoptic device (Fig. 1). After deconvolution of the concentration time signals the mean transit time can be obtained from the resulting coronary transport function (9). Coronary blood flow per 100 g myocardial tissue was derived from coronary sinus outflow and left ventricular heart weight, assuming coronary sinus drainage to represent 75% of left ventricular blood flow (6).

Determination of coronary venous blood volume

Compared to resting myocardial perfusion, the oxygen content of the coronary vessels is augmented when myocardial blood flow is increased by vasodilating drugs, such as adenosine. During coronary vasodilation the oxygen extraction of the heart is reduced, the venous oxygen saturation increases and therefore the amount of oxygen within the venous compartment is elevated. This effect can be used to estimate the intravascular coronary venous blood volume. The amount of oxygen which enters and leaves the coronary venous compartment during a transient vasodilation after a bolus injection of adenosine can be determined if kinetic measurements of myocardial oxygen uptake are possible. Since the same fiberoptic devices which were used for the determination of the dye concentration time courses are also suitable for in vivo measurements of blood oxygen saturation, continuous measurements of the myocardial oxygen uptake are possible within the same experimental set-up. The oxygen uptake can be calculated for each heartbeat from coronary sinus outflow and coronary venous oxygen saturation by the microcomputer system. Since large doses of adenosine are accompanied by hemodynamic side effects, the resulting effects on myocardial oxygen uptake do not necessarily represent loading and unloading of myocardial oxygen stores, but, could as well be due to changes in myocardial oxygen consumption. The separation of these two effects can be made by independent measurement of the energy demand per stroke, which can be derived from hemodynamic parameters (2, 7). The amount of oxygen, which is loaded into the coronary venous compartment during a transient coronary vasodilation is then the difference between the oxygen uptake and the energy demand of the heart. Figure 2 shows a typical example for the effects of an adenosine bolus injection on left ventricular pressure (P_{syst}), maximal left ventricular pressure rise (dP/dt_{max}), myocardial blood flow (MBF), coronary venous oxygen saturation ($SO_{2 CV}$), myocardial energy demand (E_t) and myocardial oxygen uptake (MVO_2). The lower two curves show the difference between the latter values and the total amount of oxygen transiently loaded into the venous compartment, which corresponds to the peak value of the lowest curve. Since E_t determines the energy demand of the heart per 100 g tissue, a constant k is introduced, which adjusts the measured coronary sinus outflow and the measured myocardial oxygen uptake to the size of left ventricular muscle draining into the coronary sinus. This constant was determined for each experiment individually by balancing E_t and MVO_2 under control conditions.

117

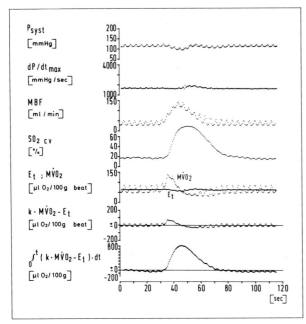

Fig. 2. Effects of an adenosine bolus injection on myocardial oxygen uptake (MVO$_2$) and myocardial energy demand (E$_t$). Each point of the recording corresponds to a single heart stroke. A bolus of adenosine (4 mg) leads to a transient vasodilation of the coronary system with consecutive increase of myocardial blood flow (MBF) and coronary oxygen saturation (SO$_2$ CV). Since the increase in blood flow precedes the increase in venous oxygen saturation a transient increase in MVO$_2$ can be observed, which is due to an elevation of the oxygen content within the venous compartment of the coronary vessels. The accompanying peripheral vasodilation leads to a slight reduction in left ventricular systolic pressure (P$_{syst}$) followed by a slight elevation of maximal left ventricular pressure rise (dP/dt$_{max}$). The calculated energy demand per beat (E$_t$) is slightly decreased. The amount of oxygen which enters or leaves the venous compartment during one heartbeat results from the difference between the myocardial energy demand and myocardial oxygen uptake (k*MVO$_2$ – E$_t$). The exchange of oxygen within the venous compartment can therefore be derived from integration of the latter curve: the total amount of oxygen which was loaded into the venous vessels during the vasodilation period corresponds to the peak value of the lowest curve.

Results

In 5 dogs 31 measurements of total coronary blood volume were performed under control conditions (n = 17) and during coronary vasodilation by adenosine infusion (n = 14). During control conditions, with an average myocardial blood flow of 55.2 ± 6.7 ml/min*100 g, an average mtt of 12.0 ± 2.0 sec was observed. The corresponding values for the intracoronary blood volume were 10.5 ± 0.8 ml/100 g tissue. During adenosine infusion the blood flow increased to 180 ± 53.0 ml/min*100 g, the mean transit time of the dye tracer was shortened to 5.4 ± 1.1 sec. The coronary vasodilation was accompanied by a slight increase in total coronary blood volume, which amounted 15.3 ± 2.0 ml/100 g under these conditions.

In 14 measurements after bolus injections of adenosine in different doses (0.6–6.0 mg) varying degrees of coronary vasodilation could be observed. As expected, the amount of oxygen which was loaded into the venous compartment exhibited a direct relation to the elevation of the coronary sinus oxygen content (Fig. 3). Due to the linear regression fit of the experimental data an augmentation of coronary venous oxygen content of 1 vol% causes an increase of 0.10 ml O$_2$/100 g left ventricular weight within the venous compartment. The average volume of the venous vessels has therefore to amount to 10 ml/100 g under these conditions.

118

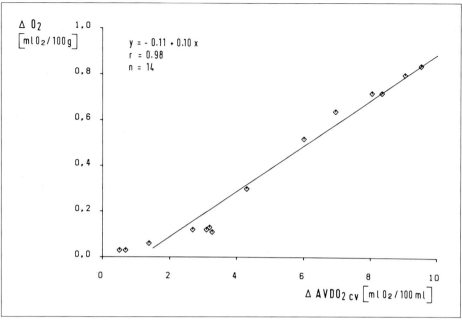

Fig. 3. Relation between elevation of coronary sinus oxygen content (ΔAVDO$_2$) and additionally loaded oxygen into the coronary venous compartment (ΔO$_2$).

Data result from kinetic measurements of myocardial oxygen uptake and myocardial energy demand after transient vasodilation by bolus injections of adenosine (0.6–6.0 mg). The elevation of coronary sinus oxygen content was calculated from baseline and peak values of fiberoptically measured coronary oxygen saturation (see Fig. 2). The amount of oxygen which is loaded into the venous compartment during vasodilation (ΔAVDO$_2$) corresponds to the peak value of the lowest curve in Fig. 2. Linear regression of the data yields a high correlation coefficient (r = 0.98) and an average increase of 0.1 ml oxygen/100 g myocardial tissue, if the coronary sinus oxygen content is increased by 1 vol%. The resulting size of the venous compartment has therefore to amount to 10 ml/100 g myocardial tissue under these conditions.

Since the coronary venous blood volume was determined during coronary vasodilation by adenosine, the corresponding values for the total coronary blood volume should be those which were measured during adenosine infusion within the first group of dogs. The resulting relation between total coronary blood volume and venous coronary blood volume is therefore approximately 3 : 2, or 1 : 2 between the arterial and venous part of the coronary vascular tree.

Discussion

The experimental results demonstrate that under in vivo conditions and resting myocardial blood flow the amount of the intracoronary blood volume is within the range of 11 ml/100 g, of which two thirds belong to the venous vessels. Since the average human left ventricle weight is approximately 200 g, a synchronized retrograde perfusion ought, therefore, to deliver approximately 14–16 ml within each diastole into the coronary sinus in order to be effective. This is considerably more than the less than 1 ml per distole usually used. However, it has to be considered that in the present study the venous compartment includes a half of the capillary vessels as well as all epicardial veins. If the perfusion catheter could be advanced more selectively into epicardial veins smaller volumes might work as well, because the drainage area and therefore the necessary perfusion volumes would decrease. Corresponding morphometric data of the coronary vascular tree, which describe the volume distribution within the branching system and could help to derive a more appropriate estimation of the neccessary perfusion volumes, are not available. But, based on the experimental results of the present study and on additional data which have been published about the structure of the capillary vessels, it is possible to develop a model of the coronary vascular tree by Strahler's law for natural branching systems (10, 11). Two different models of the coronary tree, for vasodilation and under resting conditions, were derived for a left ventricle weighing 150 g, which corresponds to the average weight of the experimentally investigated hearts. The model consists of an arterial and a venous branching system with 6 orders, the lowest corresponding to functional

Table 1. Coronary vascular tree under vasodilation.

Vessels	Order	Number	Diameter (mm)	Length (mm)	Volume (ml)
Arteries	5	$3.0 * 10^0$	$1.5 * 10^0$	$2.0 * 10^1$	0.1
	4	$1.2 * 10^2$	$4.8 * 10^{-1}$	$1.1 * 10^1$	0.2
	3	$4.9 * 10^3$	$1.5 * 10^{-1}$	$6.4 * 10^0$	0.6
	2	$2.0 * 10^5$	$4.9 * 10^{-2}$	$3.6 * 10^0$	1.3
	1	$7.9 * 10^6$	$1.6 * 10^{-2}$	$2.1 * 10^0$	3.1
Capillaries	0	$3.0 * 10^8$	$5.0 * 10^{-3}$	$1.2 * 10^0$	7.3
Veins	1	$9.2 * 10^6$	$1.8 * 10^{-2}$	$2.1 * 10^0$	4.5
	2	$2.6 * 10^5$	$6.2 * 10^{-2}$	$3.6 * 10^0$	2.8
	3	$7.6 * 10^3$	$2.2 * 10^{-1}$	$6.4 * 10^0$	1.7
	4	$2.1 * 10^2$	$7.6 * 10^{-1}$	$1.1 * 10^1$	1.1
	5	$6.0 * 10^0$	$2.7 * 10^0$	$2.0 * 10^1$	0.7

Total volume = 23.4 ml/150 g = 15.6 ml/100 g

The dimensions of the coronary tree model were derived by the law of Strahler for natural branching systems. Due to the experimental results and data from the literature the following assumptions were made:
1) Heart weight of 150 g
2) Six arterial and venous orders
3) Three arterial vessels of fifth order with a diameter of 1.5 mm and two accompanying venous vessels
4) A total coronary blood volume of 15.6 ml/100 g and a relation of 1 : 2 between arterial and venous vessels
5) Capillary density of $2500/mm^2$
6) Capillary diameter of 0.005 mm
7) An average capillary blood velocity of 0.75 mm/sec when coronary blood flow is 200 ml/min * 100 g

Table 2. Coronary vascular tree during resting blood flow.

Vessels	Order	Number	Diameter (mm)	Length (mm)	Volume (ml)
Arteries	5	$3.0 * 10^0$	$1.3 * 10^0$	$2.0 * 10^1$	0.1
	4	$1.2 * 10^2$	$4.1 * 10^{-1}$	$1.1 * 10^1$	0.2
	3	$4.9 * 10^3$	$1.3 * 10^{-1}$	$6.4 * 10^0$	0.4
	2	$2.0 * 10^5$	$4.2 * 10^{-2}$	$3.6 * 10^0$	1.0
	1	$7.9 * 10^6$	$1.3 * 10^{-2}$	$2.1 * 10^0$	2.3
Capillaries	0	$1.6 * 10^8$	$5.0 * 10^{-3}$	$1.2 * 10^0$	3.6
Veins	1	$9.2 * 10^6$	$1.5 * 10^{-2}$	$2.1 * 10^0$	3.4
	2	$2.6 * 10^5$	$5.3 * 10^{-2}$	$3.6 * 10^0$	2.1
	3	$7.6 * 10^3$	$2.9 * 10^{-1}$	$6.4 * 10^0$	1.3
	4	$2.1 * 10^2$	$6.5 * 10^{-1}$	$1.1 * 10^1$	0.8
	5	$6.0 * 10^0$	$2.0 * 10^0$	$2.0 * 10^1$	0.5

Total volume = 15.7 ml/150 g = 10.5 ml/100 g

The number and length of the vessels correspond to the derived values of the coronary vascular tree model under vasodilation. The diameters of the vessels were calculated according to the experimental result of a total coronary blood volume of 10.5 ml/100 g and the assumption of a capillary expansion factor of 2.

capillary units with a density of 2500/mm² and a functional length of 1.2 mm (1, 8). It was assumed that Strahler's law is valid for the vasodilated coronary tree, and that vasodilation is accompanied by a capillary recruitment with an expansion factor of 2 (3). The resulting data are shown in Tables 1 and 2. The main part of the intravascular volume is located in the capillaries and the small veins. The venous blood which is located within the vessels larger than 0.65 mm in diameter is less than 15% of the venous compartment. On the other hand, for a left ventricle of 200 g, a diastolic pump volume of 1 ml would be just sufficient to fill the venous vessels of the fifth order, which are mainly located on the epicardial surface. A reduction of the required pump volume to access the capillary vessels could be achieved by a selective perfusion of one of these venous branches draining a smaller area of myocardial tissue. However, even if a venous vessel of the fifth order could be selectively catheterized and the afflicted area were reduced to 25 g of myocardial tissue, the pump volume would still have to amount to more than 1 ml per diastole. Since the flow for retrograde perfusion techniques is limited by the catheters and the necessary driving pressures, the results of this study obviously suggest that a selective perfusion of smaller veins with a diameter less than 2.0 mm is required for a capillary perfusion. On the other hand, the size of the myocardial tissue treatable by such a technique would be less than 25 g and would therefore seem to be unsuitable for large myocardial infarctions.

References

1. Bassingthwaighte JB, Yipintsoi T, Hervey RB (1974) Microvasculature of the dog left ventricular myocardium. Microvascular Res 7: 229–249

2. Bretschneider HJ (1972) Die hämodynamischen Determinanten des myokardialen Sauerstoffver-brauchs. In: Dengler, HJ (ed) Die therapeutische Anwendung β-sympathikolytischer Stoffe. Schattauer Verlag, Stuttgart–New York, pp 45–60
3. Duran WN, Marsicano TH, Anderson RW (1977) Capillary reserve in isometrically contracting dog hearts. Am J Physiol 90: H276–H281
4. Feigl EO (1983) Coronary physiology. Physiological Reviews 63: 1–205
5. Gaethgens P (1977) Hemodynamics of the Microcirculation. In: Meessen H (ed) Handbuch der allgemeinen Pathologie, Mikrozirkulation Band III, Teil 7. Springer-Verlag, Berlin Heidelberg New York, pp 231–287
6. Heiss HW, Hensel I, Kettler D, Tauchert M, Bretschneider HJ (1973) Über den Anteil des Koro-narsinus-Ausflusses an der Myokarddurchblutung des linken Ventrikels. Z Kardiol 62: 593–606
7. Hoeft A, Korb H, Baller D, Wolpers HG, Hellige G, Bretschneider HJ (1984) Quantification of ischemic stress during repeated coronary artery occlusion in the dog: A method for validation of therapeutic effects. I. Estimation of O_2-debt and O_2-repayment. Bas Res Cardiol 79: 27–37
8. Honig CR, Gayeski TEJ (1983) Capillary reserve and tissue O_2-transport in normal and in hypertrophied hearts. In: Tarazi RC, Dunbar JB (eds) Perspectives in Cardiovascular Research, 8. Raven Press, New York, pp 249–260
9. Korb H, Hoeft A, Hellige G (1984) Measurements of coronary mean transit time and myocardial tissue blood flow by deconvolution of intravasal tracer dilution curves. SPIE Novel Optical Fiber Techniques for Medical Applications 494: 36–41
10. Strahler AN (1957) Quantitative analysis of watersheet geomorphology. American Geophysical Union Transactions 38: 913–920
11. Woldenberg MJ (1968) Hierachical systems: Cities, rivers, alpine glaciers, bovine livers and trees. Ph D Thesis, University of Columbia

Authors' address:
A. Hoeft, M.D.
Zentrum „Physiologie und Pathophysiologie"
Universität Göttingen
Humboldtallee 23
3400 Göttingen
West Germany

Continuous recording of coronary venous potassium and pH during myocardial ischemia

G. Müller-Esch, H. Djonlagic, E. Bauer, C. von der Lühe, T. Mackenroth, B. Hackenjos, and A. Sheikhzadeh

Klinik für Innere Medizin, Medizinische Universität zu Lübeck, Lübeck (West Germany)

During experimental myocardial ischemia, rapid shifts of potassium and hydrogen ions towards the extracellular space can be observed (2–5). However, using conventional coronary venous sampling techniques in the clinical setting, these changes can scarcely be demonstrated. We therefore asked 1) if continuous measurement and recording of coronary venous potassium and pH during atrial pacing test might detect such ischemia-related transient dynamic responses with greater reliability and 2) if this technique may prove to be a reliable tool for the evaluation of drug effects in ischemic heart disease.

Methods

Eighteen patients with recurrent chest pain were studied. A 7F gauge multipurpose bipolar electrode catheter was placed into the coronary sinus. Coronary venous potassium and pH were measured and recorded continuously by means of a flow-measuring unit (Analysator D, Eschweiler Laboratories, Kiel, F.R.G.). Incremental atrial pacing was performed. In 5 patients with pacing-induced ischemic ECG changes, the procedure was repeated after intravenous administration of nifedipine (bolus injection of 0.5 mg followed by an infusion rate of 1 mg/h).

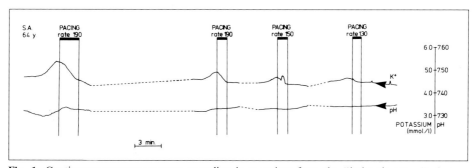

Fig. 1. Continuous coronary venous recording in a patient from the "ischemic group", demonstrating "washout" of potassium and hydrogen ions. These transient ion shifts depend on the frequency and duration of atrial pacing. Note that direction of recording is from right to left. ---- = flow interrruption (blood sampling: technical problems)

Results

In 10 patients ("ischemic group") ischemic ST-T-wave changes developed and a marked transient rise in coronary venous potassium together with (8 cases) a simultaneous pH decrease occurred (Table 1). The degree of these reproducible changes in each subject depended on the frequency and duration of atrial pacing (Fig. 1). Intravenous administration of nifedipine diminished the "washout" of potassium and hydrogen ions (Figs. 2 and 4).
In 8 patients ("non-ischemic group") atrial pacing induced neither angina nor ischemic ECG changes. Coronary venous potassium increase during prolonged pacing was rather small and a slight pH-decrease was only observed in 2 cases (Table 1 and Figs. 3 and 4).

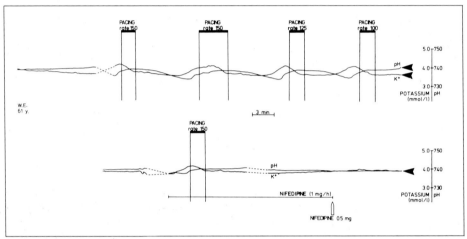

Fig. 2. Continuous coronary venous recording in another patient who developed ischemic ECG changes. Intravenous administration of nifedipine diminishes potassium increase and pH decrease following atrial pacing. Again, recording direction is from right to left, starting at the upper right part of the figure.

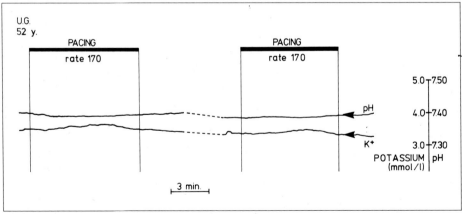

Fig. 3. Continuous coronary venous recording in a patient from the "non-ischemic" group. Prolonged atrial pacing (480 sec) only results in a slight pH decrease. The initial potassium increase turns to basal values despite on-going pacing.

124

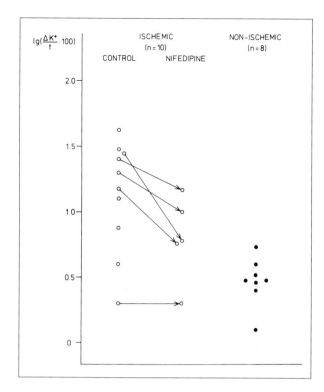

Fig. 4. Graph demonstrating the relation between potassium increase (K$^+$(mmol/l)) and pacing time (t(min)) on a logarithmic scale in patients with ("ischemic group") and without ("non-ischemic group") ischemic ST-depression. The effect of intravenous nifedipine administration in 5 cases is also shown.

Discussion

Our results indicate that pacing-induced myocardial ischemia is accompanied by a transient intracellular loss of potassium and hydrogen ions which can be detected in coronary venous blood.

By means of a continuous automated sampling technique, Parker et al. (8) demonstrated earlier that coronary venous potassium increase during the atrial pacing test was clearly more pronounced in patients with ischemic ST-wave changes than in subjects without such ECG changes. Recently, Webb et al. (10), using catheter tip ion selective electrodes, reported the "washout" of accumulated potassium after brief periods of coronary arterial occlusion induced by percutaneous transluminal coronary angioplasty. A similar mechanism may be reflected by our findings of a time- and frequency-dependent coronary venous pH decrease.

In 4 cases, intravenous nifedipine administration deminished the coronary venous increase of potassium and hydrogen ions. Perhaps this points to a direct myocardial effect of calcium channel blockers independent of their recognized vasodilating actions.

The pitfalls of coronary venous sampling notwithstanding (1), our preliminary data suggest that continuous coronary venous recording of potassium and pH may be a sensitive method for the detection of myocardial ischemia as well as for the evaluation of drug effects in ischemic heart disease. Likewise, our approach may be useful for the investigation

Table 1. Clinical data and results of continuous coronary venous recording during atrial pacing in patients with ("ischemic group") and without (,,non-ischemic group") ischemic ST segment changes. In 5 cases pacing was repeated after intravenous administration of nifedipine ("control" and "nifedipine", respectively). * = respiratory alkalosis due to hyperventilation.

Case	Age (years)		Pacing period (sec.)	Pacing rate (per min.)	K^+-increase (mmol/l)	pH-decrease
Ischemic group (n = 10)						
W.E.	61	Control	120	150	0.5	0.035
		Nifedipine	120	150	0.3	0.025
Z.E.	61	Control	180	125	0.6	0.05
		Nifedipine	240	125	0.4	0.035
K.G.	47	Control	120	170	0.3	0.01
		Nifedipine	210	170	0.2	± 0
B.H.	54	Control	120	175	0.55	0.01
		Nifedipine	300	175	0.3	± 0
B.H.	67	Control	600	155	0.2	± 0
		Nifedipine	600	155	0.2	± 0
B.M.	70		90	180	0.45	0.02
O.W.	62		120	175	0.25	0.01
S.A.	64		120	190	0.85	0.03
F.G.	51		240	125	0.3	0.02
H.W.	56		600	185	0.4	± 0
					$\bar{x} \pm$ SD 0.44 $\pm$ 0.20	
Non-ischemic group (n = 8)						
U.G.	52		480	170	0.2	0.01
F.H.	62		270	150	0.25	–*
K.H.	71		600	150	0.3	± 0
H.R.	63		420	165	0.2	± 0
M.R.	45		480	175	0.1	± 0
L.H.	45		600	160	0.3	0.01
L.K.	39		360	155	0.2	± 0
R.D.	49		300	150	0.2	± 0
					$\bar{x} \pm$ SD 0.22 $\pm$ 0.07	

of different interventions via the coronary sinus route, both in cardiology and in cardio-vascular surgery. Further studies should compare coronary venous monitoring with other indicators of myocardial ischemia such as lactate or hypoxanthine (6, 7, 9).

References

1. Brachfeld N (1976) Characterization of the Ischemic Process by Regional Metabolism. Am J Cardiol 37: 467–473

2. Cobbe SM, Parker DJ, Poole-Wilson PA (1982) Tissue and Coronary Venous pH in Ischemic Canine Myocardium. Clin Cardiol 5: 153–156
3. Corday E, Heng MK, Meerbaum S, Lang T-W, Farcot J-C, Osher J, Hashimoto K (1977) Derangements of Myocardial Metabolism Preceding Onset of Ventricular Fibrillation after Coronary Occlusion. Am J Cardiol 39: 880–889
4. Kleber AG (1983) Resting Membrane Potential, Extracellular Potassium Activity, and Intracellular Sodium Activity during Acute Global Ischemia in Isolated Perfused Guinea Pig Hearts. Circ Res 52: 442–450
5. Obeid A, Smulyan H, Gilbert R, Eich R (1972) Regional Metabolic Changes in the Myocardium Following Coronary Artery Ligation in Dogs. Am Heart J 83: 189–196
6. Opie LH, Owen P, Thomas M, Samson R (1973) Coronary Sinus Lactate Measurements in Assessment of Myocardial Ischemia. Comparison with Changes in Lactate/Pyruvate and Beta-Hydroxybutyrate/Acetoacetate Ratios and with Release of Hydrogen, Phosphate and Potassium Ions from the Heart. Am J Cardiol 32: 295–305
7. Parker JO, Chiong MA, West RO, Case RB (1969) Sequential Alterations in Myocardial Lactate Metabolism, S-T Segments, and Left Ventricular Function During Angina Induced by Atrial Pacing. Circulation 40: 113–131
8. Parker JO, Chiong MA, West RO, Case RB (1970) The Effect of Ischemia and Alterations of Heart Rate on Myocardial Potassium Balance in Man. Circulation 42: 205–217
9. Remme WJ, de Jong JW, Verdouw PD (1977) Effects of Pacing-Induced Myocardial Ischemia on Hypoxanthine Efflux From the Human Heart. Am J Cardiol 40: 55–62
10. Webb SC, Canepa-Anson R, Poole-Wilson PA (1984) Timing of Myocardial Potassium Loss During Coronary Arterial Occlusion. Eur Heart J 5: 453 (Abstr)

Authors' address:
Dr. med. Gert Müller-Esch
Klinik für Innere Medizin
Medizinische Universität zu Lübeck
Ratzeburger Allee 160
D-2400 Lübeck 1
West Germany

Continuous monitoring of coronary venous lactate in transient ischemia

G. Tommasini and F. Tamagni

Divisione di Cardiologia, Ospedale Maggiore di Lodi, Lodi (Italy)

Summary: We developed a new technique of continuous aspiration, coupled to electrochemical determination of lactate in whole blood. A Gorlin catheter is positioned in the coronary sinus, and blood is continuously withdrawn (1 ml/min) by a Sage 375A multichannel peristaltic pump, along with a pH 7.4 Triton/buffer solution, with a volume ratio of 1 : 7.5.
Carry-over is minimized by air bubbles; complete hemolysis occurs within a few seconds after mixing. Continuous determination of blood lactate is performed by a commercially available Roche 640 Lactate Analyzer, slightly modified to allow for a continuous mode.
Immobilized enzyme-electrochemical detection of first order lactate-to-pyruvate conversion is used, the output being proportional to dynamic lactate concentration from 0 to 10 mM/l. The overall response is adequate for the measurements of biological variations: 1) sensitivity 0.01 mM/l, 2) linearity better than 99%, 3) baseline drifts less than $\pm$ 2%, 4) with-drawal time less than 120 sec, 5) time constant (10 to 90%) less than 60 sec.
Myocardial ischemia can be recognised with a mean delay of 120 sec with respect to the original event.

Introduction

Myocardial lactate metabolism is conventionally studied by discrete sampling of arterial and coronary sinus blood. Inherent limitations of this approach are delayed information and incomplete description of the metabolic events.
In this paper we describe a continuous sampling technique, coupled to electrochemical determination of whole blood lactate, which operates in quasi-real time.

Methods

a) Continuous sampling

Blood is continuously aspirated from the coronary sinus via a 7F, two platinum electrode Gorlin catheter (USCI Corp.), which also allows for pacing and flow measurements (4). A Sage 375 A four-channel peristaltic pump is connected to the catheter through a 1.5 mm ID rubber tubing, which provides a flow of 1 ml/min at a dial setting of 40%. A pH 7.4 buffer containing 750 mg/l hexacyanoferrate-(III) is aspirated in parallel (4.0 mm ID tubing) at 6.5 ml/min.
For whole blood lactate monitoring, the buffer is simply added to the blood via a T connector, thorough mixing being provided by an 11 cm micro glass bead Adeplat tubing (see Fig. 1). Hemolysed blood monitoring is also possible, but requires a slightly different approach. Rapid (less than 10 sec) hemolysis is obtained by adding Triton 1 : 250 (final concentration) to the buffer solution. A third channel of the peristaltic pump is used to convey air,

129

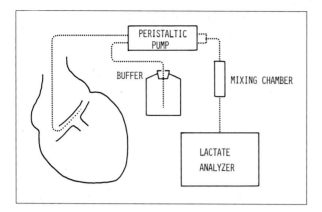

Fig. 1. Whole blood lactate monitoring assembly.

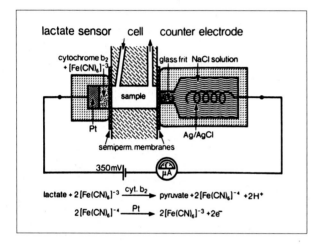

Fig. 2. Lactate sensor.

which is injected into the system immediately downstream the T connector. The fractionating air bubbles serve two-fold. They assure thorough mixing and greatly reduce system carry-over. Excess fluid and air bubbles are removed by an air trap immediately before entering the Analyzer. A 15 cm mixing coil is substituted for the glass bead tubing in this assembly, since erythrocyte ghosts will eventually lead to its obstruction.

b) Lactate assay

This is accomplished by a commercially available Roche 640 Lactate Analyzer, slightly modified in our laboratory to allow for a continuous mode. The schema of the measuring assembly is shown in Fig. 2. The sensor consists of a platinum electrode coated with a thin layer of the enzyme cytochrome b_2. The enzyme is separated from the blood/buffer solution by a semi-permeable membrane, which passes the low molecular weight compounds participating in the reaction (lactate, pyruvate, hexacyanoferrate), but is impermeable for the enzyme. A second electrode made of chloridized silver wire is utilized as a

130

potential reference and as a counter electrode. The platinum electrode of the lactate sensor is biased at 350 mV against this electrode.

The reactions involved are: 1) enzymatic oxidation of lactate, 2) electrochemical oxidation of the hexacyanoferrate-(II) formed. For each lactate oxidized, two electrons are collected on the platinum electrode. Hence a current can be measured which is related to lactate concentration (3).

Since the instrument operates in first order kinetics, it can be used to measure time-varying concentrations of lactate in flowing fluids. Accordingly, the instrument has been slightly modified in order to operate in continuous mode, by inhibiting the automatic stop-rinse cycle and providing an analog DC output for recording and on-line processing of the signal.

Results

a) In vitro experiments

The system has been validated in vitro with heparin-anticoagulated human blood. There is excellent correlation between lactate concentrations measured in the continuous mode, and the corresponding plasma values by discrete measurements (Fig. 3). This holds for plasma, hemolysed and whole blood. The lower concentration found in whole blood probably reflects a hematocrit effect, since only extracellular lactate is being measured in this assay.

The instrument has an intrinsic sensitivity of 0.01 mM/l and a linearity better than 99%. In continuous mode operation, baseline drifts are within ± 2% at 1 mM/l. Information

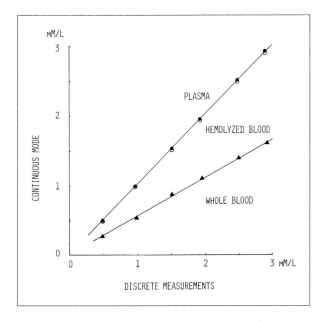

Fig. 3. Correlations between lactate concentration as measured in the continuous mode (ordinate) and plasma values by discrete measurements (abscissa).

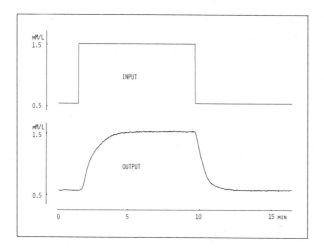

Fig. 4. Square wave response of the whole system.

delay is about 2 minutes at 1 ml/min, and the overall time constant (10–90% of full response) is less than 45 seconds (Fig. 4).

This appears adequate for describing biological variations in the setting of myocardial ischemia (2).

b) In vivo application

Continuous monitoring of coronary sinus lactate has been carried out in 17 patients submitted to provocative tests for myocardial ischemia. Tests included atrial pacing (n = 14), dipyridamole administration (n = 3) and ergonovine (n = 2).

Analog output from the Analyzer was digitized at 1 Hz and stored along with a representative ECG lead, which was then processed to obtain actual heart rate, ST shifts and QRS

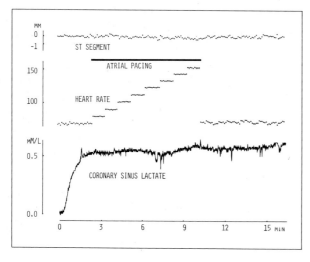

Fig. 5. Typical lactate response to atrial pacing with no evidence of ischemia.

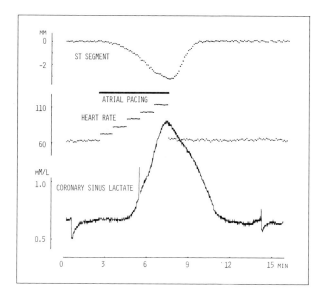

Fig. 6. A positive pacing test. Maximal lactate release occurs at the peak ST changes.

amplitude. Lactate data were corrected for time delay before replotting. Typical examples of negative and positive responses to pacing are shown in Figs. 5 and 6. Artifacts due to pacing and static charges were subsequently minimized by proper earthing of the patient. Monitoring has been carried out for as long as 60 minutes; systemic heparinization (50 mg at the beginning of the procedure) was required, however, in order to prevent catheter clotting. The whole procedure had no untoward side effect.

Discussion

The technique described above has several advantages over discrete sampling. A complete description of the metabolic event is obtained within two minutes of real time, and this permits analysis of both threshold and rate of lactate production. Uniform handling of samples assures stable baseline and easy detection of significant deviations. Furthermore, blood loss is minimized. The main disadvantage is probably the need for systemic heparinization, which could be overcome by use of heparin-bonded catheters. System carry-over was a problem with the whole blood technique, but this is much less the case with fractionating air bubbles. It can be avoided by using specially designed double lumen catheters and injecting fractionating air bubbles immediately below the tip. Moreover, distortion due to carry-over and sensor response can be corrected by mathematical procedures such as deconvolution or harmonic analysis (1).

The continuous aspiration technique can be applied to other metabolites as well. In our last studies, continuous monitoring of coronary venous PO_2 was performed by inserting an intravascular O_2 sensor in the blood line via a T connector. The possibility of operating in cascade on multiple metabolic parameters is probably a major advantage over catheter-tip miniaturized sensors.

References

1. Case R, Felix A, Castellana F (1979) Rate of rise of myocardial PCO_2 during early myocardial ischemia in the dog. Circulation Res 45: 3, 324
2. Parker J, Chiong M, West R, Case R (1969) Sequential alterations in myocardial lactate metabolism, ST segments and left ventricular function during angina induced by atrial pacing. Circulation 40: 113
3. Racine P, Klenk H, Kochsiek K (1975) Rapid lactate determination with an electrochemical enzymatic sensor: clinical usuability and comparative measurements. Z Klin Chem Klin Biochem 13: 533
4. Tommasini G, Tamagni F, Poluzzi C, Oddone A, Orlandi M, Cornalba C, Malusardi R (1985) Coronary sinus hemodynamics in transient ischemia. Computers in Cardiology, in press

Authors' address:
Giorgio Tommasini, M.D.
Cardiovascular Division
Ospedale Maggiore di Lodi
20075 Lodi (Mi), Italy

134

Myocardial temperature mapping after cold cardioplegia

A. Leguerrier, C. Rioux, P. Rosat, E. Marcade, H. Le Couls, J. Boulvard,
C. Mottez, and Y. Logeais

Cardiovascular and Thoracic Unit, University Hospital, Rennes (France)

Summary: Myocardial wall temperatures (T.) have been controlled during aorta crossclamping, into cardioplegic hypothermia, obtained by coronary perfusion (through a separated roller pump) of 2 liters of a cold (4 °C) cristalloid solution, in three groups (GR) of patients:
– GR   I: antegrade perfusion (A.P.) (via the aortic root) in 24 patients undergoing valvular surgery.
– GR II: antegrade perfusion (A.P.) in 26 patients undergoing aorto coronary bypass grafting (coronary stenoses).
– GR III: retrograde perfusion (R.P.) through the coronary sinus in 25 patients undergoing valvular surgery.
The ventricular temperatures (controlled at three different locations of the heart's surface) were analyzed by a computer (I.B.M.).
The rewarming curves are comparable in the three groups (T. = T.o + K log t); at the end of the cardioplegic perfusion, marked temperature discrepancies between the different locations of the ventricles are noted (whatever the method used for cardioplegic perfusion may be): the thermic gradients decrease during the control period.
In GR II (all patients presenting a LAD significant stenosis), the apical portion of the LV is warmer than in the two other groups free from coronary stenosis. In these two groups (GR I and GR III), the LV is colder than the RV (the left lateral wall of the LV remaining the colder site).

Introduction

An experimental study (24 dogs) showed us that there are large discrepancies in myocardial temperatures after cold cardioplegia (7).
This study was carried out on a group of 75 patients to control the variability of the final myocardial temperature (at the end of the cold perfusion) and the importance of intramyocardial gradients between different locations of the heart.

Material and methods

Seventy-five patients underwent myocardial temperature mapping during extra-corporeal circulation for valvular or coronary surgery.
The heart was cannulated with a standard ascending aortic cannula and separated cavas cannulas. Total cardiopulmonary bypass was instituted and the left ventricle was vented (during valvular surgery) via the right superior pulmonary vein. Core body temperature (as determined by a nasopharyngeal temperature probe) was lowered to 28 °C.
Subepicardial temperature was continuously monitored by needle temperature probes (Ellab AK 20). Inserted into three different sites of the heart (Fig. 1): anterior wall of the right ventricle (RV), postero-lateral wall of the left ventricle (LV) and apex of the LV.
An aorta cross-clamp was then applied, just below the aortic cannula. 2 liters of cold (4 °C) cardioplegic solution (Ringer's solution to which was added 20 meq potassium

135

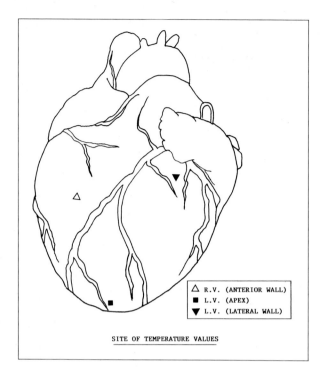

Fig. 1. Site of temperature values.

△ R.V. (ANTERIOR WALL)
■ L.V. (APEX)
▼ L.V. (LATERAL WALL)

SITE OF TEMPERATURE VALUES

chloride) was infused through a separated roller pump either via the aortic root or via the coronary sinus.

Patients were divided into three groups:

Group I (GR I): antegrade perfusion (A.P.) via the aortic root in 24 patients (free from coronary stenoses) undergoing valvular surgery: single valve replacement (16), double valve (6) and triple valve (2) replacement.
Group II (GR II): A.P. in 26 patients undergoing aorto-coronary bypass grafting (A.C.B.G.); mean 2.3 grafts per patient (left anterior descending (LAD) in every case).
Group III (GR III): retrograde perfusion (R.P.) through the coronary sinus in 25 patients (free from coronary stenoses) undergoing valvular (and/or) aortic surgery: 13 single valve replacement, 8 double or triple valve surgery, 4 combined (ascending aorta and valvular) surgery.

Results

Large differences in the cooling (4.5 °C to 14.5 °C) are observed at the end of the infusion of cardioplegic solution (2 liters); this variability is noted in the three groups; to compare the different rewarming curves, it becomes necessary to consider the initial mean temperature of each heart (class A: mean 4.6 °C; class B: 7.4 °C; class C: 9.5 °C; class D: 14.1 °C), this repartition being the same in the three groups of patients (Fig. 2).

136

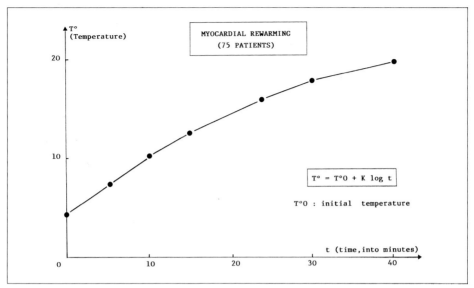

Fig. 2.

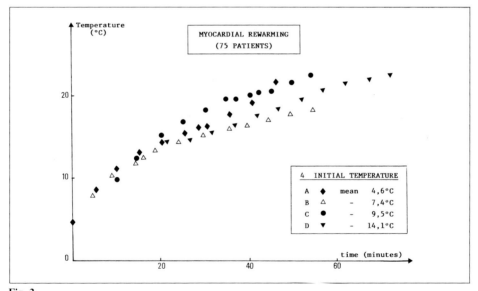

Fig. 3.

The rewarming curves (for each site of each heart) are illustrated in Fig. 3; the rewarming of the RV is comparable to that of the LV (lateral wall and apical region); there are no differences between A.P. and R.P.

It is important to consider the gradients which exist between the three ventricular sites (of each heart) and their evolution (during the rewarming time):

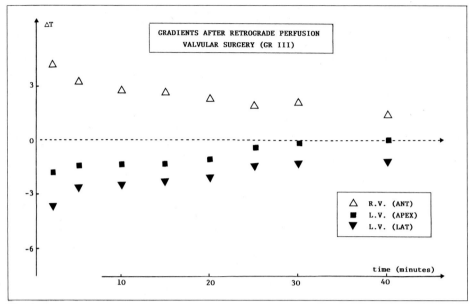

Fig. 4.

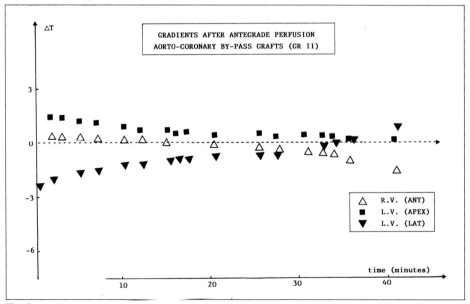

Fig. 5.

138

- in GR I (Fig. 4), just after the cardioplegic infusion, the RV is significantly warmer than the LV (the postero-lateral wall being colder than the apical region); then, the gradients are decreasing.
- in GR II (Fig. 5), the apical region of LV is the warmer place (all these patients have, at least, a significant stenosis of the LAD).
- in GR III (Fig. 6), the gradients are not different from those of GR I (the RV seems to be warmer, but the difference is not significant).

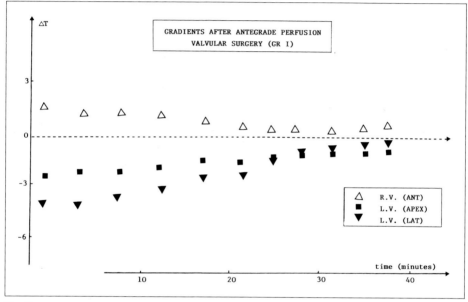

Fig. 6.

Conclusion

When performing valvular surgery (coronary arteries being free from stenoses), myocardial cooling (using a cristalloid solution) is not uniform whatever the method of cardioplegic perfusion may be (antegrade or retrograde): the lateral part of the LV is colder than the apical part (which is itself colder than the RV). Retrograde perfusion can be safely used, especially in cases of aortic incompetence, and for iterative coronary perfusion when the aortic root is opened (multiple valvular replacement, ascending aorta surgery).

In hearts with compromised coronary circulation, there are large discrepancies in myocardial temperatures; retrograde perfusion (R.P.) may reduce the thermic gradients distal to a coronary artery lesion; we are establishing a myocardial mapping after R.P. in a new group of patients undergoing aorto-coronary bypass grafts.

References

1. Bessou JP, Jarry G, Loisance D, Bui Mong Hung, Lautier A (1981) Températures myocardiques regionales au cours du refroidissement lors de la perfusion hypothermique sélective. Ann chir: Chir Thorac Cardio-Vasc 35, No 3: 183–186
2. Daggett WM, Jacocks MA, Coleman WS, Johnson RG, Lowenstein E, Vander Salm TJ (1981) – Myocardial temperature mapping. Improved intraoperative myocardial preservation. J Thorac Cardiovasc Surg 82: 883–888
3. Fabiani JN, Romano M, Chapelon C, Theard M, Bensasson D, Carpentier A (1984) La cardioplégie rétrograde: étude expérimentale et clinique. Ann Chir: Chir Thorac Cardio-Vasc 38, No 7: 513–516
4. Grover FL, Fewel JG, Ghidoni J, Trinkle JK (1981) Does lower systemic temperature enhance cardioplegic myocardial protection? J Thorac Cardiovasc Surg 81: 11–20
5. Heineman FW, MacGregor DC, Wilson GJ, Ninomiya J (1981) Regional and transmural myocardial temperature distribution in cold chemical cardioplegia. Significance of critical coronary cold chemical cardioplegia. Significance of critical coronary arterial stenosis. J Thorac Cardiovasc Surg 81: 851–859
6. Logeais Y, Rioux C, Leguerrier A, Marcade E, Scordia P, Lebettre O, Le Couls H (1979) La protection myocardique peropératoire par cardioplégie hypothermique. Etude Clinique et évolution du protocole. Coeur XI, No 3: 749–769
7. Marcade E, Logeais Y, Leguerrier A, Rioux C, Le Couls H (1984) Répartition et évolution des températures myocardiques au cours de la cardioplégie hypothermique. Etude expérimentale chez le chien. Ann Chir: Chir Thorac Cardio-Vasc 38, No: 174–179
8. Silverman NA, Schmitt G, Levitsky S, Feinberg H (1984) Optimal intraoperative protection of myocardium distal to coronary stenoses. J Thorac Cardiovasc Surg 88: 424–431
9. Steven RG, Marvin MK (1982) A comparison of retrograde cardiodioplegia versus antegrade cardioplegia in the presence of coronary artery obstruction. Circulation 66 (Suppl II): October

Authors' address:
Prof. A. Leguerrier, M.D.
Cardiovascular and Thoracic Unit
University Hospital
35033 Rennes Cedex
France

Thebesian veins in the human hearts with atherosclerotic lesions in the coronary arteries

Ewa Ratajczyk-Pakalska

Department of Normal Anatomy, Institute of Biology and Morphology Medical Academy in Łódź (Poland)

Summary: The anatomy and physiology of the Thebesian veins have not been hitherto completely elucidated. The role of the Thebesian veins in pathology, especially in coronary disease, is also unknown. Our previous observations conducted on human hearts have shown a great number of cardiac veins in the myocardium of the ventricles in hearts where atherosclerotic lesions in the coronary arteries were present. The main aim of the studies was to examine the venous side of the coronary circulation (with special reference to the Thebesian veins) in human hearts with atherosclerotic lesions in the coronary arteries. The studies were carried out on 30 dead human hearts (with atherosclerotic lesions in the coronary arteries) using the microhistoangiographic method. Particular attention was paid to the origin, course, kind of tributaries, and orifices of Thebesian veins. On the microhistoangiographs obtained from cross sections of the ventricular walls, in 67% of hearts the uniform and rich venous vascularization in the internal zone of the ventricular myocardium was noted compared with the medial and external zones of the ventricular myocardium previously observed in the normal hearts.

Introduction

Until recently the venous drainage of the coronary circulation has been ignored by anatomists and other members of the scientific community whereas the knowledge of the venous vascularization is particularly important not only in normal hearts but also in hearts where atherosclerotic lesions in the coronary artery were present. The use of the coronary sinus or its venous tributaries by a variety of techniques by the cardiac surgeon and cardiologist has great promise in the protection of the ischemic myocardium (1).

Our previous observations conducted on human hearts (2, 3, 6) have shown a great number of cardiac veins of ventricular myocardium with the atherosclerotic lesions in the coronary arteries.

The main aim of the present studies was to examine the veins of the ventricular myocardium (with references to the Thebesian veins) in hearts where atherosclerotic lesions in the coronary arteries were present.

Material and methods

A total of 30 hearts from patients who died aged 48–78 years were evaluated with respect to their venous outflow. The hearts came from patients with a history of coronary heart disease. The cardiac veins were injected retrograde via the coronary sinus and also via anterior right ventricular veins as soon as possible with Microfil MV-122 Silicon rubber injection compounds (Canton Biomedical Products, Inc. Boulder, Colo., U.S.A.). After fixation, the hearts were sectioned into uniform slices c. 500 μm thick, from the apex up

141

to just below the atrioventricular valves. Afterwards the hearts went through the routine examination using the microhistoangiographic method (4, 7). The microhistoangiographs-cross sections of the ventricular myocardium were observed at 16 to 40 times magnifications.

Results

The Thebesian veins contrary to the other veins of the heart outflow blood from the myocardium to the ventricular cavities towards to the endocardium, escaping throughout the orifices of Thebesian veins. The Thebesian veins arise either directly from the capillary vessels (Figs. 1 and 2) or indirectly from the venules (Fig. 3 – which constitutes from the capillary vessels) – tributaries of the Thebesian veins.

In their course the Thebesian veins may have tributaries which are characterized by instability of the course, number, size and length. The tributaries (the venules or the capillary vessels) enter the Thebesian veins either at an acute angle (70%) or at a right angle (30%). The number of tributaries opening into the main trunk of the Thebesian vein is 3 to 9.

On the basis of previously made observations (3, 5) concerning the venous layers of the ventricular walls, and taking into consideration the depth at which the Thebesian vein were formed together with their course, superficial and deep Thebesian veins have been singled out. Superficial Thebesian veins run parallel to the endocardial surface and out-

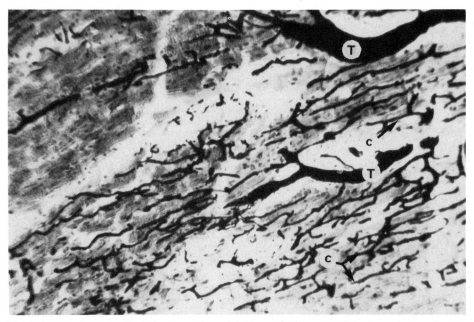

Fig. 1. Histologic preparation of cross section of right ventricular wall. Thebesian vein (canaliculate type) emptying into the right ventricular cavity (H-E*))
T – Thebesian vein
c – capillary vessel
*) (H-E) – staining with Hematoxylin-eosin

142

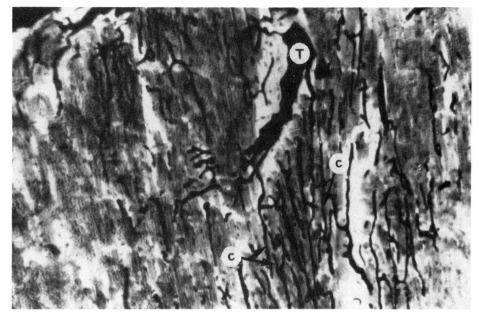

Fig. 2. Histologic preparation of cross section of left ventricular wall. Thebesian vein (canaliculate type) emptying into the left ventricular cavity (H-E)

T – Thebesian vein
c – capillary vessel

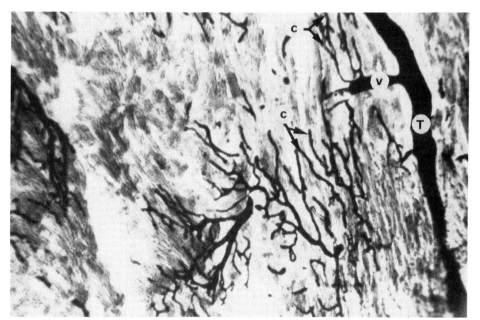

Fig. 3. Histologic preparation of cross section of left ventricular wall. Thebesian vein (canaliculate type) emptying into the left ventricular cavity (H-E)

T – Thebesian vein
c – capillary vessel
v – venula

flow at a right angle to the heart cavity whereas deep Thebesian veins run perpendicu-
larly to the endocardial surface and outflow at a right angle to the heart cavities.

It has been noted that Thebesian veins begin in various venous layers of the ventricular
walls:

I) as deep Thebesian veins in the medial venous layers in the walls of the left ventricle
or more seldom as superficial Thebesian veins in the internal venous layer,

II) as superficial and deep Thebesian veins in the internal venous layer in the walls of the
right ventricle.

Our previous observations conducted on normal hearts (2, 3, 5) have shown several types
of Thebesian veins. In the present explorations only arboriform type (73%), sinusoidal
type (7%), canaliculate type (13%) and also thread-like (or "connecting Thebesian veins"
– 7%) were found.

Distribution of the above mentioned types of Thebesian veins in the heart walls is as follows: arboriform, canaliculate and thread-like Thebesian veins were observed in the anterior and posterior walls of both ventricles. All these Thebesian veins that occur in the
ventricular septum outflow through Thebesian veins – orifices in the endocardium of the
appropriate ventricle, belong to Thebesian veins of arboriform, canaliculate and sinusoidal types. Only Thebesian veins of arboriform and canaliculate types appear in the papillary muscles of the ventricles (Fig. 4).

On the microhistangiographs obtained from the cross sections of the ventricular myocardium, in 67% of hearts, in the internal-subendocardial zone (of both right and left ventricles and also in the 1/4 part of the ventricular septum facing left and right ventricular
cavities) we noted uniform and rich venous vascularization, as compared with the medial

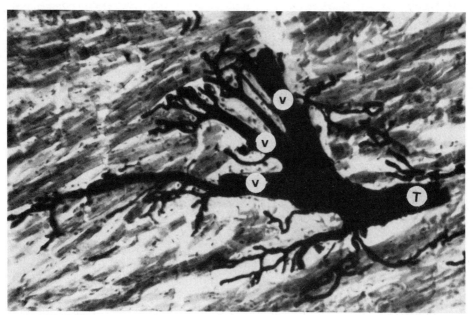

Fig. 4. Histologic preparation of cross section of ventricular septum. Thebesian vein (arboriform
type) emptying into the right ventricular cavity (H-E)
T – Thebesian vein
v – venula

144

and external zones, previously described (3) in the normal hearts. The density of venous vascularization in the internal-subendocardial zone also depends on the Thebesian veins which are easy to recognize because of their size and connections with the lumen of the ventricles.

A greater number of small veins and Thebesian veins in the ventricular walls of the atherosclerotic hearts are in agreement with the previous observations of Pakalska (2, 3, 6) and Samojłowa (8).

A special study connected with the number of Thebesian veins estimated in the ventricular myocardium (in atherosclerotic hearts) using an automated image analyser (Quantimet 720) will be published in a separate article.

Conclusions

1. Depending on the course and tributaries of Thebesian veins four types of these veins (previously described in normal hearts) have been distinguished i.e., arboriform, sinusoidal, canaliculate and thread-like types.
2. According to topography and the course of the Thebesian veins with relation to the surface of the endocardium superficial and deep (also observed in normal hearts) Thebesian veins have been described.
3. More rich venous vascularization and Thebesian veins in the internal-subendocardial zone of the ventricular myocardium have been noted.

References

1. Faxon D, Mohl W (1984) Summarizing Statement of the Panel of Working Groupsf. In: Mohl W, Wolner E, Glogar D (eds) The Coronary Sinus. Steinkopff Verlag, Darmstadt, pp 549–550
2. Pakalska E (1977) Retrograde oxygenation of myocardium through the veins. The American Society for Artificial Organs (Asaio), 23rd Annual Meeting, Montreal Canada (Abstr)
3. Pakalska E, Gołab B (1980) Coronary circulation on the venous side in the human hearts with the special references to the venae cordis minimae. In: Reinis Z, Pokorny J, Linhart J (eds) Adaptability of Vascular Wall. Springer-Verlag, Berlin Heidelberg New York, pp 679–681
4. Ratajczyk-Pakalska E, Kolff WJ (1984) Anatomical Basis for the Coronary Venous Outflow Verlag. In: Mohl W, Wolner E, Glogar D (eds) The Coronary Sinus. Steinkopff-Verlag, Darmstadt, pp 40–46
5. Ratajczyk-Pakalska E, Kolff WJ (1981) Types of the smallest cardiac veins. Folia Morphol (Warsz) 15: 345–355
6. Ratajczyk-Pakalska E, Moll J, Edelman M, Chetkowska E (1974) Venous vascularization of the ventricular myocardium after ligation of the coronary arteries. Kard Pol 17: 133–141
7. Ratajczyk-Pakalska E, Wagiel J, Kamiński M, Kolff WJ (1984) Automated image analysis for measurement of area of the smallest cardiac veins in ventricular myocardium. In: Mohl W, Wolner E, Glogar D (eds) The Coronary Sinus. Steinkopff Verlag, Darmstadt, pp 33–39
8. Samojlowa SV (1970) Anatomy of the Cardiac Blood Vessels. Medicina, Leningrad

Author's address:
Associate Professor Ewa Ratajczyk-Pakalska, M.D.
Department of Normal Anatomy
Institute of Biology and Morphology
Medical Academy in Łódź
Narutowicza 60
90-136 Łódź
Poland

Congenital occlusion of the coronary sinus

A. Lechleuthner, and M. v. Lüdinghausen

Anatomische Anstalt der Universität München, Munich (West Germany)

Introduction

Congenital occlusion of the coronary sinus (C.S.) is a very rare malformation. It may be asymptomatic or symptomatic and can be combined with other cardiac failures. It was observed and published first by Marshall (5), Gruber (3) and Siding (6).

Description of the case

A 70 year old man showed cirrhosis of the liver and a few massive gastrointestinal bleedings. During dissection of gross anatomy course we noticed a persistent left superior cava vein (v. cava superior sinistra) (Fig. 1) and a large Thebesian valve (Valvula sinus coronarii) (Fig. 2), which was completely fixed in its surroundings. Besides this there was a remarkable collateral circulation by many ectatic left atrial veins between C.S. and right atrium (Fig. 3).

Discussion

Bankl (1) found congenital occlusion of the C.S. combined with:
A) Persistence of v. cava sinistra;
B) Abnormal communication from C.S. to left atrium (arterio-venous fistula);
C) Drainage of C.S. only by multiple Thebesian veins (vv. cardiacae minimae);
D) Persistence of left anterior cardinal vein.

Occlusion of the C.S. may be associated with other anomalies (2):
A) Transposition of great arteries;
B) Univentricular heart;
C) Ebstein's malformation of tricuspidal valve (valva tricuspidalis);
D) Partial anomalous pulmonary venous connection;

Other variations and malformations of the C.S. were classified by Mantini et al. (4):
A) Enlargement of the coronary sinus
    a) Without left-to-right shunt into the coronary sinus
        1. Persistent left superior vena cava;
        2. Partial anomalous hepatic venous connection to the C.S.;
        3. Continuity of inferior vena cava with left superior vena cava through hemiazygos vein;
    b) With left-to-right shunt into the coronary sinus
        1. Low pressure shunts: communication of coronary sinus with left atrium; pulmonary venous connection to the coronary sinus
        2. High pressure shunts: coronary artery-coronary sinus fistula.

147

B) Absence of coronary sinus
   a) Atrial septal defect localized to the position normally occupied by the coronary sinus;
   b) Atrial septal defect involving entire lowermost portion of septum;
      1. Persistent common atrioventricular canal;
      2. Asplenia with congenital cardiac disease.
C) Atresia of the right atrial coronary sinus with left atrium
   a) Persistent left superior vein;
   b) Gross communication of the coronary sinus with left atrium;
   c) Multiple communications between the coronary sinus and related atria.
D) Hypoplasia of the coronary sinus.

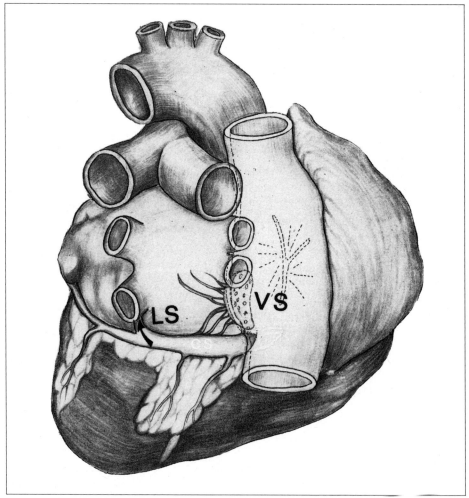

Fig. 1. Back view of described heart. LS = persistent left superior vena cava. CS = coronary sinus. VS = venous pot in the wall of the atrial septum, which receives ectatic veins from the left atrium.

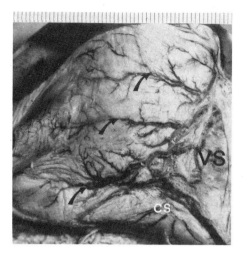

Fig. 2. Interior of the right atrium. Small arrows = foramina to the venous pot of the atrial septum. Large arrows = valvula Thebesii and closed coronary sinus. T = orifices of Thebesian veins, which drain to the right atrium.

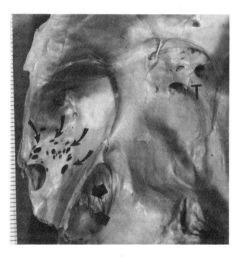

Fig. 3. VS = venous pot. CS = coronary sinus. Black arrows = left atrial veins and connection veins to the coronary sinus.

Conclusions

Congenital occlusion of the C.S. is associated with persistent left superior vena cava and therefore is to be mentioned as an individual developed malformation in combination with a persistence of embryonal structures for hemodynamic use. Nevertheless, important collateral circulation with atrial veins is noticed.

Acknowledgments

We thank Mrs. E. Mayer (Anatomische Anstalt der Universität München) and M. Spiess for excellent technical assistance.

149

References

1. Bankl H (1977) Congenital Malformations of the Heart and Great Vessels. Synopsis of Pathology, Embryology and Natural History. Urban & Schwarzenberg, Baltimore Munich
2. Gerlis LM, Gibbs JL, Williams GJ, Thomas GDH (1984) Coronary Sinus Orifice Atresia and Persistent Left Superior Vena Cava. Br Heart J 52: 648–653
3. Gruber W (1885) Duplicität der Vena cava superior (II. Fall eigener Beobachtung) bei Verschluß der Mündung der Vena cava superior sinistra in das Atrium dextrum und deren Auftreten als Abführungskanal der Herzvenen in die Vena anonyma sinistra (sicherer I. Fall). Archiv für pathologische Anatomie und Physiologie und für klinische Medicin 99: 492–497
4. Mantini E, Grondin CM, Lillehei CW, Edwards JE (1966) Congenital Anomalies Involving the Coronary Sinus. Circulation 33: 317–327
5. Marshall J (1850) On the Development of the Great Anterior Veins in Man and Mammalia; Including an Account of Certain Remnants of Foetal Structure Found in the Adult, a Comparative View of these Great Veins in different Mammalia, and an Analysis of their Occasional Peculiarities in the Human Subject. Philosophical Transactions of the Royal Society of London 141: 133–170
6. Siding A (1896) Über den Abschluß des Sinus coronarius gegen den rechten Vorhof. Anatomischer Anzeiger (Jena) 12s: 274–277

Authors' address:
Alex Lechleuthner
Anatomische Anstalt der Universität München
Pettenkoferstraße 11
8000 Munich 2
West Germany

Reduction of myocardial blood volume during regional ischemia

H. Korb, A. Hoeft, J. Böck, HG. Wolpers, and G. Hellige

Zentrum "Physiologie und Pathophysiologie" der Universität Göttingen
(West Germany)

Summary: This study was designed to estimate the effects of total and partial coronary artery occlusion on the transport characteristics and the intravascular blood volume of the coronary vascular system.

Experiments were carried out on anaesthetized mongrel dogs in open chest preparation. Measurements of coronary transport function were obtained by a transcoronary dye dilution technique.

Compared to control, no significant changes of the transport function were observed after total occlusion of the LAD artery, but intracoronary blood volume was markedly reduced. With partial occlusion, as well, the intravascular blood volume decreased significantly, but under these conditions the coronary transport function exhibited two separable compartments.

The observed reduction of coronary blood volume under total occlusion, as well as during regionally reduced coronary blood flow, leads to the question whether the therapeutic effects of PISCO could be explained on the basis of redistribution phenomena.

Introduction

A major disadvantage of conventional indicator dilution techniques lies in the fact that a quantitative analysis of perfusion inhomogeneities of the myocardium remains impossible due to recirculation of the tracer in the circulatory system. The problems involved in recirculation phenomena can be avoided by a simultaneous measurement of the concentration time courses of the indicator in front of and behind the organ and by a description of the passage of the indicator which is based on a stochastic analysis of the arterial and coronary venous indicator dilution curves (6). This analysis yields the coronary transport function which reflects, independent of the arterial concentration time course of the tracer, the distribution of the transit times of the indicator through the vascular bed of the myocardium (3). The technique provides qualitative and quantitative information on the distribution of the coronary perfusion and allows the calculation of the intracoronary blood volume assuming that myocardial blood flow is simultaneously measured.

The aim of this study was to clarify the question whether an evaluation of pathophysiological perfusion inhomogeneities of the myocardium can be achieved on the basis of the coronary transport function and intracoronary blood volume.

Methods

Methods are described in detail in (1) and (4).

Experiments were carried out in open chest mongrel dogs under piritramide anaesthesia and artificial respiration with nitrous oxide and oxygen. Coronary artery occlusion was induced by acute ligation of the LAD artery, coronary artery stenosis by a constrictor.

The coronary transport function and the intracoronary blood volume were determined by a dye dilution technique. After central venous bolus injections of indocyanine green the resulting aortic and coronary venous dye dilution curves were obtained by fiberoptic catheters and digitized on-line by a microcomputer. After completion of measurements data were stored on floppy disk, numerically deconvoluted and coronary blood flow computed by the same device (for theory and computations see (1)).

The intracoronary volume per 100 g of left ventricular weight (V_d) resulted from the product of coronary blood flow (MBF) and coronary mean transit time ($\bar{t}$) of the intravascular tracer indocyanine green: $V_d = MBF \cdot \bar{t}$.

For direct measurement of coronary blood flow a coronary sinus bypass system with an extracorporeal flow probe was installed (for details see (2) and (5)). At the end of the experiments the heart was arrested with potassium, excised and dried to constancy of weight. The ideal wet weight of the left ventricle was calculated with a dry / wet weight ratio of 0.21 and all directly measured flow values were converted to blood flow per 100 g left ventricular weight.

Results

Experiments were carried out in 6 mongrel dogs. In one group (n = 3) the LAD artery was occluded totally for 3 min (n = 14), in the other group low flow ischemia was produced by partial stenosis of the LAD artery (n = 15) with a constrictor.

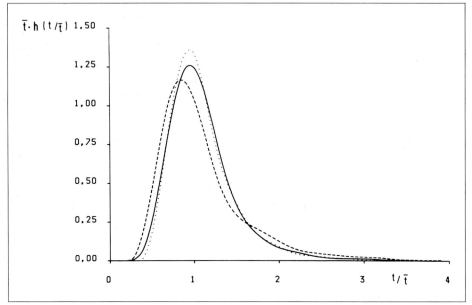

Fig. 1. Mean coronary transport functions under control conditions, during coronary artery occlusion and during coronary artery stenosis. For the analysis of the transport functions all individual curves obtained under control conditions (n = 25; ·····), during total occlusion (n = 14; —) and during partial stenosis (n = 15; ----) of the LAD artery were transformed on a normalized time axis ($t/\bar{t}$)) and mean values calculated ($\bar{t} \cdot h (t/\bar{t})$).

Figure 1 shows the mean coronary transport functions under control conditions, during coronary artery occlusion and during coronary artery stenosis. The mean coronary transport functions result from a normalization of the individual curves to the corresponding transit times. On the basis of these normalized curves with dimensionless abscissa, mean value curves can be formed which describe the transport behaviour of the coronary vasculature under the chosen experimental conditions, independent of the mean transit times, and therefore of myocardial blood flow and intracoronary blood volume.

Under total occlusion no significant changes can be observed when compared to control. On the other hand, coronary artery stenosis results in a marked skewness of the coronary transport function.

Figure 2 shows the corresponding values of the intracoronary blood volume given in relation to the coronary vascular resistance (W_{cor}). Under control conditions, a decrease of W_{cor} is accompanied by a marked increase of intracoronary blood volume. The mean value is 11.2 ± 1.5 ml/100 g tissue at a mean W_{cor} of 1.4 ± 0.36 mm Hg $\cdot$ min $\cdot$ 100 g/ml. During coronary artery occlusion the intracoronary blood volume decreases to 10.1 ± 0.8 ml/100 g, during coronary artery stenosis to 9.2 ± 1.1 ml/100 g tissue.

It is of decisive importance that with respect to coronary vascular resistance all values for intracoronary blood volume differ significantly from the corresponding values under control conditions.

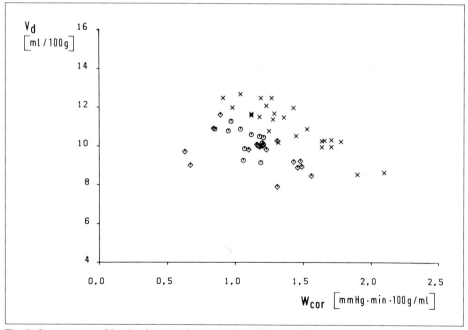

Fig. 2. Intracoronary blood volume under control conditions, during coronary artery occlusion and during coronary artery stenosis. Measurement of coronary vascular resistance (W_{cor}; mmHG $\cdot$ min $\cdot$ 100 g/ml) and of intracoronary blood volume (V_d; ml/100 g tissue) under control conditions (n = 25; x), during total occlusion (n = 14; □) and during partial stenosis (n = 15; ○) of the LAD artery. Compared to control, the intracoronary blood volume is significantly reduced during coronary artery occlusion and stenosis.

Discussion

A regional reduction of myocardial perfusion induced by occlusion or stenosis is accompanied in both cases by a decrease of total intracoronary blood volume but with different effects on the coronary transport function.

Low flow ischemia after coronary artery stenosis leads to a marked increase of the skewness of the coronary transport function. This form of myocardial perfusion inhomogeneity is characterized by the existence of two separable perfusion compartments which can be clearly demonstrated by a compartmental analysis of the curve (data not shown). It is remarkable that under these circumstances the intracoronary blood volume is significantly reduced. Compared to total occlusion, this reduction cannot be explained by a lack of indicator passage through the afflicted area (see below). Obviously, this suggests a reduction of intravasal blood volume in the sense of a decrease of the cross-section of the vascular bed. This phenomenon might be explainable by the post-stenotic fall of blood pressure. The stenosis causes a reduction of arterial driving pressure in the underperfused area resulting in smaller transmural pressure gradients which lead to a decrease of the vessels' diameter at a given vascular tone. Another possible explanation would be the systolic increase of the intramyocardial pressure which could cause a successive "pump-out" phenomenon of the vascular bed, whenever blood inflow is impeded during diastole. In this case, mainly the coronary venous part of the intramyocardially located vessels should be afflicted.

Compared to control, the coronary transport function remains unchanged after total occlusion of the LAD artery. This result can be explained by the fact that the perfusion area of the ligated artery cannot be reached by the indicator and therefore, the ischemic zone becomes "invisible" to the indicator dilution technique. Such a lack of indicator passage would also be compatible with the reduction in observed intracoronary blood volume. Primarily, acute occlusion will lead to a decrease of myocardial blood flow but the mean transit time of the indicator through the non-ischemic myocardium will remain unchanged. Mathematically this situation should result in a reduction of the distribution volume of the tracer whereby the percentual decrease of the intracoronary blood volume should be as great as the percentual portion of the perfusion volume of the left ventricle. However, intracoronary blood volume was reduced to a lesser degree as expected from the size of the ischemic zone which was determined in the same experimental set-up by intravital staining of the perfusion area of the ligated artery with Evans-blue (2, 5). This could be attributed to collateral flow but, with respect to the results with coronary stenosis, another explanation for this discrepancy seems to be possible. The reduction of intracoronary blood volume could be attributed in part to a lack of indicator passage, in part to a decrease of the intravascular blood volume in the ischemic area due to the above mentioned "pump-out" phenomenon.

Our results clearly show a reduction of intracoronary blood volume during coronary artery occlusion and stenosis. With respect to possible underlying causes, i.e. loss of transmural pressure gradients or systolic "pump-out" phenomenon of the coronary vessels during impeded diastolic blood inflow, it would be conceivable that therapeutic interventions which can increase the coronary venous "back pressure", i.e. PISCO, could be of protective value under these circumstances. These interventions could counteract an emptying of the coronary venous vascular bed and could even lead to a retrograde refilling of the vessels in the ischemic zone.

154

References

1. Hoeft A, Korb H, Wolpers HG, Hellige G (1984) Determination of myocardial blood flow with transcoronary dye dilution. In: Mohl W, Wolner E, Glogar E (eds) The Coronary Sinus. Steinkopff Verlag, Darmstadt, pp 106–112
2. Hoeft A, Korb H, Baller D, Wolpers HG, Hellige G, Bretschneider HJ (1984) Quantification of ischemic stress during repeated coronary artery occlusion in the dog. A method for validation of therapeutic effects. I. Estimation of O_2-debt and O_2-repayment. Basic Res Cardiol 79: 27–37
3. Knopp TJ, Dobbs WA, Greenleaf JF, Bassingthwaighte JB (1976) Transcoronary intravascular transport functions obtained via a stable deconvolution technique. Ann Biomed Eng 4: 44–59
4. Korb H, Hoeft A, Hellige G (1984) Measurements of coronary mean transit time and myocardial tissue blood flow by deconvolution of intravasal tracer dilution curves. SPIE Novel Optical Fiber Techniques for Medical Applications 494: 36–41
5. Korb H, Hoeft A, Baller D, Wolpers HG, Hellige G, Bretschneider HJ (1984) Quantification of ischemic stress during repeated coronary artery occlusion in the dog. A method for validation of therapeutic effects. II. Reproducibility of the release and uptake of electrolytes and substrates. Basic Res Cardiol 79: 38–48
6. Lassen NA (1979) Tracer kinetic methods in medical physiology. Raven Press, New York

Authors' address:
Harald Korb, M.D.
Zentrum „Physiologie und Pathophysiologie" der Universität Göttingen
Humboldtallee 23
3400 Göttingen
West Germany

155

Retrograde myocardial protection during surgery

Ultrastructural differences in intraoperative myocardial protection using cardioplegic solutions in antegrade or retrograde perfusion

P. Kirchner, J. Schaper, and P. Walter*

Max-Planck-Institute, Department of Experimental Cardiology, Bad Nauheim (West Germany); * Department of Cardiac Surgery, University Hospital Antwerp (Belgium)

Intraoperative cardiac arrest as induced with cardioplegic solutions produces ischemic injury of the myocardium. Different types of solutions, in combination with topical cooling of the heart and whole body hypothermia of approximately 28 °C, are in use to minimize the extent of ischemic injury. Electron microscopy is well suited to evaluate the quality of myocardial protection, since it allows for an analysis of ischemic injury of all myocardial ultrastructural components.

The evaluation process is the same for all forms of cardioplegia analysed: myocardial tissue biopsies taken intraoperatively are prepared for electron microscopy and the ultrastructural state is documented by a representative series of micrographs. Using a well standardized semiquantitative evaluation system described in detail in earlier publications (6, 7), the degree of ischemic injury of any given biopsy is determined. Besides being of normal ultrastructural appearance, myocardial tissue can suffer slight, moderate, and severe ischemic injury – these 3 forms being of reversible nature – and irreversible ischemic injury. Figure 1 shows the appearance of normal myocardium, Figures 2, 3, and 4 show slight, moderate, and severe ischemic injury, respectively.

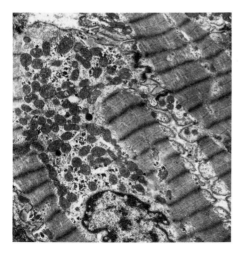

Fig. 1. Normal nonischemic myocardium. Note numerous mitochondria containing an electron dense matrix and numerous cristae. Magn. X 4 050

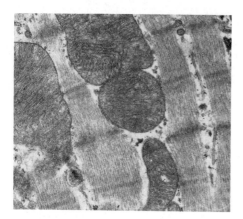

Fig. 2. Slight ischemic injury. The dark matrix granules – characteristic for normal nonischemic myocardium – have disappeared. Magn. X 30 000.

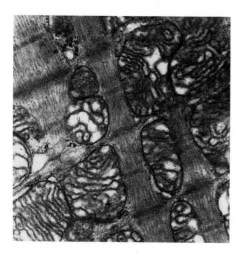

Fig. 3. Moderate ischemic injury. Mitochondrial matrix shows clearing and a decrease in the amount as well as fragmentation of the cristae. Magn. X 24 000.

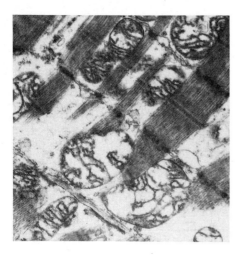

Fig. 4. Severe ischemic injury. The figure shows extreme clearing of the mitochondrial matrix and extensive destruction of cristae. Magn. X 30 000.

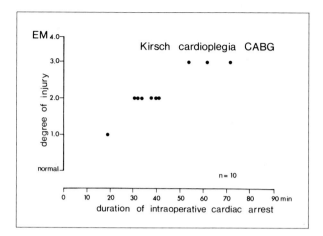

Fig. 5. Degree of ischemic injury and duration of intraoperative ischemic injury during coronary artery bypass graft surgery using Kirsch cardioplegia.

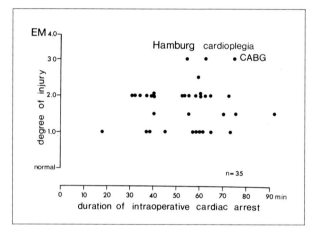

Fig. 6. Degree of ischemic injury and duration of intraoperative ischemic injury during coronary artery bypass graft surgery using Hamburg cardioplegia.

The methods described beforehand are used to analyse the qualities of myocardial protection offered by different forms of cardioplegia.

As an example, Figures 5 and 6 show the effects of 2 different types of cardioplegia on the degree of ischemic injury.

The abscissa shows the duration of ischemia as induced by cardiac arrest during coronary artery bypass graft surgery, the ordinate the degree of ischemic injury as indicated by a score (0 = normal, 1 = slight, 2 = moderate, 3 = severe, 4 = irreversible ischemic injury). Each biopsy from a particular patient is represented by a dot. Figure 5 shows the results of the use of Kirsch cardioplegia: a clear correlation exists between the degree of ischemic injury and the duration of the ischemic interval. Figure 6 demonstrates the effects of cardioplegia with Hamburg solution. The time dependent deterioration of myocardial ultrastructure is far less pronounced. Following the beginning of ischemia severe ischemic injury occurs as early as after 55 min and as late as 75 min. Most ischemic injury is, however, of slight to moderate nature, even after as much as 90 min of ischemia. Similar observations were made with St. Thomas or Bretschneider cardioplegia (8). Irreversible ischemic injury was never observed.

It is obvious, however, that even though the quality of myocardial protection can be improved by use of a different solution (Kirsch cardioplegia being less protective than the others), improvements are still desirable since the occurrence of ischemic damage cannot be entirely prevented, i.e. some degree of damage always occurs.

As a potential method of improvement, the application of cardioplegic solution in a retrograde perfusion via the coronary sinus instead of antegrade perfusion via the aorta was evaluated. Favorable effects of retrograde coronary perfusion in global ischemia during open-heart surgery have been described previously by several authors (2, 4, 9).

In a study involving 48 patients undergoing coronary artery bypass graft surgery, 28 received Bretschneider cardioplegia in an antegrade perfusion. In 14 patients cardiac arrest was induced by antegrade perfusion of Bretschneider cardioplegia but then continued by retrograde perfusion via the coronary sinus.

Table 1 shows the 2 groups of patients and the method of application of cardioplegia as well as the number of bypasses, duration of the ischemic interval, the volumes of solution used, the perfusion pressure and the duration of perfusion.

Figure 7 shows the results of the 2 groups. Again ischemic injury is depicted against duration of ischemia. It is clearly visible that the degree of ischemic injury suffered by the myocardium is significantly less severe when cardioplegia is administered via the coronary sinus.

These positive findings of protection of the myocytes from ischemic damage are, however, upset by the observation of damage in the vascular endothelium and the occurrence of extracellular edema. These changes are to be seen only in patients who have undergone retrograde perfusion and are documented in Figures 8 and 9. Figure 8 shows extracellular edema as well as thinned and swollen endothelium, and Figure 9 shows damaged vascular endothelium with swollen endothelium and disappearance of pinocytotic vesicles.

The reason for these adverse effects of retrograde perfusion of a cardioplegic solution are not entirely understood. Commonly used crystalline cardioplegic solutions lack a colloid-osmotic carrier. This could be one reason since experimental perfusion of isolated hearts with an aqueous solution for prolonged periods of time has been described to cause these hearts to become edematous (1, 3, 5).

Table 1. Retrograde coronary perfusion using Bretschneider's solution. Different patient groups and methods involved in this study.

Group I n = 28 antegrade		Group II n = 14 retrograde
2.7	n bypass	2.6
58	ischemic interval (min)	55
2000	solution volume (ml)	2000 +2160 (1300–3600)
100 40–50	hydrostatic pressure (mmHg)	30–40
8–1	perfusion duration (min)	48–82

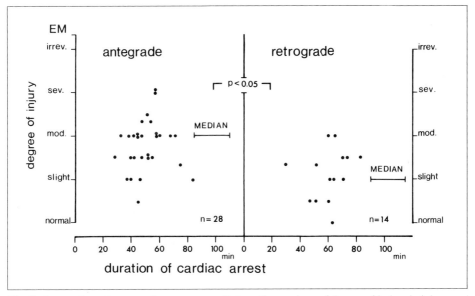

Fig. 7. Antegrade and retrograde coronary perfusion. Comparison of degree of ischemic injury and duration of cardiac arrest in both groups of patients.

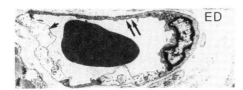

Fig. 8. Damaged blood vessel containing an erythrocyte. Note swollen (←) as well as thinned (↑↑) endothelium and extracellular edema (ED). Magn. X 7 900.

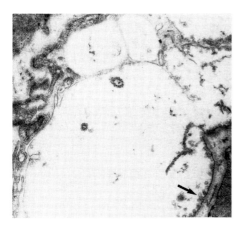

Fig. 9. Damaged vascular endothelium showing extreme swelling and rarification of pinocytotic vesicles some of which are seen at tip of arrow. Magn. X 19 500.

Also, edema of the vascular endothelium and the extracellular space could be caused by the perfusion pressure of 30 mm Hg used for retrograde perfusion – a pressure which is unusually high for venules or capillaries.

In conclusion it can be said that retrograde perfusion of a cardioplegic solution via the coronary sinus has clear advantages over antegrade perfusion via the aorta when considering myocardial protection against ischemic damage during induced cardiac arrest in open heart surgery. However, damage of the vascular endothelium and the occurrence of extracellular edema represent serious drawbacks of this method which, therefore, requires further improvement.

References

1. Bünger R, Haddy FJ, Querengasser A, Gerlach E (1975) An isolated guinea pig heart preparation with in vivo like features. Pflügers Arch 353: 317–326
2. Fabiani JN, Relland J, Carpentier A (1984) Myocardial protection via the coronary sinus in cardiac surgery: Comparative evaluation of two techniques. In: Mohl W, Wolner E, Glogar D (eds), The Coronary Sinus. Steinkopff Verlag, Darmstadt, pp 305–311
3. Fallen, EL, Elliott WC, Gorlin R (1967) Apparatus for study of ventricular function and metabolism in the isolated perfused rat heart. J Appl Physiol 22: 836–839
4. Gundry SR (1982) Modification of myocardial ischemia in normal and hypertrophied hearts utilizing diastolic retroperfusion of the coronary veins. J Thorac Cardiovasc Surg 83: 659–669
5. Ono Y, Schraven E, Gruber C, Schaper J (1979) Extracellular edema and homogeneity of tissue perfusion in the isolated working rat heart. J Mol Cell Cardiol 11 (Suppl 2): 43
6. Schaper J, Mulch J, Winkler B, Schaper W (1979) Ultrastructural, functional, and biochemical criteria for estimation of reversibility of ischemic injury: A study on the effects of global ischemia on the isolated dog heart. J Mol Cell Cardiol 11: 521–541
7. Schaper J (1979) Ultrastructure of the myocardium in acute ischemia. In: Schaper W (ed) The Pathophysiology of Myocardial Perfusion. Elsevier/North-Holland Biochemical Press, Amsterdam New York Oxford, pp 581–673
8. Schaper J, Scheld HH, Schmidt U, Hehrlein F: Ultrastructural study comparing the efficacy of five different methods of myocardial intraoperative protection in the human heart. J Thorac Cardiovasc Surg, in press
9. Solorzano J, Taitelbaum G, Chiu R (1978) Retrograde coronary sinus perfusion for myocardial protection during cardiopulmonary bypass. Am Thorac Surg 25: 201–211

Authors' address:
P. Kirchner
Max-Planck-Institute
Department of Experimental Cardiology
Benekestraße 2
D-6350 Bad Nauheim
West Germany

Effects of reperfusion on global versus regional ischemia

H. L. Lazar*, H. M. Spotnitz+, and A. J. Roberts*

* Department of Cardiothoracic Surgery, Boston University Medical Center, and
+ Division of Chest Surgery, College of Physicians and Surgeons, Columbia
University New York, N.Y. (U.S.A.)

The development of percutaneous transluminal angioplasty and the introduction of fibrinolytic agents into clinical practice has renewed interest in the reperfusion of
acutely ischemic myocardium. Unfortunately, previous methods for assessing left ventricular (LV) volume, mass, and shape have limited the clinician's ability to accurately determine the effects of reperfusion following regional and global ischemia. The development of two-dimensional echocardiography allows the clinician to measure changes in
LV compliance and mass following ischemia and avoids the manipulation and distortion
of the ventricle inherent in other methods. Accordingly, this study was undertaken to define the changes in LV mass and volume during periods of regional ischemia, and following reperfusion of regional and global ischemia using two dimensional echocardiography.

Methods

Preparation

Twenty-two adult mongrel dogs (18–25 kg) were anesthesized with intravenous
sodium pentobarbital (30 mg/kg) and placed on cardiopulmonary bypass (CPB)
with drainage catheters in the left atrium and right ventricle. A piezo-electric
Mikro-tip catheter pressure transducer (Millar Products, Houston, Texas) was inserted
through a stab wound in the LV apex to measure LV end-diastolic pressure (LVEDP).
Systemic arterial pressure was recorded with a fluid-filled left femoral arterial catheter.
Arterial blood gases and hematocrit were monitored and regulated so that acidosis (average pH 7.40 ± 0.04) and excessive hemodilution (Hct 26–33%) were avoided.

Measurements

Two-dimensional echocardiographic images were obtained using a hand-held 3.5 mH$_z$
ultrasound transducer and a V-3000 ultrasonograph (Varian Associates, Palo Alto, California). LV end-diastolic volume (EDV) was obtained by videotape recording of two per-
pendicular long axis sections and a short axis section. Echocardiographic sections
of LVEDV were recorded at stable levels of LVEDP (0–15 mm Hg). LV volume analysis
was performed on videotaped images using the Varian Microprocessor light pen system
and a Simpson's Rule Algorithm. LVEDV was plotted against LVEDP and data were an-

alyzed by exponential curve fitting to the relation $EDP = \alpha\beta EDV$ where α and β are derived constants. The same sections used to measure LVEDV were also used to measure LV mass by the equation LV mass = (epicardial volume − endocardial volume) × 1.050, where endocardial volume = LVEDV, epicardial volume = total volume contained by the epicardial boundary, and 1.050 represents the specific gravity of myocardium. Changes in LV shape were assessed from alterations in the eccentricity of the endocardial volume, and were derived from plenimetered long and short axis sections at equal end-diastolic volumes.

Protocol

To assess changes following *global ischemia,* 10 dogs were subjected to a 45 minute period of normothermic ischemic arrest followed by 45 minutes of reperfusion on CPB. Echo sections were obtained prior to arrest and following the period of reperfusion. Changes in regional ischemia were studied in another group of 12 dogs. Following control echo measurements, the left anterior descending coronary artery (LAD) was occluded with a snare for 45 minutes during which time echo measurements were repeated. Following this period of ischemia, the LAD occlusion was released and hearts received a 45 minute period of reperfusion on CPB after which final echo measurements were made. Statistical analysis was performed using an analysis of variance. A p value < 0.05 was considered significant.

Results

Global ischemia

The results following global ischemia are summarized in Table 1. There was a marked shift of the pressure-volume curve to the left accompanied by a significant increase in the ventricular stiffness constant (B) from 0.02 ± 0.01 to 0.05 ± 0.01 (p < 0.02). Calculated LV mass increased significantly from 105 ± 7 g to 128 ± 9 g (p < 0.001) in the postischemic period. Analysis of LV shape derived from echo sections at matched LVEDV revealed no significant effect of ischemic injury in the long axis: short axis ratio (L1/L2 = 1.43 ± 0.05 preischemia vs. 1.46 ± 0.06 postischemic; NS). In summary, global isch-

Table 1. LV mass, exponential constants, and ventricular shape following regional ischemia.

	Preischemia	Postischemia	P value
LV Mass (g)	105 ± 7	128 ± 9	p < 0.001
α	0.61 ± 0.06	0.49 ± 0.11	NS
β	0.020 ± 0.01	0.050 ± 0.01	p < 0.02
L1/L2	1.43 ± 0.05	1.46 ± 0.06	NS

Note: All values are mean $\pm$ SEM; α, β are exponential constants. L1/L2 = long axis; shor axis rati derived from echo sections.

emia resulted in a stiff, less compliant ventricle without any significant change in ventricular shape.

Regional ischemia

The results during and following regional ischemia are summarized in Table 2. The ischemic period was characterized by a small but significant decrease in LV mass (95 ± 5 vs. 85 ± 4 g p < 0.05), and a slight shift in the pressure-volume curve upward and to the right. However, there was no statistical difference in either then α or β constants. The calculated long axis : short axis ratio (L1/L2) decreased (1.61 ± 0.04 vs. 1.36 ± 0.03 p < 0.05), and the ratio of endocardial circumference (AL1/AL2) increased (1.04 ± 0.007 vs.

Table 2. LV mass, exponential constants, and ventricular shape following regional ischemia.

	Preischemia	Ischemia	Postischemia
LV Mass (g)	95±5	85±4*	104±5+*
β	0.036±0.004	0.053±0.010	0.074±0.010*
α	0.408±0.05	0.430±0.08	0.440±0.09
AL1/AL2	1.04 ±0.007	1.07 ±0.010*	1.05 ±0.008
L1/L2	1.61 ±0.04	1.36 ±0.03*	1.39 ±0.08*

Note: All values are mean ± SEM. * p < 0.05 from preischemia; + p < 0.05 from ischemia; α, β are exponential constants. AL1/AL2 = ratio of endocardial circumference; L1/L2 = long axis – short axis ratio.

1.07 ± 0.010 p < 0.05). The decrease in LV mass and changes in L1/L2 and AL1/AL2 ratios were reflected in the long axis echo sections which showed thinning of the septal wall and the appearance of a bulge. Upon reperfusion, LV mass increased significantly above preischemic and ischemic levels (Table 2) and the pressure-volume curve shifted to the left. There was a significant increase in the B constant from control (0.036 ± 0.004 vs. 0.074 ± 0.010 p < 0.05). The L1/L2 ratio remained unchanged from ischemia, but was still decreased from preischemic levels (1.61 ± 0.04 vs. 1.39 ± 0.03 p < 0.05) while the AL1/AL2 ratio returned toward control (1.04 ± 0.007 vs. 1.05 ± 0.008 NS). These changes were reflected in the postischemic echo sections which showed a thicker septal wall, smaller end-diastolic volumes at matched LVEDP, and loss of the "bulge" effect.

Discussion

The development of two-dimensional echocardiography has allowed the clinician to assess changes in ventricular volume, mass and shape without manipulation or distortion of the ventricle. Using this technique, this study shows that regional and global ischemia may have different effects on LV compliance, mass, and shape. Following global normothermic ischemia, there was an increase in LV mass, an increase in wall stiffness (β), and a shift in the pressure-volume curve to the left. The echo sections showed that the

167

LV wall was thicker, the end-diastolic volume was smaller at matched LVEDP, and there was no change in ventricular shape. In contrast, during periods of regional ischemia, LV mass actually decreased and the pressure volume curve shifted to the right. Echo sections showed that LVEDV was increased at matched LVEDP and that the shape of the ventricle was altered because of aneurysmal "bulging" of the thinned septum. Upon reperfusion, mass increased and the pressure-volume curve shifted to the left with an increase in wall stiffness (β). The echo sections now showed the characteristic changes seen following global ischemia; increased wall thickness, decreased end-diastolic volume with no change in LV shape.

A possible explanation for the observed increase in end-diastolic volume and the shift of the pressure-volume curve to the right during ischemia may be the development of "stress relaxation" (1). This term refers to a decrease in stress or force that occurs over a period of time when a constant stretch is applied to the muscle. After coronary occlusion, the ischemic muscle becomes non-contractile and is subjected to repeated stretch during systole. This ultimately results in "creep" which implies a permanent deformation of the muscle fibers due to changes and rearrangements of viscus and elastic elements. These changes may be responsible for the aneurysmal bulging and the changes seen in ventricular shape during the ischemic period. The decrease in LV mass and thinning of the septum during ischemia may be explained by the decrease in blood flow beyond the occlusion (3). The changes in mass and compliance seen following reperfusion of both global and regional ischemia probably reflect the development of myocardial edema and ischemic contracture (2).

We conclude that global and regional ischemia have different effects on LV mass, compliance and shape. These changes may help the clinician to better understand and interpret the effects of reperfusion following periods of global and regional ischemia.

References

1. Grossman W, McLaurin LP (1984) Diastolic properties of the left ventricle. Ann Int Med 84: 316–326
2. Jennings RB, Ganote CE (1974) Structural changes in myocardium during acute ischemia. Circ Res 34, 35 (Suppl 3): 156–172
3. Kerber RE, Martins JB, Marcus ML (1979) Effect of acute ischemia, nitroglycerin and nitroprusside on regional myocardial thickening, stress and perfusion. Circ 60: 121–129

Authors' address:
Harold L. Lazar, M.D.
Department of Cardiothoracic Surgery
Boston University Medical Center
Boston, MA 02118
U.S.A.

Improving myocardial metabolism and ventricular function following cardioplegia and reperfusion*

R. D. Weisel, K. H. Teoh, J. C. Mullen, G. T. Christakis, S. E. Fremes,
M. M. Madonik, J. Ivanov, P. R. McLaughlin, and D. A. G. Mickle

Divisions of Cardiovascular Surgery, Nuclear Cardiology and Clinical Biochemistry, University of Toronto, Toronto General Hospital, Toronto, Ontario (Canada)

Summary: Current methods of myocardial protection for cardiac surgery may result in delayed myocardial metabolic recovery and incomplete recovery of right ventricular function. Perioperative coronary sinus interventions may reverse these defects.

In our studies blood cardioplegia provided better myocardial protection for elective coronary bypass surgery than crystalloid cardioplegia. However, myocardial adenosine triphosphate concentrations fell after cardioplegia and again after reperfusion in both groups. In addition, myocardial oxygen consumption and lactate utilization recovered slowly postoperatively. The etiology of the defective postoperative myocardial metabolism remains obscure. Cardiac platelet and leukocyte deposition may induce heterogeneous cardiac perfusion. Intermittent coronary sinus occlusion may permit more homogeneous reperfusion following cardioplegic arrest.

Although blood cardioplegia produced better left ventricular function after elective coronary bypass surgery, right ventricular function was better after crystalloid cardioplegia. Blood cardioplegia resulted in warmer right atrial and right ventricular temperatures, persistent right atrial activity, and a fall in right ventricular high energy phosphates which may have induced postoperative right ventricular dysfunction. Right atrial retrograde coronary sinus cardioplegia may provide better right ventricular protection. Coronary sinus interventions may have a beneficial impact on the results of cardiac surgery.

Introduction

Current methods of myocardial protection provide excellent results for elective cardiac surgery. Patients who require urgent revascularization because of unstable angina and those with poor ventricular function requiring combined coronary bypass and valvular heart surgery face an increased risk of surgery. Improved methods of perioperative myocardial protection may improve the results in high risk patients.

We found that myocardial metabolic recovery was delayed after elective coronary bypass surgery despite apparently adequate protection. Delayed myocardial metabolic recovery may account for the increased risk in patients undergoing urgent revascularization. The etiology of the myocardial metabolic derangements after cardioplegia remain obscure. Coronary sinus interventions may improve metabolic recovery in patients undergoing elective surgery and may reduce the risks of cardiac surgery for those who require urgent revascularization.

* Supported by the Heart and Stroke Foundation of Ontario and the Canadian Heart Foundation

Current methods of cardioplegic delivery adequately protect the left ventricle but may not adequately protect the right ventricle or the right atrium. Coronary sinus interventions may improve right ventricular function in patients undergoing elective surgery and reduce the risks of surgery in patients with ventricular dysfunction who require combined coronary and valvular procedures.

Delayed myocardial metabolic recovery

We have previously demonstrated that blood cardioplegia provided better myocardial protection for elective coronary bypass surgery than crystalloid cardioplegia (3). Blood cardioplegia reduced postoperative CK-MB release and improved postoperative left ventricular function. In addition, blood cardioplegia improved myocardial metabolic recovery. Figure 1 demonstrates that myocardial adenosine triphosphate (ATP) concentrations were higher after blood than crystalloid cardioplegia. However, the figure also demonstrates that ATP concentrations decreased during cardioplegia administration and again during the first 30 minutes of reperfusion following both blood and crystalloid cardioplegia. We also found that myocardial oxygen consumption and lactate utilization increased slowly after both blood and crystalloid cardioplegia. A recent study using carbon-14 labelled substrates (palmatate and lactate) confirmed the depression in myocardial oxidative metabolism during reperfusion after apparently adequate cardioplegic protection with both blood and crystalloid cardioplegia.

The etiology of the delayed recovery of myocardial metabolism following elective surgery remains obscure. We have previously demonstrated that platelets and leukocytes were de-

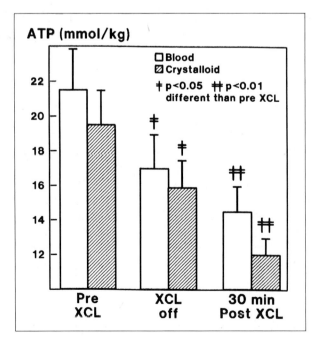

Fig. 1. Myocardial adenosine triphosphate (ATP) concentrations were measured on bypass prior to the application of the crossclamp (XCL), immediately following crossclamp removal and 30 minutes after crossclamp removal in 60 patients undergoing elective coronary bypass surgery (3). Twenty-eight patients were randomized to receive blood cardioplegia and 32 to receive crystalloid cardioplegia. ATP concentrations fell in both groups despite apparently adequate myocardial protection suggestive of inadequate metabolic recovery.

posited in the myocardium during reperfusion after elective surgery (10). We found that the heart released prostacyclin (6 keto $PGF_{1\alpha}$) for approximately 30 minutes following crossclamp release. Cardiac endothelial prostacyclin may have been stimulated by cardioplegia and ceased after reperfusion. The myocardial release of thromboxanes ($Tx B_2$) persisted for 3 hours after crossclamp release. Platelet and leukocyte deposition and the release of vasoconstrictive substances may induce heterogeneous perfusion despite adequate revascularization in the first few hours after coronary bypass surgery. Intermittent coronary sinus occlusion may permit homogeneous reperfusion after cardioplegia and permit immediate myocardial metabolic recovery.

Delayed metabolic recovery may be due to a defect in postoperative mitochondrial function following ischemia or cardioplegia (4, 5). The defect may result from inadequate Krebs cycle intermediates. Buckberg and colleagues have suggested that the addition of glutamate and aspartate to a warm terminal cardioplegic infusion may restore Krebs cycle intermediates after ischemia and cardioplegia and permit rapid recovery of mitochondrial function (8). Postoperative mitochondrial dysfunction may result from inadequate substrate availability. Increasing substrate concentrations may improve oxidative metabolism during reperfusion. Finally, the restoration of ATP following ischemia or cardioplegia may be limited by the availability of diffusable intermediates. Ribose has been demonstrated to improve ATP preservation during ischemia (7). Each of these interventions are being investigated and may permit more rapid recovery of myocardial metabolism after cardioplegic arrest.

Patients undergoing elective coronary bypass surgery have excellent results. However, improved techniques of myocardial preservation for elective surgery may reduce the risks of patients who require urgent surgery. In a recent study, we compared blood to crystalloid cardioplegia in patients undergoing urgent revascularization (1). We found that blood

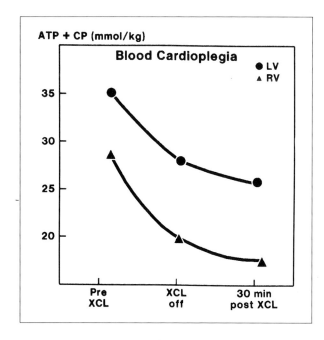

Fig. 2. High energy phosphate concentrations (the sum of adenosine triphosphate, ATP and creatine phosphate, CP) were found to be lower in the right ventricle (RV) than the left ventricle (LV) before the application of the crossclamp (XCL), immediately following crossclamp removal, and 30 minutes after crossclamp removal in 28 patients undergoing elective coronary bypass surgery with blood cardioplegia. In addition, right ventricular high energy phosphate concentrations decreased more during cardioplegic arrest and reperfusion than left ventricular concentrations.

cardioplegia reduced CK-MB enzyme release, ECG abnormalities, postoperative ventricular dysfunction and mortality. Patients who require urgent surgery for unstable angina have inadequate myocardial metabolic reserve prior to revascularization. Better methods of preparation or preservation may improve their results.

Postoperative right ventricular dysfunction

Current methods of cardioplegic delivery provide excellent protection for the left ventricle but inadequate protection for the right ventricle. We have recently demonstrated that warmer right atrial and right ventricular temperatures were found in patients who received blood cardioplegia compared to those who received crystalloid cardioplegia (6). Postoperative left ventricular function was better after blood cardioplegia, but right ventricular systolic function was better after crystalloid cardioplegia. Figure 2 demonstrates results of myocardial biopsies taken from the right and left ventricles after elective revascularization with blood cardioplegia.

The biopsies demonstrated that high energy phosphates (the sum of the adenosine triphosphate and creatine phosphate measurements) were higher in the left than the right ventricle and the fall in high energy phosphates was significantly greater in the right ventricle. Therefore, both right ventricular function and metabolism were incompletely protected with current methods of blood cardioplegic delivery.

We have recently investigated right atrial retrograde cardioplegic delivery (Figure 3). The technique was originally described by Fabiani and colleagues (2). We have modified their technique somewhat. We employed double caval cannulation and crossclamped both the aorta and pulmonary artery as described by the group from Paris. However, we gave cardioplegia antegrade for warm induction, an initial cold infusion and a terminal warm infusion (hot shot). We employed right atrial retrograde cardioplegia to maintain the cold temperatures of both the left and right ventricles. During retrograde cardioplegia, we

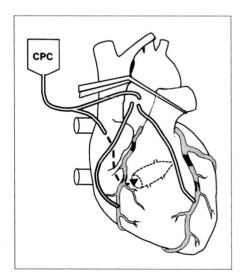

Fig. 3. The technique of right atrial retrograde cardioplegia is demonstrated in a patient undergoing double coronary bypass grafting. Double caval cannulation was employed and both the aorta and pulmonary artery were crossclamped. Cardioplegia was administered antegrade for induction. Cardioplegia was then administered into the right atrium and a pressure between 10 and 20 mm Hg to sustain the arrest.

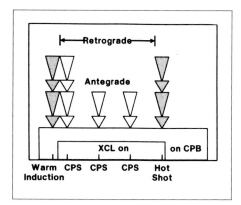

Fig. 4. The protocol for the comparison between antegrade and retrograde blood cardioplegic delivery is illustrated. In both groups, cardioplegia was delivered antegrade first for a warm induction and then cold blood was infused. A terminal warm infusion was employed prior to crossclamp release (hot shot). In the antegrade group intermittent doses of cold blood cardioplegia were employed following each bypass graft. In the retrograde group, right atrial retrograde blood cardioplegia was infused continuously during construction of coronary bypass grafts.

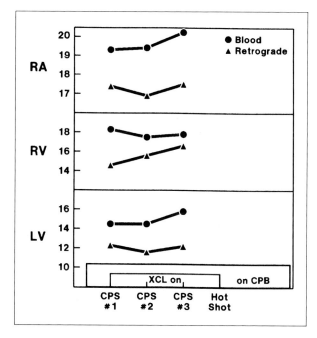

Fig. 5. The preliminary results of the comparison between antegrade and right atrial retrograde blood cardioplegia are illustrated. Systemic temperatures were lower (20 °C) in those who received retrograde cardioplegia than those who received antegrade blood cardioplegia (25 °C). Right atrial (RA), right ventricular (RV) and left (LV) temperatures were lower with retrograde delivery. Right atrial and left ventricular temperatures remained lower during cardioplegic administration with retrograde cardioplegia. The right ventricular temperature tended to be lower with retrograde cardioplegia.

monitored right atrial pressure which was maintained between 10–20 mm Hg. We vented the cardioplegic solution from the ascending aorta. Figure 4 demonstrates the protocol we have employed to compare antegrade and retrograde blood cardioplegia. A warm induction was followed by a cold blood cardioplegic infusion to induce cardiac arrest in both groups. With the antegrade delivery, infusions of cold blood cardioplegia were given intermittently during the crossclamp period. A terminal warm blood cardioplegic infusion was employed prior to crossclamp release in both groups as previously described (9). Our initial results are shown in Figure 5. Right atrial retrograde cardioplegia resulted in significantly colder right atrial and right ventricular temperatures during cardioplegic delivery. This technique may improve right ventricular preservation and improve right ventricular metabolic and hemodynamic recovery.

Coronary sinus interventions may reduce postoperative complications in patients at high risk of perioperative ischemic injury.

References

1. Christakis GT, Fremes SE, Weisel RD, Tittley JG, McDonough JH, Mickle DAG, Madonik MM, Ivanov J, Mickleborough LL, Goldman BS, Baird RJ (1986) Reducing the risk of urgent revascularization for unstable angina: a randomized clinical trial. J Vasc Surg (in press)
2. Fabiani JN, Relland J, Carpentier A (1984) Myocardial protection via the coronary sinus in cardiac surgery: Comparative evaluation of two techniques. In: Mohl W, Wolner E, Glogar D (eds) The Coronary Sinus. Steinkopff Verlag, Darmstadt, pp 305–311
3. Fremes SE, Christakis GT, Weisel RD, Mickle DAG, Madonik MM, Ivanov J, Harding R, Seawright SJ, Houle S, McLaughlin PR, Baird RJ (1984) A clinical trial of blood and crystalloid cardioplegia. J Thorac Cardiovasc Surg 88: 726–741
4. Fremes SE, Weisel RD, Mickle DAG, Ivanov J, Madonik MM, Seawright SJ, Houle S, McLaughlin PR, Baird RJ (1985) Myocardial metabolism and ventricular function following cold potassium cardioplegia. J Thorac Cardiovasc Surg 89: 531–546
5. Kanter KR, Glower DD, Schaff AV, Gardner TJ (1981) Mechanism of defective oxygen extraction following global ischemia. J Surg Res 30: 482–488
6. Mullen JC, Weisel RD, Fremes SE, Christakis GT, Ivanov J, Madonik MM, Houle S, McLaughlin PR (1986) Right ventricular function: A comparison between blood and crystalloid cardioplegia. Ann Thorac Surg (in press)
7. Pasque MK, Spray TL, Pellon GL, Wechsler AK (1982) Ribose-enriched myocardial recovery following ischemia in the isolated working rat heart. J Thorac Cardiovasc Surg 83: 390–398
8. Rosenkranz ER, Buckberg GD, Laks H, Mulder DG (1983) Warm induction of cardioplegia with glutamate-enriched blood in coronary patients with cardiogenic shock who are dependent on inotropic drugs and intraaortic balloon support. J Thorac Cardiovasc Surg 86: 507–518
9. Teoh KH, Christakis GT, Weisel RD, Fremes SE, Mickle DAG, Romaschin AD, Harding R, Ivanov J, Madonik MM, Ross IM, McLaughlin PR, Baird HRJ (1986), Accelerated myocardial metabolic recovery with terminal warm blood cardioplegia (Hot Shot). J Thorac Cardiovasc Surg (in press)
10. Teoh KH, Christakis GT, Weisel RD, Mullen JC, Madonik MM, Ivanov J, Henderson MJ, Warbick-Cerone A, Johnston LG, Mee AV, Wongd PY, Reilly PA, Glynn MFX (1986) Prevention of myocardial platelet deposition and thromboxane release with dipyridamole. Circulation (in press)

Authors' address:
Richard D. Weisel, M.D.
Toronto General Hospital,
200 Elizabeth Street, 13 EN-224,
Toronto, Ontario M5G 2C4
Canada

Retroinfusion versus antegrade delivery of cardioplegic solutions

P. Menasché and A. Piwnica

Service de Chirurgie Cardio-vasculaire, Hôpital Lariboisière, Paris (France)

For most cardiac surgeons, the technique of cardioplegic delivery during aortic cross-clamping is infusion of arresting solution into the aortic root or by direct cannulation of the coronary ostia. Although these techniques of antegrade cardioplegia have yielded overall satisfactory results, their limitations are now well recognized and primarily include the potential hazard of catheter-related coronary arterial damage, the nuisance of having perfusion cannulas present within a limited operative field and a non-homogeneous distribution of cooling and cardioplegia distal to coronary artery occlusions or stenoses. To obviate these shortcomings, we started, five years ago, to use the coronary sinus as a route of cardioplegic delivery, primarily in patients undergoing aortic valve procedures. Based upon our results and those of several experimental studies, the present report is aimed at reviewing the main features of coronary sinus cardioplegia in an attempt to better define its status comparatively with the antegrade approach.

Technical feasibility

Retrograde cardioplegia is a simple technique to deal with. For the sake of safety, the coronary sinus should be cannulated under direct vision, which requires double caval cannulation and snaring. The right atrium is then entered parallel to the atrio-ventricular groove, and a balloon-tipped catheter (Peters Laboratories, Aubervilliers, France) is introduced into the terminal portion of the coronary sinus. The balloon is gently inflated until it occludes the coronary sinus orifice, and cardioplegic infusion is initiated. Adequate drainage of retroperfused cardioplegic solution is provided by right atriotomy and the opened ascending aorta. The catheter, which is self-secured by means of balloon inflation and crimping of the balloon material, is maintained in the coronary sinus throughout the cross-clamp period. Immediately before removal of the aortic clamp, the balloon is deflated, the catheter is withdrawn and the right atriotomy is closed with a running suture.
We have no experience with retrograde cardioplegia through the right atrium since we are concerned about the distension of right-sided cardiac cavities that is associated with this approach.

Safety

Coronary sinus cardioplegia is a safe technique provided the perfusion pressure is not allowed to rise above 40 mm Hg (4, 6). Like others (4, 6), we have found that under conditions of cold cardioplegic arrest, the pressure/flow relationship in the venous system was fairly constant from one heart to the next. Consequently, we have now discontinued to monitor perfusion pressure and simply fix the flow rate of the cardioplegia delivery system to approximately 50 ml/min, which ensures that distal perfusion pressure is kept within the safety range.

Thus, in our experience, not only is coronary sinus retroperfusion as safe as antegrade perfusion by means of direct intra-coronary cannulation, but it is less iatrogenic since it does not carry the risk of catheter-related or perfusion-related arterial injury which may lead to the development of a life-threatening coronary ostial stenosis. Actually, it is because we, as others (10), have encountered such cases of coronary ostial stenosis following intermittent intra-coronary cannulation for delivering cardioplegic solution that we looked for an alternative approach and started to use coronary sinus cardioplegia. Obviously, this statement on the greater safety of coronary sinus retroperfusion compared with the antegrade route does not hold true for patients undergoing mitral valve or coronary artery bypass grafting procedures in whom cardioplegic solution can be delivered through the aortic root (or the completed vein grafts).

Efficacy

There is a growing body of experimental evidence that retrograde cardioplegia affords a level of intra-operative myocardial protection that is at least equal to that provided by techniques of antegrade cardioplegic delivery (1, 2, 4, 8, 9, 11).

This view is supported by our initial clinical study dealing with aortic valve procedures (7). Looking at two groups of patients that were matched for pre- and intra-operative data, we were unable to detect any significant difference in the postoperative course, as assessed by serial hemodynamic measurements, between patients who were given cardioplegic solution directly into the coronary ostia and those receiving the same perfusate retrogradely through the coronary sinus.

More recently, a similar study design has been used by Guiraudon and associates (3) for evaluating the effects of coronary sinus cardioplegia in patients undergoing coronary artery bypass grafting procedures. Their results show that intra-operative ischemic injury, as evidenced by enzymatic and functional indexes, was similar in all patients regardless of the route of cardioplegic delivery.

The efficacy of the coronary sinus approach to achieve adequate myocardial protection during cardioplegic arrest is not unexpected since the extensive venous network of the heart (5) results in venous channels being highly suitable conduits for delivering cooling and cardioplegic ingredients throughout the thickness of the myocardium.

One step further, several investigators (1, 4, 8, 11) have recently claimed that retrograde cardioplegia could be a more effective technique of myocardial preservation in patients with coronary artery disease because it would circumvent the difficulty of achieving homogeneous distribution of cooling and cardioplegic solution that is associated with the use of antegrade techniques of cardioplegic delivery. However, it is important to emphasize that, at the present time, this assumption is exclusively based upon results obtained in animal models of myocardial ischemia. There is no question that these studies convincingly demonstrate that retrograde cardioplegia provides better preservation to myocardial areas supplied by obstructed coronary arteries than antegrade cardioplegia does.

These findings contrast, however, with those of Guiraudon (3) who, as previously mentioned, was unable to disclose any superiority of coronary sinus cardioplegia over the aortic root approach in *patients* undergoing revascularization procedures. Although one might argue that the criteria used in Guiraudon's study for assessing results were too rough for detecting potential between-group differences, a more likely explanation for this discrepancy lies in the well-known observation that data on coronary flow patterns cannot be readily extrapolated from normal dog hearts (even if a coronary artery occlusion has been artificially created) to diseased human hearts. This statement does not deny any room for coronary sinus cardioplegia in coronary patients but simply points out that only some of them are likely to benefit from retrograde techniques.

Advantages

While preserving global cardiac performance to the same extent as antegrade cardioplegia does, coronary sinus cardioplegia offers some additional advantages which can be of clinical relevance.

First, cardioplegic infusions can be repeated as often as required without interrupting the surgical procedure because the retroperfusion catheter is kept away from the aortic root. Thus, if one uses multidose cardioplegia, the nuisance of having coronary artery perfusion cannulae intermittently obscuring the operative field is avoided. Further, since one single size of catheter (12 F in adults) fits all coronary sinus orifices, the requirement for matching the size of the cannula to that of the native coronary ostia is avoided, which contributes to earlier initiation of cardioplegic infusion after the aorta has been cross-clamped.

Secondly, the prolonged period of cardioplegic delivery due to the low flow rate of retroinfusion is expected to enhance washout of harmful byproducts of anaerobic metabolism. Similarly, diffusion of cardioplegic ingredients into ischemic cells is likely to be more effective than after a short period of antegrade perfusion.

Thirdly, coronary sinus cardioplegia seems to result in better atrial hypothermia than aortic root cardioplegia. Thus, in a recent study (data not yet published), we have found that the rate of atrial rewarming between cardioplegic infusions was $8.1 \pm 5.5\,°C$ (m $\pm$ SD) in mitral valve patients subjected to antegrade cardioplegia versus $2.9 \pm 3.2\,°C$ in aortic valve patients undergoing coronary sinus retroperfusion ($p < 0.001$). We speculate that this effect of retrograde cardioplegia could be due to a more prolonged bathing of right atrial structures with cold cardioplegic solution egressing into right-sided cardiac chambers. This observation is of clinical relevance since augmented atrial hypothermia is known to correlate with a reduced incidence of supra-ventricular arrhythmias postoperatively (12).

Limitations

Although there are some concerns with the use of coronary sinus cardioplegia, our experience suggests that they can be easily met, so that the potential limitations of retrograde techniques do not overwhelm their aforementioned advantages.

Coronary venous injury can be prevented by avoiding excessive balloon inflation and perfusion pressures in excess of 40 mm Hg. In a five-year period that encompasses approximately 500 patients subjected to coronary sinus cardioplegia, we have encountered

3 cases of venous injury, all three during our early experience. Guiraudon (3) reported no complication in his series of patients which consists of 40 coronary cases and over 100 aortic valve procedures. Increased safety should be further provided by the pear-shaped balloon design of our newly developed retroperfusion catheter, which enables the inflated balloon to fit the funnel-like configuration of the coronary sinus orifice, thereby reducing trauma to the underlying venous wall.

Delayed onset of asystole and increased myocardial edema that might be anticipated from the low flow rate of infusion and the related duration of cardioplegic delivery have been shown not to be a significant problem, either in the laboratory setting (1), or clinically.

Finally, one could infer from the drainage flow patterns of the heart that coronary sinus cardioplegia results in poor protection of the right ventricle. None of the experimental studies that have addressed this issue (1, 11) supports this assumption, a finding that is consistent with the observation that injection of dye into the coronary sinus results in staining of the right ventricle (1, 11). In the clinical setting, we have been concerned, by the time we were using a Foley catheter for retroperfusing cardioplegic solution, that because of its spherical shape, the balloon, once inflated, would occlude distal branches of the coronary sinus. This prompted us to develop a pear-shaped balloon design that prevents the distal tributaries being excluded from cardioplegic retroperfusion, and hence should improve distribution of cooling and protective solution to right-sided cardiac structures. Alternatively, Guiraudon and associates (3) have used a Foley catheter without inflating the balloon. The disadvantage with the latter technique is that it requires an additional maneuver, i.e. the placement of a purse-string around the rim of the coronary sinus orifice in order to keep the catheter properly secured in place into the sinus. Presently, we are looking specifically at right ventricular function in patients subjected to coronary sinus cardioplegia. Although the study is still under progress, we have not yet seen patterns of postoperative right ventricular dysfunction that could be ascribed to the use of the retrograde approach. However, it is also likely that the simultaneous use of topical hypothermia significantly contributes to preserving the right ventricle which, because of its ventral position, is particularly well cooled by topical lavage.

Conclusion

Whenever direct cannulation of the coronary ostia has to be performed, i.e. during aortic valve procedures, we consider that retrograde cardioplegia is more appropriate than the antegrade technique. This statement thus applies to patients with major aortic insufficiency and, more generally, to those in whom the ascending aorta has been opened, thereby making direct ostial cannulation mandatory for reinfusion of cardioplegic solution in the course of the aortic cross-clamp period.

The problem is different for patients operated upon for mitral valve disease since cardioplegic solution can be instilled directly into the aortic root, thus eliminating the risk of postperfusion coronary ostial stenosis. From a theoretical standpoint, coronary sinus cardioplegia could have two distinct advantages over aortic root cardioplegia in these patients: (1) avoidance of coronary air embolism that may result from repeated infusions of perfusate into an air-filled aorta, and (2) better atrial cooling. However, clinical studies are warranted to assess the practical relevance of these considerations.

Regarding revascularization procedures, we have already emphasized that data based upon experimental studies could not be readily extrapolated to the clinical setting. We assume that, in a significant number of patients with coronary artery disease, the extensive development of collateral channels makes antegrade techniques of cardioplegic delivery effective in ensuring adequate preservation of the myocardial areas in jeopardy. Future clinical studies should therefore be specifically directed towards identification of patients in whom anatomical patterns of coronary artery disease may render coronary sinus cardioplegia a superior technique of myocardial protection. We speculate that this subset primarily consists of patients who demonstrate *totally occluded* coronary arteries and *poor collateral circulation* since such patterns are likely to make antegrade cardioplegia really unable to induce adequate cooling and effective electro-mechanical arrest in the corresponding myocardial areas.

References

1. Bolling SF, Flaherty JT, Bulkley BH, Gott VL, Gardner TJ (1983) Improved myocardial preservation during global ischemia by continuous retrograde coronary sinus perfusion. J Thorac Cardiovasc Surg 86: 659–666
2. Goldstein JP, Salter DR, Abd-Elfattah AS, Murphy CE, Morris JJ, Wechsler AS (1985) Efficacy of coronary sinus cardioplegia without topical hypothermia during two hours of cardiac arrest. Proceedings of the International Symposium on Myocardial Protection, Boston, May 1985, p 59
3. Guiraudon GM, Campbell CS, McLellan DG, Kostuk WJ, Purves PD, McDonald JL, Cleland AG, Tadros NB (1985) Retrograde coronary sinus versus aortic root perfusion with cold cardioplegia. A randomized study using cardiac enzymes in 40 patients. Ann Thorac Surg (submitted for publication)
4. Gundry SR, Kirsk MM (1984) A comparison of retrograde cardioplegia versus antegrade cardioplegia in the presence of coronary artery obstruction. Ann Thorac Surg 38: 124–127
5. Hochberg MS, Austen WG (1980) Selective retrograde coronary venous perfusion. Ann Thorac Surg 219: 578–588
6. Lolley DM, Hewitt RL (1980) Myocardial distribution of asanguineous solutions retroperfused under low pressure through the coronary sinus. J Cardiovasc Surg 21: 287–294
7. Menasché P, Kural S, Fauchet M, Lavergne A, Commin P, Bercot M, Touchot B, Georgiopoulos G, Piwnica A (1982) Retrograde coronary sinus perfusion: a safe alternative for ensuring cardioplegic delivery in aortic valve surgery. Ann Thorac Surg 34: 647–658
8. Mori F, Ivey TD, Misbach GA, Tabayashi K, Thomas R, Breazale DG (1985) Regional myocardial protection by retrograde coronary sinus infusion of cardioplegic solution. Circulation 72: Supp III-376 (Abstr)
9. Okike ON, Phillips D, Chi C, Gore JM, Vandersalm TJ, Marsicano TH, Alpert JS (1985) Efficacy of coronary sinus cardioplegia (CSCP) during two hours of hyperkalemic arrest of hypertrophied left ventricle. Circulation 72: Supp III-394
10. Pennington DG, Dinger B, Bashiti H, Barner HB, Kaiser GC, Tyras DH, Codd JE, Willman VL (1982) Coronary artery stenosis following aortic valve replacement and intermittent intracoronary cardioplegia. Ann Thorac Surg 33: 576–584
11. Solorzano J, Taitelbaum G, Chiu RCJ (1978) Retrograde coronary sinus perfusion for myocardial protection during cardiopulmonary bypass. Ann Thorac Surg 25: 201–208
12. Smith PK, Buhrman WC, Levett JM, Ferguson TB, Holman WL, Cox JL (1983) Supraventricular conduction abnormalities following cardiac operations. A complication of inadequate atrial preservation. J Thorac Cardiovasc Surg 85: 105–115

Authors' address:
Philippe Menasché, M.D.
Service de Chirurgie Cardio-vasculaire
Hôpital Lariboisière
2, rue Ambroise Paré
75010 Paris
France

Metabolic differences of retrograde cardioplegia

A. S. Wechsler, D. R. Salter, C. E. Murphy, J. P. Goldstein, L. A. Brunsting, and A. S. Abd-Elfattah

The Department of Surgery, Duke University Medical Center Durham, North Carolina (U.S.A.)

Administration of cardioplegia through the coronary sinus has been demonstrated to provide good functional recovery following global myocardial ischemia (3). However, it has been demonstrated that functional recovery may precede metabolic recovery following injury. Diminished metabolic recovery, even with demonstrated functional recovery, would provide a lesser reserve in instances of prior myocardial injury in myocardium that was to be again stressed during the course of a cardiac operation. Therefore, there are two immediate reasons for examining retrograde cardioplegia from a metabolic viewpoint. The first is to determine whether or not something related to the continuous, as compared with the intermittent, nature of cardioplegia administration might alter metabolic recovery and the second aspect would be to determine if retrograde cardioplegia provided the same metabolic preservation as antegrade administration.

Despite clinical application of retrograde cardioplegic techniques, few studies have examined the metabolic consequences of this form of cardioplegia administration. In 1981, Catinella studied two groups of dogs comparing continuous cold blood cardioplegia given intermittently every thirty minutes for a total of 120 minutes of ischemia with a second group of dogs given continuous antegrade cold blood cardioplegic solution (2). When functional, endocardial to epicardial ratios, myocardial oxygen consumption and adenosine triphosphate levels were examined, there were no important differences between the two groups. Thus, in this experimental model, there did not appear to be significant differences between continuous and intermittent antegrade administration of cardioplegia. Olin, in the same year, in Stockholm, compared three groups of patients given cardioplegia during aortic valve replacements (4). Of the three groups, two are worthy of mention. One group of patients received single dose antegrade blood cardioplegia and the second group received continuous antegrade blood cardioplegia. The crossclamp time for the two groups was approximately the same (about 60 minutes). Minimal differences were noted with respect to perioperative enzyme release and functional recovery although the group receiving continuous blood cardioplegia had the fastest return to normal levels of ventricular performance. Gardner later demonstrated in dogs that in the presence of an acute experimental anterior coronary occlusion, antegrade cardioplegia failed to cool or metabolically protect the region of myocardium supplied by the acutely ligated vessel (1). Silverman on the other hand, demonstrated that retrograde coronary sinus cardioplegia cooled and protected myocardium metabolically better than antegrade administration of

Supported by NIH Grant = HL26302

cardioplegia in a similar model of acute coronary ligation followed by ischemia (15). No significant differences were observed between groups with or without a patent left anterior descending coronary artery when the cardioplegia was administered in a retrograde fashion. However, in their studies baseline levels of left ventricular and right ventricular adenosine triphosphate were lower at the end of ischemia and following 30 minutes of reperfusion than when compared with control levels in all groups. This was felt to be due to the slower arrest times obtained in dogs administered retrograde cardioplegia. Thus, prior to our own investigations, there appeared to be no specific disadvantage to administering cardioplegia in a retrograde fashion. Continuous, as compared with intermittent, administration of cardioplegia also did not seem specifically to injure myocardium.

To assess the metabolic protection afforded by retrograde cardioplegia, we designed a more stringent test in a group of dogs. Initially, we compared "optimal" cardioplegia by combining retrograde coronary sinus cardioplegia with the use of topical hypothermia provided by iced saline slush. In subsequent tests, we utilized only retrograde coronary sinus cardioplegia during a two hour period and global ischemia. In addition to examining both the left and right ventricles of normal hearts, two additional sets of dogs were prepared. The first group had obliteration of the noncoronary sinus while puppies, and were studied 6–9 months later in the presence of severe valvular, subcoronary stenosis. This model has been demonstrated to provide intense and severe concentric left ventricular hypertrophy. The second group of dogs was prepared by banding the pulmonary artery to produce right ventricular outflow tract obstruction and was studied 2–3 months ollowing operation. Biopsies of both the right and left ventricles were obtained prior to ischemia ("control"), following two hours of ischemia, prior to reperfusion, and following sixty minutes of reperfusion. The metabolic results are presented in Table 1. No significant differences as a consequence of the ischemia or following reperfusion were noted in the experimental groups with the exception of the right ventricular biopsies in normal heart at the end of sixty minutes of reperfusion. These data were not replicated in the studies of right ventricles from hearts with left ventricular hypertrophy or right ventricles from hearts with right ventricular hypertrophy and although the difference was sta-

Table 1. ATP concentrations following two hours of global ischemia. Even in the absence of topical hypothermia, perfusion of retrograde cardioplegia preserves ATP concentration both in the right and left ventricles. This was also true of hypertrophied ventricles.

		μmoles ATP/mg protein		
		Control	2 hrs. ischemia	60 min reperfusion
Normal hearts (Topical)		29.5 ± 2.1	29.5 ± 2.2	27.6 ± 3.0
Normal hearts (No Topical)	LV	31.1 ± 1.9	35.1 ± 1.8	33.3 ± 2.1
	RV	30.4 ± 2.0	30.0 ± 1.5	$25.0 \pm 1.7^*$
LVH (No Topical)	LV	35.1 ± 2.8	30.9 ± 2.9	27.0 ± 2.6
	RV	28.3 ± 3.7	23.0 ± 2.2	26.8 ± 1.4
RVH (No Topical)	LV	31.2 ± 2.1	30.7 ± 2.1	27.8 ± 1.8
	RV	24.7 ± 2.9	26.7 ± 2.6	23.3 ± 2.7

* $p < 0.05$ NS Control, ANOVA

182

tistically significant, we do not believe that it was of biologic significance. At each of these time intervals, sophisticated evaluation of functional differences was also made utilizing the linear relationship between stroke work and varying end-diastolic lengths. This method of analysis provides a highly sensitive estimate of contractile function of the ventricle in a manner that is essentially free from the influence of afterload. Heart rates were carefully controlled and in every instance no functional left or right ventricular differences were observed. Therefore, we concluded that retrograde coronary sinus cardioplegia is a highly effective method for providing myocardial protection even in the absence of topical hypothermia and in pathologic as well as normal ventricles. Most prior studies have demonstrated increased sensitivity of hypertrophied ventricles to ischemia and excellent preservation of metabolic and functional integrity in our studies was highly encouraging.

Optimal cardioplegic techniques have not been determined for acutely ischemic and acutely injured ventricles in the evolving field of medical and surgical revascularization and acute myocardial infarction. Therefore, we created an additional experimental model. In this model, dogs were subjected to twenty minutes of warm (37 °C) global ischemia prior to the administration of retrograde cardioplegia. This model was designed to deliberately create myocardial injury for the purpose of allowing breakdown products of adenosine triphosphate to accumulate. The study examined the extent to which continuous administration of retrograde cardioplegia would result in washout of soluble precursors when compared with antegrade intermittent administration of cardioplegia. Biopsies were obtained prior to ischemia, immediately following the twenty minutes of global ischemia, and at multiple intervals during the ischemic period while cardioplegia was being administered. After a total of 120 minutes of ischemia (20 minutes warm, 100 minutes of cardioplegia) the crossclamp was released and biopsies were obtained after 30 and 60 minutes of reperfusion. During the cardioplegic administration, samples were collected from the aortic root in the retrograde group, and from the right atrium in the coronary sinus group to examine the qualitative content of myocardial washout. During the experiment, both cavae were cannulated and snares placed around the cannulae to prohibit

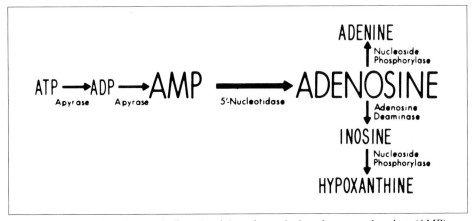

Fig. 1. Adenosine nucleotide catabolism. Breakdown beyond adenosine monophosphate (AMP) generates ATP percursors that diffuse across cell membranes and are lost during reperfusion.

venous blood from entering the right atrium. The pulmonary artery was occluded to allow capture of all right sided coronary sinus return. The left ventricle was vented and perfusion was maintained through the ascending aorta.

Adenosine triphosphate catabolism is shown in Figure 1. The transition from adenosine monophosphate to adenosine is an extremely important step since the action of 5'nucleotidase initiates conversion of relatively non-diffusable adenosine monophosphate to precursors that are highly soluable, move easily across cell membranes and result in subsequent loss to the cell of substrates for resynthesis of high energy phosphates using the salvage pathway following reperfusion. Full presentation of the data acquired is beyond the scope of this manuscript. However, several salient characteristics are shown. Figure 2 illustrates adenosine triphosphate concentrations for the left ventricle in the antegrade and retrograde groups. Both groups demonstrated highly significant ($p < 0.001$) losses when the data were analyzed by two way analysis of variance. This was predictable since the experiment was designed to cause adenosine triphosphate loss during the first twenty

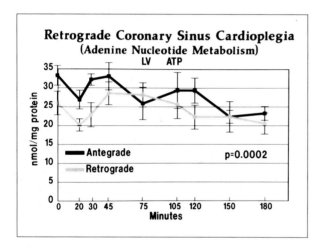

Fig. 2. ATP concentration during the experimental protocol. The twenty minute period of warm ischemia was associated with predictable decline in ATP concentrations. A second loss of ATP was associated with warm blood reperfusion following the ischemic interval.

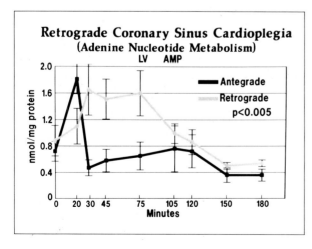

Fig. 3. Adenosine monosphosphate concentrations during the study interval. AMP accumulation is generally seen during ischemic injury to the extent that generation proceeds faster than breakdown by 5'nucleotidase. No obvious explanation is apparent for the different pattern of accumulation in the antegrade as compared with the retrograde cardioplegia groups.

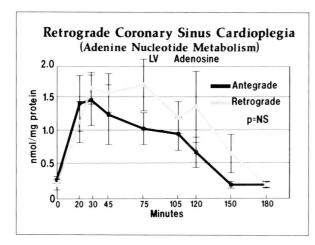

Retrograde Coronary Sinus Cardioplegia
(Adenine Nucleotide Metabolism)

Fig. 4. Adenosine concentrations in the two study groups. Rapid accumulation of adenosine occurred during warm ischemia in both groups. It was surprising that infusion of cold cardioplegic solution did not wash adenosine out of the myocardium whereas warm blood reperfusion decreased levels significantly.

minutes of ischemia. There were not, however, significant differences in the patterns of adenosine triphosphate loss or magnitude of adenosine triphosphate loss between the group administered cardioplegia antegrade and the group administered cardioplegia retrograde. Significant differences were observed in the adenosine monophosphate concentrations in the two groups (Figure 3), with accumulation of adenosine monophosphate in the retrograde group as compared with initial reduction, then stabilization in the antegrade treated group. In both groups, thirty minutes of reperfusion was associated with a fall in adenosine monophosphate levels. Figure 4 illustrates left ventricular adenosine levels. No differences were observed between the two groups with rapid accumulation of adenosine within the myocardium during the twenty minutes of warm ischemia, relative preservation of adenosine levels in the myocardium during cardioplegic administration interval, and marked washout of adenosine associated with reperfusion.

Table 2 demonstrates concentrations of various adenine nucleotide fractions recovered from the aortic root of the coronary sinus during cardioplegia administration. Most significant are the observations that evidence of significant myocardial ischemia is manifest by high concentrations of hypoxanthine associated with the initial cardioplegic administration in both groups and a secondary with concentration of hypoxanthine associated with reperfusion. Washout of hypoxanthine following the twenty minutes of ischemia confirms significant breakdown of high energy phosphate products during the period of warm global ischemia.

From these data and those currently available in the literature several conclusions may be drawn regarding metabolic consequences of retrograde cardioplegia.

1. Retrograde cardioplegia may not be as effective for maximal high energy phosphate preservation due to the delayed onset of arrest associated with administration of retrograde cardioplegia. This observation is garnered from the literature. Our own studies suggest that this may be a relatively trivial difference.

2. Despite continuous flow, high energy phosphates are not washed out from the myocardium. Specifically, high levels of adenosine and inosine within the myocardium do not appear to be markedly reduced during continuous cardioplegic infusion. This observation is noteworthy, since on the basis of known responses of these agents to warm re-

Table 2. Qualitative content of myocardial washout during cardioplegia. Values are given as a percent of the total adenine nucleotide metabolites present in the effluent. Significant myocardial injury and ATP loss is manifest by the high percentage of adenine nucleotide appearing as hypoxanthine and xanthine.

	ATP	ADP	HX	X	AMP	NAD	INO	CAMP	ID
Antegrade									
20I	1.71	1.67	53.38	19.94	0.63	0.70	17.12	1.81	1.30
	±0.91	±1.06	±8.63	±8.11	±0.11	±0.16	±7.25	±1.31	±0.59
R	0.78	0.86	49.57	44.03	1.05	0.44	2.17	0.95	0.31
	±0.37	±0.16	±8.20	±7.43	±0.26	±0.07	±1.24	±0.17	±0.18
	NS	NS	NS	NS	NS	NS	NS	NS	NS
Regrograde									
20I	0.53	0.40	54.97	29.35	1.02	0.33	11.66	1.14	0.07
	±0.24	±0.29	±12.97	±10.38	±0.49	±0.16	±6.09	±0.40	±0.05
R	0.82	0.45	50.84	41.0	1.50	1.04	2.18	1.44	0.73
	±0.29	±0.28	±8.52	±6.4	±0.40	±0.68	±1.30	±0.59	±0.59

perfusion (corroborated by our own studies), we suggest that either antegrade or retrograde cooling of the heart produces a fundamental change in the cell membrane and alters its permeability characteristics to these substances. Thus, further efforts to entrap these precursors during warm blood reperfusion seem a highly fruitful area for further investigation.

3. As a consequence of our observations presented in this manuscript, further studies designed to understand alterations in membrane physiology during hypothermia appear highly warranted.

4. With the knowledge that retrograde cardioplegia effectively cools and preserves adenine nucleotide substrates within ischemic myocardium, further efforts should be directed towards minimizing washout of these precursors during reperfusion or to examine further the effects of including high concentrations of substrates during the reperfusion period to favor myocellular influx rather than egress flow of precursors during warm blood reperfusion.

References

1. Bolling SF, Flaherty JT, Bulkley BH, Gott VL, Gardner TJ (1983) Improved myocardial preservation during global ischemia by continuous retrograde coronary sinus perfusion. J Thorac Cardiovasc Surg 86: 659–666
2. Catinella FP, Cunningham JN, Scungaram RK, Nathan IM, Knopp EA, Paone G, Bajumann FG, Adams PX, Spencer FC (1981) Blood potassium cardioplegia administration. Arch Surg 116: 1509–1515
3. Hochberg M, Austen W (1980) Selective retrograde coronary venous perfusion. Ann Thorac Surg 29: 578–588
4. Olin CL, Bomfim V, Bendz R, Kaijser L, Strom SJ, Sylven CH, Bjork VO (1981) Myocardial protection during aortic valve replacement, J Thorac Cardiovasc Surg 82: 837–847
5. Silverman NA, Schmitt G, Levitsky S, Feinberg H (1985) Effect of coronary artery occlusion on myocardial protection by retroperfusion of cardioplegic solutions. J Surg Res 39: 164–171

Authors' address:
Andrew S. Wechsler, M.D.
Department of Surgery
Duke University Medical Center
Durham, North Carolina 27710
U.S.A.

Functional differences between retrograde and antegrade cardioplegia in hearts with varying degrees of coronary artery obstruction

S. R. Gundry, M. M. Kirsh, R. March, C. Koch, P. Carmen, and R. Long

Section of Thoracic Surgery, Department of Surgery, University of Michigan Medical Center (U.S.A.)

Summary: The best route for cardioplegia (CP) delivery in multivessel coronary lesions is not known. We compared coronary sinus (CS), right atrial (RA), and aortic root (Ao) CP in 15 dogs with temporary 80% LAD and 100% RCA lesions using temp. mapping and sonomicrometry crystals in the RV, LAD, and CIRC distributions. Five dogs were each given 4 °C, 20 mEq KCL/L blood CP every 20 minutes into the CS, the RA with caval and PA clamping, or the Ao. After 1.5 hours, the coronary lesions were removed, the dogs reperfused for 30 minutes, and weaned from bypass. Two RA and Ao dogs died. Post CP temps. and systolic shortening (SS) change from pre bypass to 1 hour post bypass appear below:

Temp.	RV	Septum	LAD	CIRC
(°C)	CS $17\pm2^{***}$	$14\pm3^{**}$	$14\pm3^{***}$	$15\pm2^{**}$
	RA 22 ± 2	23 ± 3	23 ± 3	24 ± 4
	Ao 22 ± 3	19 ± 6	21 ± 3	12 ± 2
Systolic shortening change (mm)				
	CS $-0.1\pm0.7^{***}$		$-0.3\pm0.5^*$	$+0.1\pm0.3^*$
	RA -1.7 ± 1.2		-0.9 ± 0.5	$-0.1\pm0.4^*$
	Ao -0.6 ± 2.4		-1.8 ± 1.0	-1.3 ± 1.2

* = p < 0.01 CS vs. Ao; ** = p < 0.01 VS vs. RA

We conclude that CS cardioplegia gives superior cooling and preservation of myocardium distal to both coronary artery occlusions and stenosis. Additionally, it appears that coronary sinus cardioplegia is superior to right atrial cardioplegia in preserving the function of the right ventricle.

Introduction

We and others have previously shown that retrograde cardioplegia gives superior protection to myocardium distal to acute coronary artery obstructions during aortic cross clamping (1, 3–5). Recently, Fabiani and his colleagues have demonstrated in a parallel patient population that cardioplegia infused into the right atrium with simultaneous occlusion of both cavae and the pulmonary artery (hereafter referred to as right atrial cardioplegia) gave equal or better myocardial protection than when the cardioplegia was infused via the coronary sinus (2).

The role of retrograde cardioplegia and the most effective route for its delivery in hearts with multivessel and varying degrees of coronary artery obstruction has heretofore not

189

been investigated in an experimental setting. Because changes in myocardial function may occur experimentally that cannot be measured clinically, we designed an experimental model to compare the effects of retrograde cardioplegia, delivered either via the coronary sinus or right atrium and antegrade cardioplegia, delivered via the aortic root, on myocardial function in animals with controlled degrees of coronary artery stenoses or occlusions.

Methods

Fifteen mongrel dogs (wt = 24 ± 2 kg) were anaesthesied with 120 mg/kg of chloralose and placed on a volume ventilator with ambiant FiO_2 and ventilated to maintain normal pH. A standard median sternotomy was performed, the pericardium incised and fashioned into a cradle. The left femoral artery was cannulated with fluid-filled polyvinyl chloride tubing and connected to a Statham transducer to record systolic, diastolic and mean arterial blood pressure on an eight channel Gould chart recorder. The right femoral artery was cannulated with a 14F perfusion cannula for inflow from the bubble oxygenator and roller pumps. The right external jugular vein was cannulated with a triple lumen Swan-Ganz thermodilution catheter which was passed into the distal pulmonary artery. This was connected to fluid-filled transducers to record right atrial, pulmonary artery, and pulmonary artery capillary wedge pressures. Cardiac outputs were determined via thermodilution and the mean of three separate determinations used for calculations. The left atrial appendage was cannulated and a fluid-filled catheter advanced into the left ventricle to measure and record left ventricular end-diastolic pressure.

Three pairs of 2 mm piezo-electric ultrasound crystals were implanted approximately 1.5 cm apart within the mid myocardium in the anterior and posterior surfaces of the left ventricle and the anterior free wall of the right ventricle and aligned in the free wall to septal axis of major fiber shortening in zones supplied by the left anterior descending coronary artery (LAD), circumflex (CIRC) and right coronary arteries (RCA). These were connected to an ultrasonic pulse generator of 5 KHz frequency. As previously described, ultrasonic transit time and crystal separation were recorded and electronically converted into a continuous display of regional myocardial wall motion (dl) in the LAD, CIRC and RCA coronary artery distributions (6). Adjustable snares encircled the LAD proximal to the origin of the first diagonal branch and the RCA at the right atrial-right ventricular junction.

The inferior and superior vena cavae were separately cannulated with wide bore multi-side hole cannulas via the right atrium to serve as returns to the bypass circuit. Adjustable snares were placed around each cava. Following stabilisation, baseline measurements were made with all animals at 10 mm Hg left ventricular end-diastolic pressure. The snare on the LAD was then snugged down until systolic shortening ceased in the left anterior ventricle's crystal recording, indicating an approximately 80% stenosis of the LAD (6). All animals were then immediately placed on cardiopulmonary bypass and cooled to 28 °C. The aorta was then cross clamped for 1.5 hours and the RCA simultaneously occluded with its snare.

The dogs were divided into three groups: the Ao cardioplegia group (n = 5) had 10 cc/kg of 4 °C 20 meq KCL/l blood cardioplegia infused via the aortic root at 100 mm Hg pressure. At 20 minute intervals this was supplemented with 5 cc/kg additional infusions for the one and one half hour cross clamp period; the RA cardioplegia group (n = 5) had identical amounts of the same cardioplegic solution infused into the right atrium via a catheter with simultaneous clamping of both cavae and the pulmonary artery. An aortic root vent was introduced into the ascending aorta and cardioplegia recovered by gravity drainage. Distal coronary vein pressure monitoring was done via an indwelling catheter and was not allowed to exceed 40 mm Hg. Additional infusions were performed at the same 20 minute intervals as the Ao group; the CS cardioplegia group (n = 5) had the same amounts and regimen of cardioplegic solution infused into the coronary sinus via a balloon tipped 10F catheter introduced through a purse string suture on the right atrium. Distal coronary vein pressure was kept below 40 mm Hg and the solution was recovered from the aorta root.

After each cardioplegic infusion in all three groups, myocardial temperatures were measured by microtipped thermister probes inserted in the right ventricular free wall, the mid septum, and the anterior and posterior surfaces of the left ventricle.

After 1.5 hours of aortic occlusion the LAD and RCA snares were released, the aorta unclamped, the dogs rewarmed and weaned from bypass after 30 minutes of reperfusion. Measurements of regional myocardial function were recorded at intervals up to one hour post bypass with all measurements determined at a controlled filling pressure of 10 mm Hg LVEDP. All results were tabulated and compared for statistical significance using the chi square and Student's paired t-test.

Results

Temperature

In the Ao group, myocardial temperatures consistently fell to $12 \pm 2\,°C$ in the CIRC area where no coronary lesions existed, yet LAD, septal and RCA regional temperatures were poor at 21 ± 3, 19 ± 6 and $22 \pm 3\,°C$ respectively (Table 1). RA group myocardium failed to cool significantly in any region with temperatures of $22–24\,°C$ throughout the heart. In contrast, CS group hearts had consistently excellent lowering of temperature in the zones supplied by coronary stenoses with RV temperatures of $17 \pm 2\,°C$, septal of $14 \pm 3\,°$, LAD of $14 \pm 3\,°$, and CIRC of $15 \pm 2\,°C$. Adequate cooling was thus achieved in all zones of the heart only by CS cardioplegia.

Systolic shortening

Systolic shortening of regional myocardial segments was compared in the RV, LAD and CIRC regions in all groups and plotted as change in shortening pre and one hour post bypass (Table 2). Ao group shortening was depressed in all zones, most markedly in the LAD and CIRC zones where shortening decreased by 1.8 ± 1.0 and 1.3 ± 1.2 mm respectively ($p < 0.05$ in LAD post bypass compared to baseline). RA group shortening was depressed markedly in RV segments, down 1.7 ± 1.2 mm, while only slightly depressed in LAD and CIRC regions. CS cardioplegia showed little or no depression of systolic shortening compared to pre bypass levels; RV shortening was down only 0.1 ± 0.7 mm while LAD shortening fell 0.3 ± 0.5 with CIRC shortening up 0.1 ± 0.3 mm in post

Table 1. Post cardioplegia temperatures (°C).

Cardioplegia	RV	Septum	LAD	CIRC
CS	17±2**	14±3**	14±3***	15.2**
RA	22±2	23±3	23±3	24±4
Ao	22±3	19±6	21±3	12±2

* = p < 0.01 CS vs. Ao; ** = p < 0.01 VS vs. RA

Table 2. Change in systolic shortening pre and post bypass (mm).

Cardioplegia	RV	LAD	CIRC
CS	−0.1±0.7***	−0.3±0.5*	+0.1±0.3*
RA	−1.7±1.2	−0.9±0.5	−0.1±0.4
AO	−0.6±0.4	−1.8±1.0	−1.3±1.2

* = p < 0.01 CS vs. Ao; ** p = p < 0.01 CS vs. RA

Table 3. Change in end-diastolic length (mm) pre and post bypass.

Cardioplegia	RV	LAD	CIRC
CS	0.1±1	+0.4±4	0.0±1.5
RA	+4.8±1	−0.8±0.4	+1.2±1.0
Ao	+4.1±2*	−0.7±0.7	+0.4±0.5

* = p < 0.01 Ao vs. RA or CS

bypass. CS cardioplegia showed significantly better post bypass systolic shortening in the RV compared to both Ao and RA cardioplegia and significantly better LAD and CIRC function than Ao cardioplegia (p < 0.01).

Diastolic compliance

End-diastolic length at an LVEDP of 10 mm Hg was plotted for all groups and change in pre and post bypass lengths calculated as an expression of myocardial stiffness (Table 3). Ao group length increased by 4.1 ± 2 mm in the RV versus only minimal changes in the LAD and CIRC region (−0.7 ± 0.7 and +0.4 ± 0.5 mm respectively) (p < 0.01 in RV region compared to baseline). RA cardioplegia also caused severe increases in end-diastolic length in the RV zone of 4.8 ± 1 mm (p < 0.01 compared to pre op) while also causing dilatation in the CIRC zone of 1.2 ± 1.0 mm (NS). CS cardioplegia caused no changes in end-diastolic length in any zone and this was significantly better than either Ao or RA groups in the RV (p < 0.01).

Discussion

The best method of protecting ischemic myocardium during aortic cross clamping is still not known. Although aortic root cardioplegia is known to produce excellent myocardial protection when there are normal coronary arteries, its usefulness declines whenever acute coronary artery occlusions are present (3, 4). The role of retrograde protection of the heart via the coronary veins has been delineated by ourselves and others previously (1–5, 7) but heretofore, no experimental comparison has been performed between right atrial and coronary sinus cardioplegia nor between either of these and aortic root cardioplegia in hearts with multivessel coronary artery lesions.

Our study again substantiates the notable improvement in protection of myocardial function that coronary sinus cardioplegia produces in areas of the heart supplied by acutely occluded coronary arteries. More importantly, this effect was also seen in those regions of the heart served by coronary arteries with critical stenoses. Antegrade aortic root cardioplegia again failed to produce satisfactory cooling or protection of the myocardium in these areas.

Just as importantly, right atrial cardioplegia appears to produce inadequate cooling of the myocardium and hence, inadequate myocardial protection. Although on face value, right atrial cardiplegia would appear to make excellent theoretic sense, utilising all Thebesian vessels as well as the coronary sinus to deliver cardioplegia to the right ventricle, in practice, however, this delivery is difficult to achieve.

This difference in theoretical, experimental and clinical results is best explained by considering the options for flow in the coronary and Thebesian veins during retrograde cardioplegia. During retrograde delivery via the coronary sinus, cardioplegia may egress the veins at the capillary level either by crossing the capillaries into the arterial bed and hence into the aorta where it is drained by gravity, or by connecting with other venous pathways to exit into the atrial or ventricular chambers via the Thebesian veins. When coronary artery lesions make arterial egress difficult, more flow thus most go via the Thebesian route to egress from the myocardium.

This latter method is not available when right atrial (and, by definition, right ventricular) cardioplegia is used. In this case, the pressures within the right atrial and ventricular cavities are equal to those of the coronary sinus and Thebesian venous system. Hence most flow must be by arterial routes to exit the heart. If arterial routes are blocked, insufficient flow of cardioplegia will result.

This explanation is confirmed by our experimental findings which show adequate protection of the CIRC region of the heart by RA cardioplegia since no coronary artery lesions were present, and very poor protection of the LAD and RCA regions where coronary stenoses and obstructions had been created. This theory also explains why coronary sinus cardioplegia effectively is delivered to the right ventricle despite an apparent paucity of direct venous connections with the coronary sinus.

Conclusions

Coronary sinus cardioplegia appears to offer excellent protection of myocardium served by stenotic or occluded coronary arteries. No deleterious effects of coronary sinus cardioplegia have been detected in this study. In contrast, both aortic root and right atrial cardioplegia experimentally give poor protection of the heart, most notably the right ventricle, when used in the presence of multivessel coronary artery lesions. Continued and expanded use of coronary sinus cardioplegia in patients with coronary artery disease undergoing bypass operations appears warranted.

References

1. Bolling SF, Flaherty JT, Bulkely BH, Gott VL, Gardner TJ (1983) Improved myocardial preservation during global ischemia by continuous retrograde cardioplegia. J Thorac Cardiovasc Surg 86: 659–66
2. Fabiani J, Carpentier AF (1983) Comparative evaluation of retrograde cardioplegia through the coronary sinus and the right atrium. Circulation 68 (Suppl III): 251
3. Gundry SR, Kirsh MM (1982) A comparison of retrograde cardioplegia versus antegrade cardioplegia in the presence of coronary artery obstruction. Circulation 66 (Suppl II): 142
4. Gundry SR, Kirsh MM (1984) A comparison of retrograde versus antegrade cardioplegia in the presence of coronary artery obstruction. Ann Thorac Surg 38: 124–127
5. Gundry SR, Kirsh MM (1984) Myocardial compliance following antegrade versus retrograde cardioplegia in the presence of coronary artery obstructions. In: Mohl W et al (eds) The Coronary Sinus. Steinkopff Verlag, Darmstadt, pp 270–274
6. Gundry SR, Siepps H, Solomon R, Jones M (1980) Sonomicrometry to assess regional changes in myocardial contractility. Surg Forum 22
7. Homeffer PJ, Gott VL, Gardner TJ. Retrograde coronary sinus perfusion prevents infarct extension during intraoperative global ischemic arrest. Ann Thorac Surg (in press)

Authors' address:
Steven R. Gundry, M.D.
Department of Surgery
University of Maryland Hospital
22 South Greene Street
Baltimore, MD 21201

Selective arterialization of coronary veins: Clinical experience of 55 American heart surgeons*

M. S. Hochberg, A. J. Roberts, V. Parsonnet, and D. Fisch

Summary: A survey of American heart surgeons to determine the clinical experience with coronary *venous* bypass grafting was undertaken. There have been sporadic reports of bypassing into selected coronary veins in a planned manner as an alternative to coronary artery bypass grafting. In general these were performed in desperation because conventional coronary artery bypass grafting could not be performed due to distal disease in the coronary arteries or small coronary arteries. In addition, there have been some reports of bypasses placed into the coronary venous system inadvertently – where the vein was mistaken for the artery. In an attempt to catalogue both the planned and inadvertent coronary venous bypass grafts, the membership of the Society of Thoracic Surgeons of North America was polled. Two thousand three hundred questionnaires were sent.

Fifty-five surgeons performed 117 coronary venous bypass grafts. Forty-one of these CVBGs were planned due to an anatomical situation which did not permit the standard coronary artery bypass operation. In 95% of these patients, the coronary vein was tied cephalad to the anastomosis to prevent an A-V fistula. Eighty-eight percent of the patients were symptomatically improved. Postoperative catheterization was performed in 13 of these patients with 12 or 92% of the CVBGs found to be patent. Ninety-two percent of these 41 patients are long-term survivors.

Seventy-six of the CVBGs were performed inadvertently. Forty-five percent of these patients had signs or symptoms of myocardial ischemia following operation and 65% of these patients underwent a second operation for surgical correction.

The encouraging patency rate shown at postoperative catheterization following planned coronary venous bypass graft suggests that this procedure deserves a more formal prospective clinical trial.

Introduction

Coronary artery bypass grafting (CABG) is a well established technique for the treatment of coronary artery disease (25). The operation is performed over 200,000 times per year in the United States and is the most frequent of all cardiac operations (21). However, in individuals with atherosclerosis extending distally into the coronary arteries or in individuals with small coronary arteries, coronary artery bypass grafting is unlikely to succeed. It is estimated that perhaps 10–15% of all patients with severe myocardial ischemia have this type of pathologic anatomy which make them unsuitable for the conventional CABG operation (11). In addition, many centers are now seeing increasing numbers of patients who are returning with occluded CABG years after their initial operation (17). These patients presumably have developed atherosclerosis in their CABG or distally in their native coronary arteries, or both. While we have reported coronary artery endarterectomy and concomitant grafting can be useful in some such circumstances (12), in general it is of little value for individuals with diffuse distal coronary artery disease.

There has now been extensive evidence from animal investigation that selective arterialization of a coronary vein can be successful in adequately perfusing a region of a myocar-

---

* Supported in part by a grant from the Sagamore Foundation

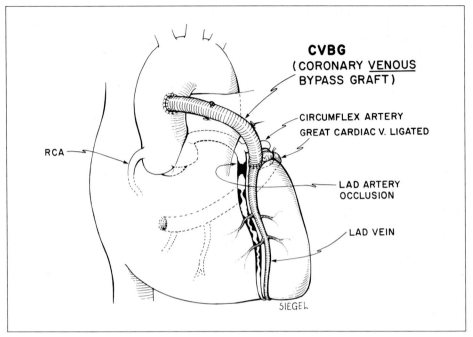

Fig. 1. Anatomic arrangement of a coronary *venous* bypass graft, performed in the circumstance of diffuse distal coronary artery disease. Note the ligature on the coronary vein cephalad to the anastomosis to prevent an arterio-venous fistula

dium (13). A review published in 1980 summarizes this work (11). Figure 1 depicts the anatomic arrangement of a coronary venous bypass graft. Note that cephalad to the anastomosis, a tight ligature must be placed on the coronary vein to prevent an arterio-venous fistula via the coronary sinus. In both short term and long term animal experiments, coronary *venous* bypass grafts (CVBG) have been proven to deliver oxygenated blood, in an adequate amounts, to the subendocardium – the most ischemically sensitive layer of the myocardium (10–14).

Sporadic reports in the literature have detailed occasional use of coronary venous bypass grafting in humans (4, 16, 24, 26). These reports deal with both planned CVBGs in which surgeons identified a vein, placed an arterialized conduit into it, and tied off the vein cephalad to prevent arterio-venous fistula, and inadvertent CVBGs in which the vein was misidentified as an artery. A few of the former and even fewer of the latter appear in the surgical literature. In order to determine more accurately the extent to which coronary venous bypass grafts have been performed, a survey was prepared.

Methods

The survey was prepared to permit reporting of all knowingly performed coronary venous bypass grafts, both planned and inadvertent (Table 1). It was mailed to the 2,300 members of the *Society of Thoracic Surgeons* based in North America. The questionnaire

Table 1. Survey mailed to 2,300 thoracic surgeons.

Aorto-coronary *venous* bypass survey

1. In your practice how many *aorto-coronary vein bypass grafts* (CVBG) have been performed (bypasses from the aorta to a coronary vein, not to a coronary artery)? _____

2. How many of these coronary vein bypasses were performed by design (unable to find coronary artery; distal coronary artery too small or too diseased to accept bypass) and how many were performed inadvertently? Planned CVBG _____ Inadvertent CVBG _____

3. Patients with *planned* CVBG
   a) How many had the coronary vein tied off proximally to prevent an A–V fistula? _____
   b) How many underwent post-op cath to determine patency? _____
   c) How many were patent? _____
   d) How many were alive? _____   _____
   e) How many were dead? _____   _____
   f) Any further information – e.g. symptomatic status, length of follow-up.

4. Patients with *inadvertent* CVBG
   a) How many had symptoms of myocardial ischemia following heart operation? _____
   b) How many were catheterized? _____
   c) How many underwent surgical correction? _____
   d) What surgical procedure was subsequently performed? _____
   e) How many were alive? _____
   f) How many were dead? _____
   g) Any further information – e.g. symptomatic status, length of follow-up.

5. How many coronary *artery* bypass operations do you perform yearly? _____

6. Would you consider performing a CVBG if, on exploration, you could not find a coronary artery or found a diffusely diseased or small coronary artery? YES _____ NO _____

7. Additional comments.

---

was specifically designed to be short, anonymous, and with pre-paid postage to encourage each recipient's reply. One section dealt with planned CVBGs and a separate one dealt with inadvertent CVBGs. Each provided room for postoperative follow-up including symptoms, catheterization, survival and additional comments.

Additional space was provided for any pertinent comments. The survey was sent to the membership of The Society of Thoracic Surgeons because its 2,300 members comprise the largest organization of cardiac surgeons.

Results

Three hundred and fifteen thoracic surgeons replied to the questionnaire. In aggregate, they perform 48,500 coronary *artery* bypass operations per year. Fifty-five of these surgeons had performed 117 coronary venous bypass procedures in their collective experience.

Planned CVBG

Forty-one of these coronary venous bypass grafts were planned. The indications (Table 2) for these 41 planned CVBGs were 1) diffuse distal coronary disease, 2) small distal coro-

Table 2. Indications for coronary *venous* bypass grafting.

1. Diffuse distal coronary artery disease
2. Small distal coronary arteries.
3. A second or "redo" coronary artery operation in which a coronary artery cannot be found.
4. Intramyocardial coronary arteries where coronary arteries cannot be located.
5. Patients with inflammatory atherosclerosis.

Table 3. Planned coronary *venous* bypass grafts.

– Total planned CVBGs	41
– Coronary vein tied cephalad to prevent A–V fistula	95% (39/41)
Symptomatic improvement	88% (22/25)
– Post-op cath to determine patency	31% (13/41)
– Patent CVBGs determined by post-op cath	92% (12/13)
– Survivors	92% (38/41)

nary arteries, 3) a second or "redo" coronary artery operation in which coronary arteries could not be found, 4) intra-myocardial coronary arteries in which the artery could not be found (especially in the circumflex distribution), and 5) inflammatory atherosclerosis in which distal coronary disease is likely to occur.

Pertinent additional data on 41 planned CVBGs is detailed in Table 3. Virtually all (95%, 39/41) had the coronary vein tied off cephalad to the CVBG anastomosis to prevent an arterio-venous fistula. Eighty-eight percent (22/25) of the patients surveyed had symptomatic improvement, and 93% (38/41) are long-term survivors. More importantly, of the 13 CVBGs studied angiographically, 92% (12/13) were patent.

Inadvertent CVBG

Inadvertent placement of a vein graft or internal mammary artery into a coronary vein was reported 76 times in the survey (Table 4). In each instance, the coronary vein was misidentified as a coronary artery. An inadvertent coronary venous bypass graft can be identified in several ways. Prior to chest closure, a thrill in the graft can be a tip-off that an arterio-venous fistula has been created. Those centers in which the team measures graft flow will note a flow in excess of 300 ml per minute in these inadvertent CVBGs.

Table 4. Inadvertent coronary *venous* bypass grafts.

– Total inadvertent CVBGs	76
– Signs or symptoms of myocardial ischemia post-op	49% (37/76)
– Catheterized post-op	46% (35/76)
– Underwent surgical correction	65% (49/76)
Survivors	93% (71/76)

Also, all adjacent epicardial veins will be pink with oxygenated blood. Following closure of the chest, an inadvertent CVBG is usually appreciated by the signs or symptoms of myocardial ischemia. In the survey, 49% (37/76) had myocardial ischemia which lead to postoperative catheterization in 46% (35/76). Ultimately, 65% (49/76) of the inadvertent CVBGs underwent surgical correction. Long-term survival of the inadvertant CVBG patients was 93% (71/76).

Discussion

At the 1st International Symposium on Myocardial Protection via the Coronary Sinus, experimental evidence was presented from our center as well as from others that in animal models, regional areas of myocardial ischemia could be successfully reversed by coronary venous bypass grafting (14). Using the multiple techniques of 1) radioactive microsphere myocardial flow studies, 2) CVBG flow probe results, 3) angiography and 4) post-mortem histologic evaluation, the efficacy of CVBG in reversing myocardial ischemia seems well established.

The purpose of the present survey is to catalogue the sporadic clinical reports and add them to the previously unreported planned and inadvertent CVBGs. We believe the collected survey data is encouraging. It should be emphasized that coronary venous bypass grafting should never be employed if a conventional coronary artery bypass graft can be successfully performed. However, for the clear indications (Table 2) in which CABG will probably fail, CVBG may be an acceptable alternative. With the experimental and occasional clinical reports of coronary venous bypass grafting now collected, it may now be appropriate to undertake a planned prospective clinical protocol to further evaluate coronary venous bypass grafting.

Conclusions

1) In a survey of American heart surgeons, 55 report 117 coronary *venous* bypass grafts. Forty-one of these grafts were planned because conventional coronary artery bypass grafting was thought to be unsuitable. Seventy-six of the reported CVBGs were placed inadvertently into a coronary vein which was mistaken for a coronary artery.

2) Of the patients with planned CVBG, 92% were patent at postoperative catheterization and 92% are long-term survivors.

3) For patients with diffusely diseased coronary arteries or small distal coronary arteries, coronary venous bypass grafting may be an appropriate procedure.

4) Further prospective clinical trials must be undertaken to determine if coronary venous bypass grafting can be a useful technique for the long-term reversal of myocardial ischemia.

References

1. Andreadis P, Natsikas N, Arealis E, Lazarides DP (1974) The aortocoronary venous anastomosis in experimental acute myocardial ischemia. Vasc Surg 8: 45

2. Arealis EG, Volder JG, Kolff WJ (1973) Arterialization of the coronary vein coming from an ischemic area (Letter). Chest 63: 462
3. Bates RJ, Toscano M, Baldermann SC, Anagnostopoulos CE (1977) The cardiac veins and retrograde coronary venous perfusion. Ann Thorac Surg 23: 83
4. Benedict JS, Buhl TG, Henney RP (1975) Cardiac vein myocardial revascularization: An experimental study and report of three clinical cases. Ann Thorac Surg 20: 550
5. Bhayana JN, Olsen DB, Byrne JP, Kolff WJ (1974) Reversal of myocardial ischemia by arterialization of the coronary vein. J Thor Cardiovasc Surg 67: 125.
6. Chiu CJ (1975) Myocardial revascularization in diffuse coronary atherosclerosis: Recent experimental progress. In: Norman JC (ed) Coronary Artery Medicine and Surgery: Concepts and Controversies. Appleton-Century-Crofts, Inc, New York
7. Chiu CJ, Mulder DS (1975) Selective arterialization of coronary veins for diffuse coronary occlusion: An experimental evaluation. J Thor Cardiovasc Surg 70: 177.
8. Demos S, Brooks H, Holland R, Balderman S, Anagnostopoulos C (1974) Retrograde coronary venous perfusion to reverse and prevent acute myocardial ischemia. Circ 49, 50 (Suppl 3): 168
9. Gardner RS, Magovern GJ, Park SB, Dixon CM (1974) Arterialization of coronary veins in the treatment of myocardial ischemia. J Thor Cardiovasc Surg 68: 273
10. Hochberg MS (1977) Hemodynamic evaluation of selective arterialization of the coronary venous system: An experimental study of myocardial perfusion using radioactive microspheres. J Thor Cardiovasc Surg 74: 774
11. Hochberg MS, Austen WG (1980) Selective retrograde coronary venous perfusion: A collective review. Ann Thorac Surg 29: 578
12. Hochberg MS, Merrill WH, Michaelis LL, McIntosh CL (1978) Results of combined coronary endarterectomy and coronary bypass for diffuse coronary artery disease. J Thor Cardiovasc Surg 75: 38
13. Hochberg MS, Roberts WC, Morrow AG, Austen WG (1979) Selective arterialization of the coronary venous system: Encouraging long-term flow evaluation utilizing radioactive microspheres. J Thor Cardiovasc Surg 77: 1
14. Hochberg MS, Gielchinsky I, Hussain SM, Norman JC, Parsonnet V (1984) Arterialization of the left anterior descending coronary vein in dogs: Successful long-term flow evaluation. In: Mohl W, Wolner E, Glogar D (eds) The Coronary Sinus. Steinkopff, Darmstadt, pp 328–335
15. Kay EB, Suzuki A (1975) Coronary venous retroperfusion for myocardial revascularization. Ann Thorac Surg 19: 327
16. Lawrie GM, Morris GC, Winters WL (1976) Aortocoronary saphenous vein autograft accidentally attached to a coronary vein: Follow-up angiography and surgical correction of the resultant arteriovenous fistula. Ann Thorac Surg 22: 87
17. Loop FD, Cosgrove DM, Kramer JR, Lytle BW, Taylor PC, Golding LAR, Groves, LK (1981) Late clinical and arteriographic results in 500 coronary artery reoperations. J Thorac Cardiovasc Surg 81: 675
18. Magovern GJ (1977) Personal communication
19. Marco JD, Hahn JW, Barner HB, Jellinek M, Blair OM, Standeven JW, Kaiser GC (1977) Coronary venous arterialization: Acute hemodynamic, metabolic and chronic anatomical observations. Ann Thorac Surg 23: 449
20. Meerbaum S, Lang TW, Osher JV, Hasimoto K, Lewis GW, Feldstein C, Corday E (1976) Diastolic retroperfusion of acutely ischemic myocardium. Am J Cardioil 37: 588
21. Miller DW, Ivrey TD, Bailey WW, Johnson DD, Hessel EA (1981) The practice of coronary artery bypass surgery in 1980. J Thorac Cardiovasc Surg 81: 423–427
22. Mohl W, Wolner E, Glogar D (1984) The Coronary Sinus. Proceedings of the 1st International Symposium on Myocardial Protection via the Coronary Sinus. Steinkopff Verlag, Darmstadt
23. Moll JW, Dziathowiak A, Rybinski K, Edelman M, Ratajczak-Pakalska E (1973) Arterialisierung des Sinus Coronarius – Indikationen, Technik, Ergebnisse. Thoraxchirurgie 21: 295
24. Moll JW, Dziatkowiak AJ, Edelman M, Iljin W, Ratajczyk-Pakalska E, Stengert K (1975) Arterialization of the coronary veins in diffuse coronary arteriosclerosis. J Cardiovasc Surg 16: 520.
25. Mundth ED, Austen WG (1975) Surgical measures for coronary heart disease (Three parts). N Engl J Med 293: 13, 75, 124
26. Park SB, Magovern GJ, Liebler GA, Dixon CM, Begg FR, Fischer DL, Dosios TJ, Gardner RS (1975) Direct selective myocardial revascularization by internal mammary artery-coronary vein anastomosis. J Thorac Cardiovasc Surg 69: 63

27. Razzuk MA (1975) In Discussion of Benedict JS, Buhl TG, Henney RP: Cardiac vein myocardial revascularization: An experimental study and report of three clinical cases. Ann Thorac Surg 20: 556
28. Williams GD, Burnett HG, Derrick BL, Miller CH (1976) Retrograde venous cardiac perfusion for myocardial revascularization: An experimental evaluation. An Thorac Surg 22: 322
29. Zajtchuk R, Heydorn WH, Miller JG, Strevey TE, Treasure RL (1976) Revascularization of the heart through the coronary veins. Ann Thorac Surg 21: 318

Authors' address:
Mark S. Hochberg, M.D.
Newark Beth Israel Medical Center
201 Lyons Avenue
Newark, New Jersey 07112, U.S.A.

Comparison of three methods of myocardial preservation: storage, intermittent and continuous perfusion

B. Walpoth[1], D. Weber[2], F. Barbalat-Rey[3], M. Schmidt[4], B. Faidutti[1], and R. Mégevand[2]

Departments of Cardiovasculuar[1] and Experimental[2] Surgery, Pharmaceutical[3] and Clinical Chemistry[4] University of Geneva, Geneva (Switzerland)

Introduction and Problems

During cardiac surgery most cases require cardiac arrest, inducing myocardial ischemia. Protection of the surgically induced ischemic myocardium can be achieved with either one of the following methods, or a combination of them: hypothermia, metabolic inhibition (cardioplegia) and perfusion. In recent years, most centres have chosen the first two, due to their simplicity, reliability and practicality. Continuous perfusion is not only more cumbersome but has some inherent risks, such as coronary dissection, inhomogeneous perfusion and myocardial edema (1, 5). Its advantages reside in an occasionally better myocardial protection due to ongoing aerobic metabolism. In recent years cold cardioplegic intermittent or continuous ante or retrograde perfusion via the coronary sinus have been advocated (2).

Basically, the same methods and principles apply to cardiac transplantation. The major difference is the lack of rewarming and washout by the non-coronary collateral circulation. For clinical applications, the safe ischemic time is around 3 to 4 hours which is a limiting factor, prohibiting an optimal donor-recipient matching and HLA typing. A longer ischemic period might also increase the number of possible donors for cardiac transplantation, who are at present very scarce. Experimentally several authors have reported good results after 24 hours of hypothermic storage or low pressure perfusion followed by successful orthopic cardiac transplantation (3, 6, 8).

Our aim was to investigate and compare all three methods under comparable experimental conditions, namely, long-term myocardial preservation with either hypothermic storage, intermittent and continuous ante and/or retrograde low pressure coronary perfusion; and to evaluate advantages and disadvantages for clinical application.

Method

Thirty-six New Zealand white rabbits were anethesized with Hypnorme (Duphar®: 10 mg Fluasion + 0.2 mg Fentanyl/ml) and ventilated via a tracheostomy. After heparinisation (3 mg/kg) hearts were removed through a sternotomy and immediately cooled by coronary flushing with a hyperkaliemic hyponatrimic, high pH and osmolality crystalloid cardioplegic solution (Stanford solution: Na^+72, K^+33, Cl^-64, HCO_3^-41 mmol/L, lidocaine

0.01%, mannitol 0.45%, dextrose 4.5%) given at 4 °C at a pressure not exceeding 40 cm of water and a flow of 10 ml/min.

Hearts were then divided into the following groups:

I. *Controls*   No ischemia, immediate evaluation

II. *Storage*   Small volume (30 ml)

III. *Storage*   Large volume (150 ml)

IV. *Intermittent perfusion*

Repeated cardioplegic flush (10 ml/kg) every six hours at 4 °C.

V. *Continuous antegrade coronary perfusion*

Via the aortic root (1 cc/kg), pressure below 25 cm of water.

VI. *Continuous retrograde coronary perfusion*

Via the coronary sinus (1 cc/kg) pressure below 25 cm of water.

Except for the control group, all hearts were flushed, stored or perfused with the same solution (Stanford cardioplegia) at 0 °C, on ice and kept ischemic for 24 hours before evaluation.

The following parameters were assessed at the beginning and at the end of the ischemic period:

● Left ventricular compliance (LV volume), the time to and the force of the ischemic contracture (after rewarming the hearts in normothermic saline) (7).

● pH, PO_2, PCO_2, glycolysis, lactate production, and cardiac enzymes (CPK, LDH) and water content.

● The high energy phosphate stores of phosphocreatine (PC) and adenosine-triphosphate (ATP) and internal pH were measured by phosphorus nuclear magnetic resonance (31P NMR: Spectrospin, 81.85 MHz).

● Perfusion parameters in the form of temperature flow and pressure were continuously recorded.

Results are expressed as means ± standard deviation (SD). Statistical analysis included unpaired T tests (Wilcoxon) and linear regressions.

Results (Consult Table 1)

Comparison of the control to the ischemic hearts showed a significant ($p < 0.05$) decrease of left ventricular compliance (LV volume), the time and force to ischemic contracture, and the high energy phosphate stores (see Figure 1 and Table 1). After 24 hours no more PC could be found by 31 P NMR and only little ATP was left. There is a loss of visible phosphate in groups V and VI (continuous perfusion) due probably to washout. In addition, the global pH was measured in each group and showed: I. 7.6, II 7.2, III 7.5, IV 7.3, V 7.9, VI 7.9 (see Figure 2).

There were no significant differences between hearts stored in small volumes as compared to hearts stored in large volumes.

Comparing the storage groups to the perfusion groups we could demonstrate a significant increase in the coronary vascular resistance (3.4 vs. 46.4 cm of H_2O; $p < 0.05$) and water content (73.1 ± 3.8 vs. 85.2 ± 4.6: $p < 0.05$). In addition, these hearts used more sugar (−3.8 ± 6.8 vs. 105.9 ± 123.8: $p < 0.02$) produced more lactate (18.4 ± 20.3 vs. 119.1 ± 203.5: $p < 0.05$) and released more cardiac enzymes (CPK: 34.1 ± 45.3 vs. 440.5 ± 702.5: $p < 0.025$ and LDH: 5.8 ± 8.1 vs. 175.8 ± 277.4: $p < 0.02$). However,

Table 1. Results of controls (I), pooled storage groups (II and III) and perfusion groups (IV–VI) for the following variables: Ti = ischemic time in minutes, Vol = left ventricular compliance (volume in μl/g w.w. heart), Force = force of LV to perform the ischemic contracture (μl/g w.w.), Te = time to perform contracture in minutes, Lac = lactate production (μmol/g w.w.), Glu = glucose utilization (μmol/g w.w.), pH, PO2, PCO2 (expressed as change from the storage solution in kPa), cardiac enzymes (CPK and LDH in UL/g w.w.) and water content (O in %). Data are expressed as mean and standard deviation (S.D.). Level of significance: * p 0.05.

Variable	Controls		Storage		Perfusion	
	Mean	SD	Mean	SD	Mean	SD
Ti	0.0	0.0	24.38	0.21	24.37	0.38
Vol	132.20	118.06	* 100.20	51.44	113.77	78.95
Force	149.13	21.43	* 79.06	103.39	* 38.39	34.83
Te	29.00	8.89	12.64	10.88	* 3.56	3.22
Lac			18.41	20.27	* 119.07	203.52
Glu			-3.81	6.87	* 105.98	123.83
pH			0.56	0.31	0.26	0.56
PO2			1.97	2.17	1.19	2.27
PCO2			-4.20	2.47	-2.09	1.64
CPK			34.19	45.32	* 440.49	702.50
LDH			5.85	8.14	* 175.83	277.39
O			73.09	3.78	85.17	4.59

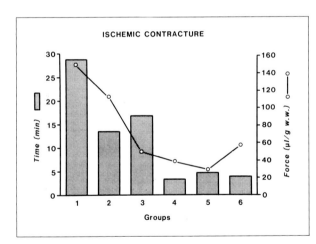

Fig. 1. Results of the ischemic contracture test for all six groups. Columns represent the time to the contracture in minutes, the line the force of contracture in μL/gm w.w. heart. There is a significant difference between the controls (I) and the storage or perfusion groups. However, the difference between the two latter groups is not significant, due to high standard deviations in groups IV, V and VI.

there were no significant differences between the antegrade or retrograde coronary perfusion groups.

No good linear correlation could be achieved between changes of pH, lactate production ($r = 0.14$) and glucose utilization.

Discussion and Conclusion

We tried to test different methods of long term hypothermic, myocardial preservation for transplantation. Our experimental set-up was designed to use standardized conditions

205

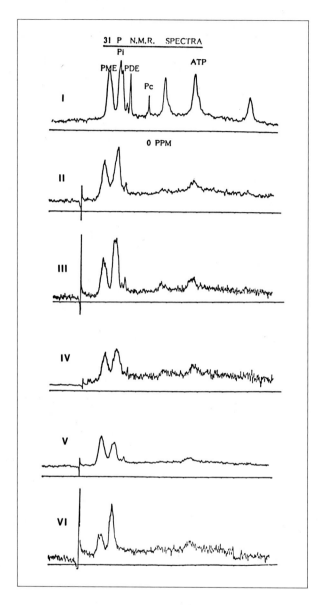

Fig. 2. Phosphorous nuclear magnetic resonance spectra (31 P NMR) of control (I) and experimental groups (II–VI). Peaks represent from left to right: phosphomonoesters, inorganic phosphorous (Pi), phosphodiesters, phosphocreatine and the three ATP peaks: γ, α, β. Each spectrum represents pooled data from each group (n = 6). The scale is in parts per million (PPM) and zeroed on the phosphocreatine peak. Note that the perfusion groups (V and VI) have lost more energy-rich phosphate compounds and even total phosphorous.

with regard to heart excision and cardioplegic arrest, using the same solution for all groups as well as identical perfusion parameters, whether ante or retro coronary perfusion was tested.

As expected, significant differences could be found between controls and ischemic groups analyzed after 24 hours. No significant differences were found between small and large volume in the storage groups, suggesting only a limited contribution of the diffusion effect, neither were there major differences between the storage and perfusion groups as regards ischemic contracture test. However, all the perfused hearts showed evidence of metabolic activity (glucose utilization) with washout of metabolites (lactate production) and enzyme release (CPK, LDH). The lack of a linear correlation between lactate production, glucose utilization and pH drop, suggests a breakdown of internal glycogen stores.

The perfused hearts required more attention and showed more differences in their results (high SD) suggesting that perfusion methods have some inherent unpredictability. Since there was evidence of a high washout rate, better results could certainly be obtained when perfusing with solutions capable of inducing a metabolic resynthesis of high energy phosphates, instead of phosphorous washout as we saw in our experiment (4).

We conclude that neither method showed significantly better results after 24 hours of hypothermic myocardial long-term preservation. The functional and metabolic results indicate more activity and possible damage in the perfused hearts and they showed more variations. In addition, no difference was found between antegrade and retrograde continuous hypothermic low pressure perfusion. Advantages of hypothermic storage are simplicity, reproducibility and fast handling for myocardial preservation and transport. We therefore think that the latter should be the method of choice in clinical, long distance heart procurement for transplantation.

References

1. Blackstone EH, Evans RH, Eckner FA, Drake A, Moulder PV (1968) Perfusion Induced Myocardial Injury. J Thorac Cardiovasc Surg 56: 689–698
2. Mohl W, Wolner E, Glogar D (1984) The Coronary Sinus. Steinkopff Verlag, Darmstadt
3. Reitz BA et al (1974) Protection of the Heart for 24 Hours with Intracellular Solution and Hypothermia. Surg Forum 25: 149
4. Rousou JH, Engelman RM, Dobbs WA, Anisimowicz L (1983) Metabolic Enhancement of Myocardial Preservation During Cardioplegic Arrest Surg Forum Vol XXXIV
5. Stemmer EA, Joy I, Aronow WS, Thibault W, McCart P, Connolly JE (1975) Preservation of Myocardial Ultrastructure. J Thorac Cardiovasc Surg 70: 666–676
6. Suzuki S, Sasaki H, Tomita E, Amemiya H (1985) Preservation of Canine Hearts for 24 Hours by Retrograde Sinus Perfusion and Orthotopic Heart Transplantation. Nippon Kyobu Geka Gakkai Zasshi 33: 139–146
7. Walpoth B, Bleese N, Modry D, Jardetzky N, Jardetzky O, Jamieson S, Shumway N (1983) Assessment of Myocardial Preservation by Ischemic Contracture and Nuclear Magnetic Resonance. Heart Transplantation Vol 2, No 4
8. Wicomb WN, Cooper DK, Novitzky D, Barnard CN (1984) Cardiac Transplantation Following Storage of the Donor Heart by a portable Hypothermic Perfusion System. Ann Thorac Surg 37 (3): 243–248

Authors' address:
Dr. B. Walpoth
Division of Cardiovascular Surgery
Department of Surgery
Hôpital Cantonal Universitaire
1211 Geneva 4, Switzerland

Efficacy of myocardial protection as reflected in blood of the right chamber during open heart surgery

I. Lengyel, E. Moravcsik, and Z. Szabó

Clinic for Cardiovascular Surgery, Semmelweis Medical University, Budapest (Hungary)

The aim of our study is to make a new approach to the pathobiochemical consequences of surgically-induced ischemia and to draw practical conclusions from it, if possible, concerning myocardial protection. Our investigations were based on 64 patients (39 male, 25 female; age: 34–53 years; mean: 41.4 years) suffering from ischemic heart disease and having undergone coronary bypass grafting. Blood samples were taken from the right heart chamber, according to our routine method (4). In each patient 24 parameters were determined involving their physiological condition, results of medical examination, surgical-technical data and laboratory values.

Patients characterized by this multifactorial system of correlations were studied further by the help of the cluster method (2), and our results were demonstrated by dendrograms (3).

Another assortment has been done according to the time the patients spent in the intensive care unit after the operation.

Thus two groups could be constructed:

1. patients who left the intensive care unit within 4 days (i.e. recovered without complication),
2. patients who spent more than 4 days in the intensive care unit (because of certain complications).

("Complications" includes anything delaying the normal course of recovery, e.g. low output syndrome, postoperative bleeding, cerebral complications, pneumonia, embolism, etc.)

Before the surgical intervention the interrelations among the several parameters (Fig. 1) are characterized by three independent clusters:

- in the first cluster the patients' anamnestic data, results of their medical examination and the therapy required are bunched together;
- the second cluster is constructed by the CK-MB activity and the myoglobin concentration in close correlation; and
- in the third cluster four laboratory parameters (CO_2, pH, lactate, glycosaminoglycan (= GAG)) are connected to each other.

In the course of the operation, components of the several clusters, as well as position and place of fusion of the objects (dendrons) change dynamically: significant differences develop between the pattern of the dendrograms representing the two groups of patients.

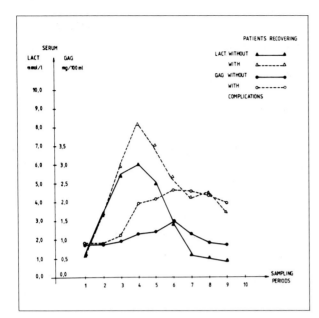

Fig. 1. Differences in lactate and GAG levels between the two groups of patients in the course of the examination.

Thus, by the end of reperfusion in group 1 (patients without postoperative complication) four surgical-technical data (aortic cross-clamping time, length of reperfusion, degree of systemic and topic hypertomia) seem to be in a good harmony with the efficacy of combined myocardial protection (Fig. 2). The laboratory values show a more moderate quantitative change than in the second group. In this stage the alterations of the O_2 level and CK-MB activity, in close correlation to the increase of the myoglobin and GAG concentrations, are supposed to be the most characteristic laboratory syndrome, which may refer to the minimal damage caused by the ischemic arrest. However, in the second group (patients with complications), only two surgical-technical factors (aortic cross-clamping time and length of reperfusion) are of great importance, and the four-fold system of pathobiochemical consequences is composed of the CK-MB, myoglobin, lactate and GAG levels (Fig. 3). Evidently, the length of aortic cross-clamping time is a direct causative factor of surgically-induced ischemia. According to the lesson of our study, the pathobiochemical response of myocardium to the challenge of global ischemia – besides the effectiveness of myocardial protection – mainly depends on the severity of the existing metabolic damage caused by chronic hypoxibiosis. While the combined hypothermic cardioplegia (1, 7), to reduce the consequences of global ischemia – and reperfusion, employed in order to wash out detrimental metabolites, are both influencing the extent of pathobiochemical response given by the myocardium, till then, the effect of persisting chronic hypoxia decreases the ischemia tolerance of the myocardium. If the balance between these two antagonistic factors, i.e. between the joint effect of chronic hypoxibiosis, plus that of acute global ischemia on the one hand, and effectiveness of myocardial protection on the other, breaks down, or cannot be evolved at all, then in all probability (0.90 > P > 0.70) complications may arise during the early postoperative period. If be-

210

cause of insufficiency of O_2 supply the citric acid cycle does not start, the metabolic process of oxidative glycolysis is interrupted at the level of pyruvate-lactate transformation. The several intermediates of the Embden-Meyerhof pathway begin to be accumulated, beginning with its end product (lactate) advancing gradually forward to the G 6-P. Thus, first the increase of the lactate concentration can be observed, followed by the concomitant exhaustion of cellular buffer capacity and the acidotic shift of the pH (8). Meanwhile the profound rearrangement of aerobic glucose catabolism involves all the possible interconnections among the various metabolic pathways (5). As a practical consequence of this the increase of lactate level in the intraoperative samples is more moderate and its return to normal is faster when patients are recovering normally; but in the case of those suffering from complications, although the ischemic increase of lactate level starts from the same level, it reaches a higher peak and remains on an elevated level if the complication persists.

When the congestion of intermediates of the Embden-Meyerhof pathway reaches G 6-P, a unique metabolic sideway may be opened up (Fig. 4): the GAG synthesis starts (6).

According to our opinion the overproduction of GAGs and their appearance in a higher concentration in the extracellular fluid may have a whole series of immediate and late pathologic consequences, concerning edema formation, distribution of bivalent cations and changing the quality and quantity of developing scar tissue in place of necrotic myocardium. Although the laboratory follow-up of lactate and GAG overproduction does not provide diagnostic information about the actual condition of the myocardium, it can be helpful in forecasting certain complications occurring in the early postoperative period.

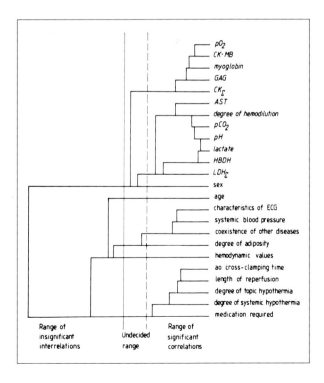

Fig. 2. Interrelations among the parameters at the end of reperfusion.

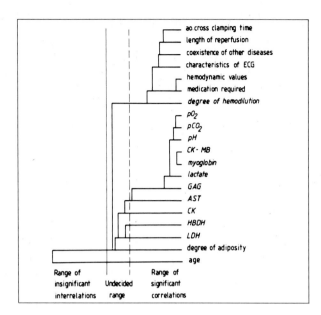

Fig. 3. Interrelations among the parameters at the end of reperfusion in patients with postoperative complications.

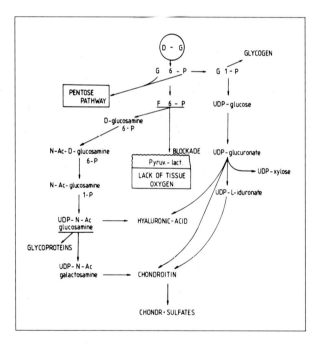

Fig. 4. Proposed scheme for GAG biosynthesis.

References

1. Bretschneider HJ (1980) Myocardial protection. Thorac Cardiovasc Surg 28: 295–302
2. Hartigan J (1975) Clustering Algorithms. Wiley, New York

3. Lance GN, Williams WT (1967) A general theory of classificatory storing strategies. 1. Hierarchical systems. Comp J 9: 373–80
4. Lengyel I, Szabó Z (1984) Myocardial protection, complex laboratory examinations and their computerized evaluation. In: Mohl W et al (eds) The Coronary Sinus. Steinkopff Verlag, Darmstadt, pp 194–201
5. Liedtke AJ (1981) Alterations of carbohydrate and lipid metabolism in acutely ischemic heart. Progr Cardiovasc Dis 23: 321–36
6. Phelps CF (1973) The biosynthesis of glycosaminoglycans. Biochem Soc Trans 1: 814–9
7. Refsum H, Jynge P, Mjös OD (1983) Myocardial Ischemia and Protection. Churchill Livingstone Edinburgh London Melbourne New York, pp 181–202
8. Taegtmeyer H (1985) Carbohydrate interconnections and energy production. Circulation 72: 1–8

Authors' address:
I. Lengyel, M.D.
Clinic for Cardiovascular Surgery
Semmelweis Medical University
Budapest XIII, Varosmajor u. 68.1122
Hungary

Retrograde coronary sinus cardioplegia – influence on fatty acid metabolism during myocardial ischemia[1]

R. M. Engelman, D. K. Das, H. Otani, J. A. Rousou, and R. Breyer

The Departments of Surgery, The University of Connecticut Health Center, Farmington, CT, and the Baystate Medical Center, Springfield, MA (U.S.A.)

Introduction

Publications abound on the success of antegrade hypothermic chemical cardioplegia on protecting myocardial function and viability during induced global ischemia (6). In recent years, benefits have been demonstrated equally for coronary sinus cardioplegia based upon comparable studies in similar models (10). The present study was designed to evaluate a completely different approach to monitoring myocardial preservation during cardioplegic arrest. It has long been known that the effects of induced ischemia on myocardial muscle inhibit fatty acid β-oxidation, thus decreasing the availability of acetyl CoA to enter the Krebs cycle and prevent regeneration of ATP (5). Additionally, long-chain acyl CoA and acyl carnitine accumulate within the cell and have been shown to have detergent properties harmful to both membrane and enzyme function (2). No work has been reported in the ischemic heart model using cardioplegic preservation to determine how hypothermic chemical cardioplegia influences the changes seen in fatty acid metabolism during ischemia. The present study was designed to evaluate this.

Methods

Twenty-four pigs, weighing between 23 and 42 kg, were placed on cardiopulmonary bypass and the hearts isolated in an in vivo perfusion apparatus previously published by our group (3). Ten animals, serving as control, had normothermic global ischemia of 40 minutes followed by 60 minutes of normothermic reperfusion. The second group of seven animals had hypothermic crystalloid cardioplegic arrest using a 35 mEq/L potassium solution based on an extracellular formulation. Cardioplegia in these animals was administered via the antegrade or coronary artery route. The cardioplegia was administered at 4–8 °C and the hearts further cooled to 10 °C by submersion in a cooled saline bath. After 40 minutes of protected ischemia, 60 minutes of normothermic reperfusion was induced. Antegrade cardioplegia was administered in a dose of 50 ml every 15 minutes during the 40 minute ischemic interval. The third group of seven animals underwent hypothermic crystalloid cardioplegic infusion in a retrograde fashion through the coronary si-

[1] Supported by NIH Grant No. 22559-05 from the Heart and Lung Institute

nus. The solution was administered at a fixed rate of 40 cc/min throughout the full duration of the 40 minute ischemic interval such that a total volume of 1.6 liters of cardioplegia was administered via the retrograde route in comparison to only about 200 ml administered in the antegrade fashion. Myocardial temperature in both groups was maintained at a hypothermic level by submersion in a cool saline bath.

Biopsies were taken from the free wall of the left ventricle using a cooled modified dental drill and immediately placed in liquid nitrogen for lipid and high energy phosphate determinations before, during and following ischemia such that a total of four samples were taken from each animal.

The biochemical methods for determination of fatty acid metabolites are enzymatic techniques which are readily performed (4, 7, 9). ATP analysis was carried out using standard HPLC methods (1).

Results

Normothermic ischemia, without the benefit of either hypothermia or cardioplegia, results in a striking and significant (p < 0.001) decrease in carnitine, acetyl carnitine, CoA, acetyl CoA, and ATP levels. These are illustrated graphically in Figures 1–8. Additionally, there is a concomitant increase in the level of long-chain acyl CoA, long-chain acyl carnitine, and the ratio of NADII/NAD.

All of these markedly detrimental metabolic changes are significantly (p < 0.001) improved when hypothermic cardioplegic preservation is employed. As can be seen in Figures 1–8, there is no significant difference between the antegrade and retrograde administration of cardioplegia and both are equally effective in preventing accumulation of the degradation products of β-oxidation. It is apparent, however, that even with hypothermic cardioplegia, electron transport as measured by the NADH/NAD ratio remains inhibited following ischemia and reperfusion, resulting in the accumulation of NADH and resultant depression of oxidative phosphorylation. Nonetheless, cardioplegia provides significantly elevated levels of carnitine, acetyl CoA and ATP compared to the normothermic

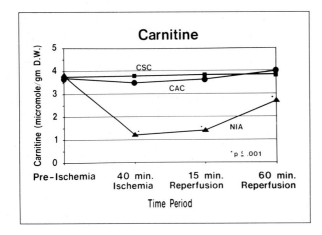

Fig. 1. Changes in intracellular carnitine level induced by 40 min of ischemia and 60 min of reperfusion, comparing normothermic ischemia (NIA) with antegrade or coronary artery cardioplegia (CAC) and retrograde or coronary sinus cardioplegia (CSC).

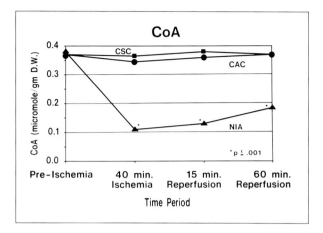

Fig. 2. Changes in intracellular Co-A level induced by 40 min of ischemia and 60 min of reperfusion, comparing normothermic ischemia (NIA) with antegrade or coronary artery cardioplegia (CAC) and retrograde or coronary sinus cardioplegia (CSC).

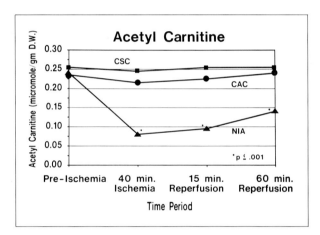

Fig. 3. Changes in intracellular acetyl carnitine level induced by 40 min of ischemia and 60 min of reperfusion, comparing normothermic ischemia (NIA) with antegrade or coronary artery cardioplegia (CAC) and retrograde or coronary sinus cardioplegia (CSC).

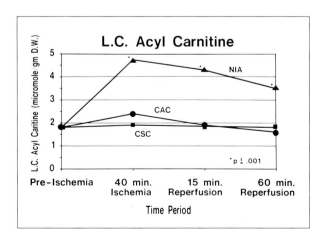

Fig. 4. Changes in intracellular long chain acyl carnitine level induced by 40 min of ischemia and 60 min of reperfusion, comparing normothermic ischemia (NIA) with antegrade or coronary artery cardioplegia (CAC) and retrograde or coronary sinus cardioplegia (CSC).

217

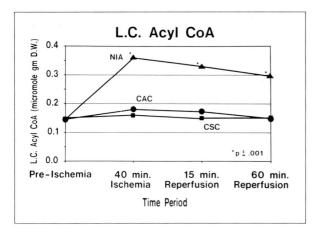

Fig. 5. Changes in intracellular long chain acyl CoA level induced by 40 min of ischemia and 60 min of reperfusion, comparing normothermic ischemia (NIA) with antegrade or coronary artery cardioplegia (CAC) and retrograde or coronary sinus cardioplegia (CSC).

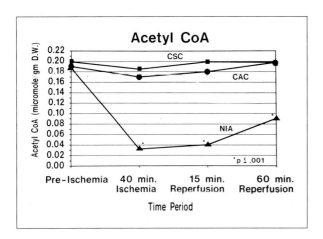

Fig. 6. Changes in intracellular acetyl CoA level induced by 40 min of ischemia and 60 min of reperfusion, comparing normothermic ischemia (NIA) with antegrade or coronary artery cardioplegia (CAC) and retrograde or coronary sinus cardioplegia (CSC).

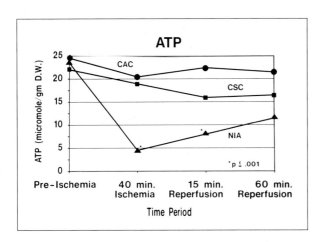

Fig. 7. Changes in intracellular ATP level induced by 40 min of ischemia and 60 min of reperfusion, comparing normothermic ischemia (NIA) with antegrade or coronary artery cardioplegia (CAC) and retrograde or coronary sinus cardioplegia (CSC).

218

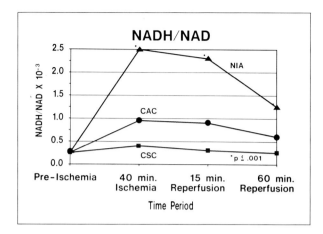

Fig. 8. Changes in the level of reducing equivalent (NADH/NAD ratio) induced by 40 min of ischemia and 60 min of reperfusion, comparing normothermic ischemia (NIA) with antegrade or coronary artery cardioplegia (CAC) and retrograde or coronary sinus cardioplegia (CSC).

ischemic arrest group. Further, there are significantly lower levels of long-chain fatty acid metabolites accumulating both during arrest and reperfusion in the cardioplegia group. It is only in the cardioplegia groups that both acyl carnitine and acyl CoA return to control levels during reperfusion. They remain significantly elevated in the unprotected, normothermic ischemic group.

Discussion

The changes in fatty acid metabolism induced by ischemia are complex and interrelated with those present in carbohydrate utilization (8). While in the normal, non-ischemic heart, fatty acid is a preferred substrate for energy utilization, during ischemia, as shown in this study, fatty acid utilization is halted because of the inhibition of β-oxidation (11). This study has shown that two differing methods of cardioplegic administration, antegrade and retrograde, both serve equally well to allow maintenance of near normal metabolite levels (acyl CoA and acyl carnitine) during protected ischemia. The fact that NADH/NAD levels rise at all during the ischemic event is, however, evidence that inhibition of β-oxidation is still a factor in the protected hypothermic heart. This is certainly to be expected from what we know about the influence of hypothermic cardioplegia on cellular metabolism and the fact that cardioplegia is not totally protective.

The importance of this study rests with the validation of the return of metabolic function following resumption of perfusion. In the unprotected group, there is evidence of continuing elevation of fatty acid intermediate metabolites after completion of the reperfusion interval. However, in the cardioplegic-protected groups, the levels of these intermediaries have all returned to normal, indicating resumption of β-oxidation in this group. This is supportive of the contention that cardioplegic preservation does preserve myocardial metabolic function. Further, there is now support that both antegrade and retrograde cardioplegia provide comparable degrees of metabolic protection during induced global ischemia.

References

1. Brown PR, Krstulovic AM, Hartwick RA (1980) Current state of the art in the HPLC Analyses of free nucleotides, nucleosides, and bases in biological fluids. In Giddings JC (ed) Advances in Chromatography. Marcel Dekker, Inc, New York and Basel, pp 101–138
2. Chien KR, Sen A, Buja LM, Willerson JT (1983) Fatty acylcarnitine accumulation and membrane injury in ischemic canine myocardium. Am J Cardiol 52: 893–897
3. Engelman RM, Rousou JH, Dobbs W, Pels MA, Longo F (1980) The superiority of blood cardioplegia in myocardial preservation. Circ Supp 62: I-64-I-66
4. Gutmann I, Wahlefeld AW (1974) L-(+)-Lactate determination with lactate dehydrogenase and NAD. In: Bergmeyer HU (ed) Methods of Enzymatic Analysis. Verlag Chemie Intl. Deerfield Beach, FL, Vol 3, pp 1464–1468
5. Liedtke AJ (1981) Alterations of carbohydrate and lipid metabolism in the acutely ischemic heart. Prog Cardiovasc Dis 23: 321–336
6. McGoon DC (1985) The ongoing quest for ideal myocardial protection. J Thorac Cardiovasc Surg 89: 639–653
7. Michal G, Bergmeyer HU (1974) Coenzyme A. In: Bergmeyer HU (ed) Methods of Enzymatic Analysis. Verlag Chemie Intl, Deerfield Beach, FL, Vol 4, pp 1967–1980
8. Neely JR, Morgan HE (1974) Relationship between carbohydrate and lipid metabolism and the energy balance of heart muscle. Physiol Rev 14: 413–459
9. Pearson DJ, Chase JFA, Tubbs PK (1969) The assay of (–)-carnitine and its O-acyl derivatives. Methods Enzymol 14: 612–622
10. Schaper J, Walter P, Scheld H, Hehrlein F (1985) The effects of retrograde perfusion of cardioplegic solution in cardiac operations. J Thorac Cardiovasc Surg 90: 882–887
11. Whitmer JT, Idell-Wenger JA, Rovetto MJ, Neely JR (1978) Control of fatty acid metabolism in ischemic and hypoxic hearts. J Biol Chem 253: 4305–4309

Authors' address:
Richard M. Engelman, M.D.
The Baystate Medical Center
759 Chestnut Street
Springfield, MA 01107
U.S.A.

Coronary sinus versus antegrade aortic cardioplegia: myocardial protection during two hours of global ischemia[1]

J. P. Goldstein, D. R. Salter, A. S. Abd-Elfattah, C. E. Murphy, J. J. Morris, and A. S. Wechsler

Duke University Medical Center, Department of Surgery, Durham, North Carolina (U.S.A.)

Hypothermic, hyperkalemic cardioplegia, infused through the aortic root, is widely used for myocardial preservation during cardiac surgery. This technique, involving multiple reinfusions of cardioplegia and application of topical cooling, has been shown to be simple and effective, allowing good myocardial preservation after two hours of ischemia (2, 6).

Antegrade aortic root cardioplegia, however, may not always be suitable in the presence of severe proximal coronary arterial stenosis or severe aortic valvular insufficiency. Moreover, in some clinical situations, such as cardiac transplantation and aortic valve replacement, antegrade cardioplegia may be technically difficult. To overcome the problem of cardioplegic solution delivery, a retrograde approach via the coronary sinus has been proposed (1).

The present study, performed on dogs, was designed to evaluate the efficacy of retrograde coronary sinus cardioplegia (CSCP), with or without topical hypothermia, as compared to classical antegrade cardioplegia. Myocardial function was evaluated using a sensitive, load-independent index of contractility and ATP levels were measured to evaluate myocardial preservation.

Materials and methods

Twenty-three dogs were subjected to two hours of global myocardial ischemia on cardiopulmonary bypass. Systemic hypothermia to 28 °C and high potassium, cold crystalloid, cardioplegia were used. The dogs were divided into three groups. In Group 1 (n = 7), antegrade cardioplegia was delivered via the aortic root (20 ml/kg as a bolus followed by 10 ml/kg every 20 minutes) in association with topical cooling. In Group 2 (n = 7), CSCP was infused continuously into the coronary sinus through a 12 French Foley catheter introduced under direct vision. The average flow ranged from 20 to 25 ml/min. Topical cooling was also used in this group. In Group 3 (n= 9), CSCP was administered using the

---
[1] Supported by NIH Grant # HL 26302

same protocol as in Group 2 but without topical hypothermia to identify the specific effect of CSCP on myocardial preservation.

To evaluate left ventricular (LV) function, a micromanometer-tipped catheter was inserted through the apex and LV minor axis dimension was measured by sonomicrometry. Following stabilization LV function was assessed using simultaneous determination of pressure and dimension. Stroke work (SW) was calculated as the area of the work loop for each cardiac cycle over a range of end-diastolic volumes obtained during gradual unclamping of the bypass pump venous cannula. LV function was described by the linear and load-independent SW/end-diastolic length (EDL) relationship (4) and was determined in triplicate before ischemia and after 30 and 60 minutes of reperfusion.

Myocardial biopsies were obtained before ischemia, at the end of ischemia, and after 60 minutes of reperfusion using Tru-cut needles. Myocardial adenine nucleotides were separated using high-pressure liquid chromatography (HPLC) and measured using ultraviolet absorbance at 254 nm. ATP concentration was expressed as μmol/g of protein.

In all groups myocardial temperatures, obtained at 10-minute intervals, were recorded using thermistor-tipped probes inserted into the anterior and posterior walls of the left ventricle.

Statistical analysis between groups was performed using analysis of variance for repeated measurements. A p-value less than 0.05 was considered significant. All results are expressed as mean $\pm$ SEM.

Results

A significant decrease in myocardial function was observed in the 3 groups after 30 minutes of reperfusion (Table 1). However, full recovery of function occurred in the 3 groups after 60 minutes of reperfusion. No significant difference in LV performance was observed between the 3 groups at any time studied.

No significant difference in ATP concentration was observed between the 3 groups (Table 2). Moreover, there was no significant difference in ATP concentration at the end of ischemia or after 60 min minutes of reperfusion.

Myocardial temperature fell rapidly in the 3 groups with the infusion of cardioplegia. The mean myocardial temperature of the LV during cardioplegic arrest was significantly higher in Group 3, where no topical cooling was used (13.2 ± 0.8 vs. 6.0 ± 1.2 °C in Group 1 and 8.4 ± 1.0 °C in Group 1, $p < 0.01$).

Table 1. Evolution of SW/EDL relationship in the three experimental groups.

	Group 1	Group 2	Group 3
SW/EDL (slope) Dynes X CM^{-2} X 10^3			
Pre-ischemia	91 ± 5	84 ± 6	106 ± 6
30 min reperfusion	75 ± 6*	61 ± 8*	86 ± 11*
60 min reperfusion	85 ± 4	83 ± 7	98 ± 10

mean $\pm$ SEM; * $p < 0.05$ vs. control

Table 2. Evolution of left ventricular ATP in the three experimental groups.

	Group 1	Group 2	Group 3
ATP (μmol/g protein)			
Pre-ischemia	28.2 ± 2.1	29.5 ± 1.9	30.0 ± 1.9
End-ischemia	28.3 ± 2.2	29.5 ± 1.9	35.0 ± 1.5
End-reperfusion	25.9 ± 1.3	27.6 ± 2.6	33.3 ± 2.1

Mean $\pm$ SEM

Discussion

Although the use of CSCP has gained clinical acceptance in Europe (3, 5), few research studies have been undertaken to compare antegrade and CSCP using functional and metabolic indices of myocardial recovery. In our study, CSCP, with or without topical cooling, preserved LV function after one hour of reperfusion using a highly sensitive, load-independent index of contractility (SW/EDL). Moreover, ATP was preserved in the three groups after ischemia and reperfusion despite a small increase in the mean LV temperature during ischemia in Group 3 (CSCP without topical cooling).

Therefore, this study demonstrates that CSCP, with or without topical cooling, is as effective as antegrade cardioplegia for preserving myocardial function and metabolism during two hours of ischemia.

References

1. Bolling SF, Flaherty JT, Bulkley BM, Gott VL, Gardner TJ (1983) Improved myocardial preservation during global ischemia by continuous retrograde coronary sinus perfusion. J Thorac Cardiovasc Surg 86: 659–666
2. Engelman RM, Rousou JM, Vertrees RA, Rohrer C, Auvil J (1980) Safety of prolonged ischemic arrest using hypothermic cardioplegia. J Thorac Cardiovasc Surg 79: 705–712
3. Fuentes M, Batanero J, Robles D, Martinez A, Garcia J, Casinello N (1984) Cardioplegia via the coronary sinus. Our experience in 331 cases. In: Mohl W, Wolner E, Glogar D (eds) The Coronary Sinus. Steinkopff Verlag, Darmstadt, pp 316–319
4. Glower DD, Spratt JA, Snow ND, Kabas JS, Davis JW, Olsen CO, Tyson GS, Sabiston DC, Rankin JS (1985) Linearity of the Frank-Starling relationship in the intact heart: the concept of preload recruitable stroke work. Circulation 71: 994–1009
5. Menasché P, Kural S, Fauchet M, Lavergne A, Commin P, Bercot M, Touchot B, Georgiopoulos G, Piwnica A (1982) Retrograde coronary sinus perfusion: a safe alternative for ensuring cardioplegic delivery in aortic valve surgery. Ann Thorac Surg 34: 647–657
6. Silverman NA, Wright R, Levitsky S, Schmitt G, Feinberg H (1985) Efficacy of crystalloid cardioplegic solutions in patients undergoing myocardial revascularization. J Thorac Cardiovasc Surg 89: 90–96

Authors' address:
A. S. Wechsler, M.D.
Duke University Medical Center
Department of Surgery
Box 3174
Durham, North Carolina 27710
U.S.A.

Myocardial protection by retroperfusion of the coronary sinus with cardioplegic solution in valve surgery

M. Botta, F. Scribani Rossi, L. Beretta, A. Morandi, and C. Santoli

Department of Thoracic and Cardiovascular Surgery, "L. Sacco" Hospital, Milan, Italy

Retroperfusion of the coronary sinus (RCSP) has recently raised interest as a means of myocardial protection. This paper reports our experience in order to test the effectiveness of the RCSP as compared to the traditional antegrade method in valve surgery.

Materials and methods

Thirty consecutive patients, undergoing operation for rheumatic valvulopathy, were divided into two groups according to the method of cardioplegic delivery:
– Group 1 included 20 patients (8 males and 12 females aged from 25 to 61 years) undergoing mitral valve replacement (4 patients), aortic valve replacement (10 patients), aortic and mitral valve replacement (4 patients), mitral valve replacement and tricuspidal valve reconstruction (2 patients). These patients received the cardioplegic solution by RCSP.
– Group 2 included 10 patients (6 male and 4 female aged from 29 to 60 years) undergoing mitral valve replacement (4 patients), aortic valve replacement (3 patients), mitral valve replacement and tricuspid valve reconstruction (2 patients), mitral and tricuspid valve reconstruction (1 patient). These patients received the cardioplegic solution by anterograde coronary perfusion (ACP).

Cardioplegic techniques

Group 1: after the aorta was clamped a Foley catheter (14–16 F) was inserted into the CS through a short right atriotomy. Once correctly positioned the balloon was inflated and secured in the proximal position of the CS, cardioplegic solution was infused at a flow rate of 150 ml/min with an initial dose of 1,000 ml. Further infusions were repeated every 20 minutes at a dose of 300 ml/m². Group 2 (ACP): the cardioplegic solution was infused at the same doses and timing as Group 1 into the ascending aorta and at a flow rate of 300 ml/m.
In both Groups the pericardial cavity was intermittently irrigated with ice saline solution for topical cooling.
The patients of both Groups were comparable by pathology, age, NYHA Class and haemodynamic pattern. The coronary arteries were normal in all the patients.
All the patients were operated on with standard techniques with regard to cardiopulmonary bypass (CPB) (cannulation of ascending aorta and both venae cavae), systemic hypothermia and haemodilution.

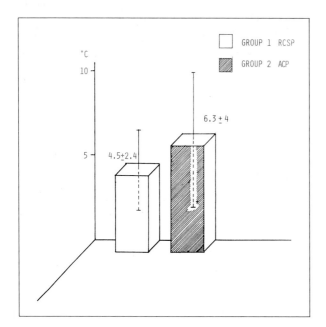

Fig. 1. Myocardial temperature: mean of all values ± S.D. (p > 0.05).

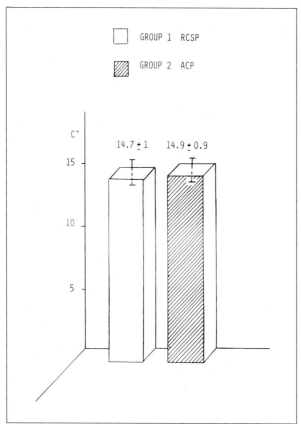

Fig. 2. Myocardial temperature: difference between maximal and minimal temperature in each case; mean value ± S.D. (p < 0.05).

Both Groups of patients were compared by aortic cross-clamping time, difficulty of weaning from CPB, postoperative complications (i.e. need of inotropic support, arrythmias, ECG change, mortality rate). In addition, the following measurements were recorded:
– myocardial temperature from interventricular septum during the entire cross-clamping time.
– myocardial lactate extraction, evaluated by arterial and coronary sinus (CS) samples taken simultaneously; just before aorta cross-clamping and again 1 and 10 minutes after coronary reperfusion. Myocardial lactate extraction was calculated by the formula: (arterial lactate – CS lactate / arterial lactate × 100). Statistical analysis was performed using Student's t-test.

Results

No death and no myocardial infarction occurred in either Group. No significant difference was found between the two Groups with respect to need of inotropic support. Aorta

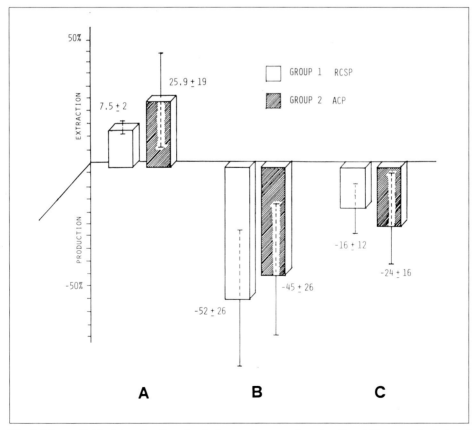

Fig. 3. Myocardial lactate extraction. A = before aortic cross clamping, B and C = respectively 1 and 10 minutes after coronary reperfusion.

227

cross-clamping time was longer in Group 1 (60.4 ± 5.8 min vs. 48.4 ± 6.2 min). In both Groups the induction of electromechanical quiescence was extended for 120 s and myocardial temperature during the whole cross-clamping time was < 20 °C. With regard to myocardial temperature the mean of all values recorded in the two Groups did not statistically differ (Fig. 1). The mean of the difference between maximal and minimal temperature recorded in each case, given as an index of uniformity of myocardial cooling was lower ($p < 0.05$) in Group 1 (Fig. 2). No significant difference was found between the two Groups with respect to myocardial lactate extraction (Fig. 3).

In one patient from Group 1 a small laceration of the CS wall occurred (probably by over-inflation of the Foley balloon) and it was easily repaired before weaning from CPB.

Conclusions

RCSP is a safe and effective method of cardioplegic delivery for the protection of ischemic myocardium. Considering the advantages provided from the technical point of view (RCSP can be repeated without interrupting the surgical procedure and avoids the selective cannulation of the coronary ostia) we recommended the use of RCSP in the aortic valve and multivalvular surgery.

References available from the author.

Authors' address:
Professor C. Santoli
Ospedale "L. Sacco"
Division di Chirurgia Toracia e Cardiovasculare
Via G. B. Grassi, 74
20157 Milan, Italy

Retrograde versus antegrade cardioplegia for myocardial protection in coronary artery bypass graft surgery

P. Fundarò, M. Salati, L. Beretta, and C. Santoli

Department of Thoracic and Cardiovascular Surgery, "L. Sacco" Hospital, Milan, Italy

The improvement of myocardial protection remains one of the most interesting current investigations in the field of cardiac surgery. We have begun to use an alternative cardioplegic technique which delivers cardioplegic solution via the coronary sinus (CS), providing retrograde coronary perfusion. This paper reports our experience in order to test the effectiveness of retrograde coronary perfusion (RCSP) as compared to the traditional antegrade method in coronary bypass surgery.

Materials and methods

Twenty-five patients undergoing coronary artery revascularization were divided into two groups according to the method of cardioplegia (CPL) delivery: 15 patients (Group 1) received the CPL solution via CS and 10 patients (Group 2) received it via antegrade coronary perfusion (ACP). The preoperative clinical characteristics were similar in the two groups (Table 1).

Table 1. Clinical characteristics of patients.

	Group 1 (n = 15) mean ± SD	Group 2 (n = 10) mean ± SD
Age	53.8 ± 8.9	56.8 ± 6.9
Sex distribution (male/female)	13/ 2	9/ 2
Type of angina		
– by effort	8	4
– mixed	7	6
Previous M.I.	11/15	7/10
Ejection fraction < 40%	3/15	1/10
Coronary disease		
– three vessels	12/15	6/10
– two vessels	3/15	4/10
– * left main	2/15	1/10

M.I., myocardial infarction; * already considered in the three vessels group

CPL Techniques

A "St. Thomas" CPL solution cooled at 4 °–6 °C was employed and the flow rate was controlled by a roller pump.

Group 1: RCSP. After the aorta was clamped, a balloon-tipped catheter was inserted into the CS through a short right atriotomy. Once the balloon was secured in the proximal portion of the CS, CPL solution was infused at a flow rate of 100 ml/min, with an initial dose of 1000 ml. Further infusions were repeated precisely every 20 min at the same flow and with a dose of 300 ml/m². The left ventricle was vented by a 16 French catheter inserted through the aortic root.

Group 2: ACP. The CPL solution was infused through the aortic root at a flow rate of 300 ml/min and with an initial dose of 1000 ml. Further infusions were repeated every 20 min, according to the surgical procedure at the same flow rate and with a dose of 300 ml/m².

Measurements

The following measurements were recorded:
– Cardiac output (CO) was measured by the thermodilution technique before the cardiopulmonary bypass institution and 30 min after its discontinuation.
– Temperature recordings were obtained from three different sites: distal interventricular septum, posterior wall of the right ventricle, midway lateral wall of the left ventricle. All measurements were taken immediately after the administration of the first dose of CPL solution.
– Arterial blood myocardial-specific creatine kinase (CK-MB) measurements were taken before anesthesia induction, at skin incision, in cardiopulmonary bypass before the aortic cross-clamping, and 1, 20, and 60 min after releasing the aortic cross-clamp. CK-MB were also measured at the 3rd, 6th, and 20th hour postoperatively. From these CK-MB determinations a myocardial injury index (MII) was derived according to Gray (2) from the formula: $MII = \sum (E \times \Delta T) \times BW \times 0.06$, where $E = CK-MB$ (IU/l), $T =$ time between consecutive blood samples (min), $BW =$ body weight (kg) and $0.06 =$ volume distribution of the enzyme.

Statistical analysis was performed by using Student's t-test, and a p value of less than 0.05 was considered significant. All the results are expressed as mean ± standard deviation of the mean.

Results

No death and no myocardial infarction occurred in either group. No significant difference appeared between the two groups with respect to number of distal coronary anastomosis, cross-clamp time, and need of peri-operative inotropic support (Table 2).

As for the cardiac index, both groups of patients exhibited a similar pattern: there was a statistically significant increase of this index after the surgical procedure: 2.6 ± 0.7 to 2.8 ± 0.4 l/min/m² (p < 0.05) in Group 1 and 2.4 ± 0.5 to 2.6 ± 0.5 l/min/m² in Group 2.

Table 2. Intra- and post-operative data of the two groups.

	Grafts/pat.	Cross-clamp time	M.I.	Inotropic support	Arrhyth-mias	Mortality
Group 1	2.5	53.8 ± 5.5	0	1	0	0
Group 2	3.0	56.3 ± 5.6	0	1	3*	0
P value	N.S.	N.S.	N.S.	N.S.	N.S.	N.S.

* atrial flutter or fibrillation

From the beginning of CPL infusion the induction time of heart electromechanical quiescence was 104.6 ± 47.7 s in Group 1, while in Group 2 it proved to be 53 ± 18.7 s ($p < 0.05$).

Temperature recordings showed that RCSP induced a deeper cooling at the level of the interventricular septum (9.8 ± 1.4 °C vs. 11.6 ± 1.9 °C; $p < 0.05$) and the posterior wall of the right ventricle (9.1 ± 2.5 °C vs. 11.1 ± 3.2 °C; $p < 0.05$) than that obtained with ACP (Fig. 1).

In the lateral wall of the left ventricle, where the lower temperatures were recorded in both groups, the antegrade CPL was a better cooler (7.5 ± 1.7 °C vs. 8.5 ± 1.4 °C; $p < 0.05$) (Fig. 1). However, the RCSP cooled better globally. In fact, the mean of the values derived from all the temperatures recorded in several sites was significantly lower in the group treated with RCSP (9.1 ± 0.9 °C vs. 10.0 ± 1.5 °C; $p < 0.05$). In order to evaluate the uniformity of cooling in the two groups, we calculate for each patient the maximal gradient between the temperatures in the three different sites: the mean of these values proved to be lower in Group 1 (2.9 ± 1.1 °C vs. 5.9 ± 2.9 °C; $p < 0.05$), thus suggesting a more uniform cooling due to RCSP.

Considering serial measurements of CK-MB the higher average value was not statistically significantly greater in Group 1 than in Group 2 (37.8 ± 5.6 IU/l vs. 34.2 ± 8.9 IU/l;

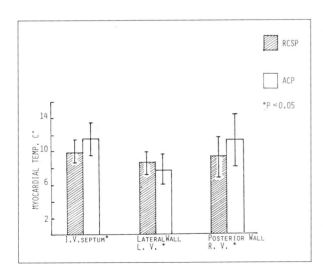

Fig. 1. Minimal myocardial temperatures: mean of the values recorded in the different sites ± standard deviation. I.V.: interventricular septum; L.V.: left ventricle; R.V.: right ventricle.

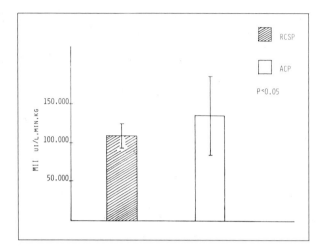

Fig. 2. Myocardial injury index (see text): mean ± standard deviation.

n.s.). The values of CK-MB elaborated as MII have shown that MII was significantly higher in Group 2 (131.008 ± 50.003 IU/l · min · kg vs. 109.328 ± 16.990 IU/l · min · kg; p < 0.05) (Fig. 2).

Discussion

Both experimental (1, 3) and clinical observations have demonstrated that RCSP provides substantial preservation of the heart during ischemic arrest. It was in order to attempt an improvement of myocardial preservation that we started this technique in coronary surgery, knowing that RCSP should avoid the maldistribution of the cold CPL solution distally to coronary artery stenosis (1, 3). In our study the clinical results and hemodynamic pattern did not show any significant difference between the two techniques. Some differences, however, have been seen. In patients of Group 1 the induction time of electromechanical quiescence was significantly longer, probably as a result of the slower rate employed with RCSP. In order to obtain a quicker electromechanical quiescence of the heart, we have progressively increased the flow rates, and at present we use flows of 150 ml/min without recording any complication.

As observed by other authors (1, 3) intra-operative myocardial temperature measurements showed that RCSP induces globally a more marked and homogeneous cooling, even if the lateral wall of the left ventricle was cooler in the group treated by ACP.

Concluding, our experience confirms that RCSP is a safe and effective method of CPL delivery. Because RCSP is more laborious to perform, it appears to be a valid alternative to the traditional ACP in patients with multiple coronary artery occlusions suggestive of maldistribution of the CPL solution.

References

1. Bolling SF, Flaherty JT, Bulkley BH, Gott VL, Gardner TJ (1983) Improved myocardial preservation during global ischemia by continuous retrograde coronary sinus perfusion. J Thorac Cardiovasc Surg 86: 659–666

2. Gray RJ, Shell WE, Conklin C, Ganz W, Shah PK, Miyamoto AT (1978) Quantification of myocardial injury during coronary artery bypass graft. Circulation 58 (Suppl 1): 38
3. Gundry SR, Kirsch MM (1984) Comparison of retrograde cardioplegia versus antegrade cardioplegia in the presence of coronary artery obstruction. Ann Thorac Surg 38: 124–127
4. Menasché P, Kural S, Fauchet M, Lavergne A, Commin P, Bercot M (1982) Retrograde coronary sinus perfusion: a safe alternative for ensuring cardioplegic delivery in aortic valve surgery. Ann Thorac Surg 36: 647

Authors' address:
Professor C. Santoli
Ospedale "L. Sacco"
Division di Chirurgia Toracia e Cardiovasculare
Via G. B. Grassi, 74
20157 Milan, Italy

Comparative study between antegrade cardioplegia and retrograde cardioplegia using intraoperative myocardial contrast echography

S. Mihaileanu, J. N. Fabiani, J. Julien, J. Viossat, G. Dreyfus, and A. Carpentier

Hôpital Broussais, Paris (France)

Introduction

Retrograde coronary sinus perfusion provides an excellent alternative for cardioplegic solution delivery in cardiac surgery (2, 6). In the presence of significant coronary stenosis, or myocardial hypertrophy, retrograde cardioplegia provides a better myocardial protection than antegrade cardioplegia (1).

Intraoperative cardioplegic delivery was found to give good myocardial echographic contrast (4). Intraoperative myocardial contrast (MC) echocardiography has been used in recent years to investigate perfusion defects after antegrade cardioplegia (AC) in coronary artery disease (CAD) patients (3, 4). Coronary venous contrast perfusion was found to reach ischaemic zones after coronary artery ligation in dogs (5).

The aim of this study was to determine if cardioplegic solutions used antegradely or retrogradely could represent a reliable echographic contrast for myocardial imaging in CAD patients and normal coronary artery (non-CAD) patients and further, if significant differences of MC exist between the two methods.

Methods

A. Patient selection

Thirty CAD patients were randomized into two groups: in group 1, 15 patients had AC followed by retrograde cardioplegia (RC), and in group 2, 15 patients had only RC. Twenty non-CAD patients were also divided into two groups: in group 1, 10 patients had AC, and in group 2, 10 patients had RC.

CAD patients had 2 to 5 vessel disease (mean value 3.2) and 7 of them exerted a myocardial infarction prior to the operation. Non-CAD patients had valvular diseases: mitral regurgitation (n = 9), mitral and aortic regurgitation (n = 6), aortic stenosis (n = 3) and mitral regurgitation plus tricuspid regurgitation (n = 2).

B. Echocardiographic technique

Intraoperative echocardiography was begun once the patient was on cardiopulmonary bypass before cardiac arrest and cardioplegic infusion. A 5 MHz transducer (Diasonics

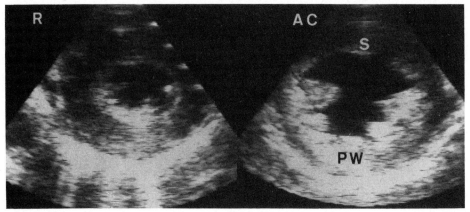

Fig. 1. 80% LAD stenosis and 90% first diagonal stenosis. Left: reference (R) short axis plane through the left ventricle. Right: lack of myocardial contrast after antegrade cardioplegia (AC) in the interventricular septum (S) and non transmural contrast in the antero-lateral segment. Intense myocardial contrast in the postero-internal segment (PW) is seen.

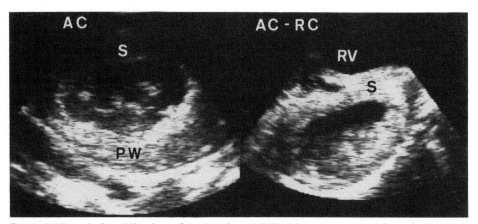

Fig. 2. LAD occlusion, 75% circumflex stenosis and 75% right coronary stenosis. Left: short axis plane through left ventricle after antegrade cardioplegia (AC). Lack of myocardial contrast in the interventricular septum (S) and the anterolateral segment is noted. 1/3 of the posterointern segment (PW) is well whitened out. Right: retrograde cardioplegia followed (AC-RC). Note the opacification of the septum (S) and the anterolateral segment. The right ventricle is dilated (RV) by the cardioplegic solution.

DRF 100 C) was directly applied on the right ventricle by the surgeon and a continuous videotape recording was started including the last 4–5 minutes before cardiac arrest and the duration of cardioplegic infusion. Echographic recording was performed in the cooling period between 37 °C and 30 °C–27 °C. When RC followed AC a second recording was obtained during the RC. A short axis plane through the left ventricle was maintained after the gain settings were carried out. Post cardioplegic images were compared for each patient to his own reference images obtained at the beginning of the examination.

C. Cardioplegic technique

1. Antegrade cardioplegia (AC): 1000 ml of cold (4 °C) hyperkaliemic solution was delivered into the aortic root by a roller perfusion pump at a high flow rate (250–350 ml/min).
2. Retrograde cardioplegia (RC): 1000 ml of cold (4 °C) hyperkaliemic solution was delivered by a roller perfusion pump directly into the right atrium according to the Fabiani technique (2), without cannulation of the sinus, after venae cava, aorta and pulmonary artery were clamped. The flow rate was also high: 250–350 ml/min. When not used alone (Group 1 CAD patients), RC immediately followed AC.

D. Echocardiographic analysis

The left ventricle was divided into 3 segments: septum, anterolateral wall and posterointern wall. LV motion before arrest and the type of arrest (systolic/diastolic) of the segments were noted.

Withing out of the myocardium after cardioplegic solution delivery was considered as echographic myocardial contrast (MC) and was compared for each patient with his own references images. A segment was considered poorly perfused if complete lack of MC was noted or if just a few patchy non-transmural contrast images occurred, not exceeding ⅓ of the segment. CAD patients had 45 segments investigated for each group and non-CAD patients had 30 segments investigated for each group.

Results

Myocardial contrast
A. CAD patients:

1. Group 1 (AC + RC): after AC only 18 segments from 45 had good MC, 27 being found with poor MC. After the RC delivery all the remaining 27 segments were well whitened out.
2. Group 2 (RC): after initial RC, 40 segments from 45 investigated had good MC and 5 segments poor MC.

B. Non-CAD patients:

1. Group 1 (AC): after AC from 30 investigated segments 24 had good MC and 6 poor MC.
2. Group 2 (RC): after RC from 30 investigated segments 27 had good MC and 3 poor MC.

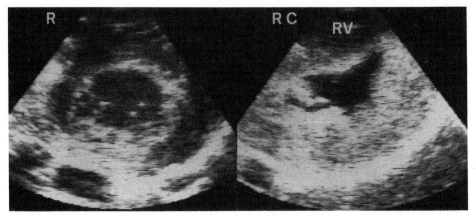

Fig. 3. Mitral regurgitation (non-CAD) patient. Left: reference (R) left ventricle short axis plane. Right: Intense whitening out of the myocardium. RV – right ventricle. Note the curved interventricular septum.

Left ventricular motion

Dyskinetic zones at the beginning of the echocardiographic recording, at 37 °–36 °C, had poor MC when AC was used. Cardiac arrest was inharmonious: some segments had a quick arrest once the temperature lowered. It seems that precocious diastolic arrest occurred in poorly perfused segments. Persistent fibrillatory movements were present in poorly whitened out zones.

When RC was used a significant dilation of the right ventricle occurred, with a secondary curving of the interventricular septum toward the left ventricle.

Discussion

Intraoperative myocardial contrast echography using cardioplegic solutions seems appropriate for myocardial imaging. However there are some limitations. In normal coronary artery patients lack of myocardial contrast occurred mainly when lower flow rates, such as 250 ml/min were used. An important question to answer is if high flow rates (Fig. 3) produced a better penetration of the fluid into the myocardium, more microbubbles or both. Probably in our model a good density of microbubbles was obtained at higher rotation of the pumping rolls, since even when poor contrast was obtained in non-CAD patients, we had good evidence of the passage of the cardioplegic solution through the myocardium. For the CAD patients, comparison of myocardial contrast after AC and after RC was performed at the same output of cardioplegic delivery in the same patient. Striking differences between AC and RC (Fig. 1 and 2), proves that in humans as in the dog experimental model (5), myocardium depending on severely stenosed coronary arteries can be reached by cardioplegic retroinfusion. The difference between our study and animal experimental studies lies in the fact that human coronary disease produces chronic myocardial changes; excellent transmural contrast obtained by retroinfusion in ischaemic zones suggests a very well maintained venular bed. When

RC was associated to AC all investigated LV segments were whitened out, demonstrating that cardioplegic retroinfusion has important advantages over AC in CAD patients. In some patients, well defined perfusion defects were found in segments with old myocardial infarctions. It is difficult to elucidate whether these defects were real avascular scars or coincidental artefacts. The cardioplegic technique by right atrial infusion provided a good and reliable left ventricular perfusion. No shunting to the right ventricular cavity occurred, due to the opposition of elevated right ventricular pressure. Dilation of the right ventricle was constant at high flow rates and associated with intense myocardial contrast. At these flow rates myocardial contrast echocardiography proved the better contrast uptake into the ischaemic myocardium when RC was used.

Unfortunately cardioplegic solutions at lower perfusion outputs do not produce a good myocardial contrast, probably due to a lower density of microbubbles. RC at lower flow rates probably has the same advantage over AC, but contrast echocardiography in this case is probably not sufficiently sensitive.

Conclusion

Intraoperative contrast echocardiography proves that in CAD patients, ischaemic zones have a much better uptake of cardioplegic solution when retrograde cardioplegia is used alone or in addition to antegrade cardioplegia.

High flow rates are important for generating a good echocardiographic myocardial contrast, giving an excellent definition between normally and poorly perfused areas. However when cardioplegic solutions are infused at lower flow rates, lack of myocardial contrast is not an argument for poor myocardial perfusion.

References

1. Chiu RCJ (1984) Cold cardioplegia via retrograde coronary sinus infusion for myocardial protection. In: Mohl W et al (eds) The Coronary sinus. Steinkopff Verlag, Darmstadt, pp 275–283
2. Fabiani JN, Relland J, Carpentier A (1984) Myocardial protection via the coronary sinus in cardiac surgery: comparative evaluation of two techniques. In: Mohl W et al (eds) The Coronary Sinus. Steinkopff Verlag, Darmstadt, pp 304–315
3. Fishbein M, Rit J, Shah PM, Corday E (1984) Verification of myocardial contrast two dimensional echocardiographic assessment of perfusion defects in ischemic myocardium. J Am Coll Cardiol 3: 34–38
4. Goldman ME, Mindich BP (1984) Intraoperative cardioplegic contrast echocardiography for assessing myocardial perfusion during open heart surgery. J Am Coll Cardiol 4: 1029–1034
5. Maurer G, Punzengruber C, Haendchen RV, Torres MAR, Meerbaum S, Corday E (1984) Penetration of coronary venous injections into ischemic myocardium. In: Mohl W et al (eds) The Coronary sinus. Steinkopff Verlag, Darmstadt, pp 167–175
6. Menasché P, Kural S, Fauchet M (1982) Retrograde coronary sinus perfusion: a safe alternative for ensuring cardioplegic delivery in aortic valve surgery. Ann Thor Surg 34: 647–659

Authors' address:
S. Mihaileanu, M.D.
Hôpital Broussais
96, rue Didot
75014 Paris
France

289 Cases of retroperfusion via the coronary sinus.
Clinical results and indications

C. Rioux, A. Leguerrier, L. Guillou, H. Le Couls, C. Mottez, J. P. Lenormand, and Y. Logeais

Department of Cardiovascular and Thoracic Surgery University Hospital, Rennes (France)

Summary: 289 patients underwent valve surgery ($\pm$ ascending aorta surgery) with myocardial protection via the coronary sinus. Comparison with 969 patients protected for the same surgery, by infusion of the same cardioplegic solution into the aortic root for the same period, shows no significant differences in terms of 1) hemodynamic improvement after bypass, 2) low cardiac output, 3) myocardial infarction, 4) mortality related with myocardial damage.
This technique seems to be very safe and the procedure of choice for:
1. isolated aortic valve replacement for aortic regurgitation,
2. multiple valve replacement,
3. valve replacement combined with multiple aorto-coronary bypasses,
4. surgery of the ascending aorta.

Between January 1st 1982 and December 31st 1985, valvular surgery was performed on 1,258 patients. For 289 patients, cardioplegic solution was administered via the coronary sinus. For the other 969 it was infused via the aortic root or in a few cases directly into the coronary ostia.

Our purpose is to compare several criteria in both groups in order to assess the effectiveness of the former technique of cardioplegic solution administration. Each patient had an initial 2000 ml infusion of the same cardioplegic solution (Ringer's lactate containing 20 meq/l of potassium chloride) with subsequent doses at 45 to 50 minute intervals of 1000 ml if necessary.

Material

The 289 patients of the "coronary sinus" series were divided into three groups, according to the number of cardioplegic infusions.

In group I, the 150 patients had one infusion only. Mean age of the patients was 58.6 years (12 to 85), and 62% of them fell within classes III and IV of the NYHA classification. Their cardiothoracic ratio (CTR) mean value was 0.56 (0.44 to 0.80). The surgical procedures comprised: 118 single, 27 double and 5 triple valve replacements, associated in 4 cases (2.7%) with plastic reconstruction of the ascending aorta or its replacement with a Dacron tube needed because of aortic aneurysm.

In group II, the 117 patients had one re-infusion. Mean age was similar, 58.2 years (9 to 77). 77.7% were in functional classes III or IV. CTR mean value was 0.57 (0.45 to 0.75).

38 single, 47 double and 26 triple valve replacements were performed, twelve of them being associated with correction of aneurysm of the ascending aorta (10.2%). 6 acute dissections, without aortic insufficiency, were treated only by replacement of the aorta with a tube.

In group III, the 22 patients had two or more re-infusions. They were older, with a mean age of 60.7 years (45 to 77). 86.4% of them fell within a critical functional class: half of them (11) in class IV and 8 in class III. However, their CTR did not differ from that of the previous group: 0.57 (0.48 to 0.71).

5 single, 3 double and 7 triple valvular replacements were performed, 5 of them combined with correction of aneurysm of the aorta (27.7%).

Emergency incidence was particularly high in this group, being 54.4% (10/20).

Mean clamping time was significantly different in the three groups: 54.8 min (28 to 91) in I; 81.4 min (45 to 118) in II and 133.8 min (99 to 194) in III.

In the "aortic root" comparison group (n = 969) patients had a better functional condition: 582 patients were in class III or IV (60%) versus 203 (70.2%) in the "coronary sinus" series (p < 0.01). There was no significant difference in age. 825 single, 121 double and 23 triple valve operations were performed, associated with surgery of the ascending aorta in 28 cases (2.9%) only.

Results

Four clinical criteria were chosen to assess the efficacy of the technique for myocardial protection.
1. Hemodynamic improvement after bypass.
2. Low cardiac output in the first postoperative days.
3. Myocardial infarction.
4. Mortality related with myocardial damage.

Hemodynamic improvement at weaning from bypass

Three grades of improvement were defined:
– grade 1: spontaneously good hemodynamic condition at weaning;
– grade 2: inotropic agents needed to restore satisfactory cardiac output level;
– grade 3: bypass assistance needed to maintain ventricular function until drugs become efficacious.

In our "coronary sinus" series, out of 289 patients, 238 (82.4%) were in grade I, 42 (14.5%) in grade 2 and 9 (3.1%) in grade 3.

In our "aortic root" series, out of 969 patients, 785 (81%) were in grade 1, 165 (17%) in grade 2, and 19 (2%) in grade 3. Statistically these results are not significantly different.

Low cardiac output

Three grades of low cardiac output (LCO) were defined, according to the presence or absence of the following criteria: either hemodynamic criteria (cardiac index < 2

242

l/mn/sqm) or clinical criteria: systolic pressure < 85 mm Hg and urine output < 20 ml/mn/sqm:
- grade 1: hemodynamic desorders are corrected in less than 6 hours with administration of inotropic agents;
- grade 2: hemodynamic insufficiency is present and needs drugs within 12 hours;
- grade 3: despite drug administration, insufficiency persists for more than 12 hours.
In our "coronary sinus" series and "aortic root" series, overall frequency of LCO was respectively:
grade 1: 7.3% (21/289) and 4.4% (43/969);
grade 2: 5.9% (17/289) and 4.4% (43/969);
grade 3: 4.5% (13/289) and 3.9% (38/969).
There is no statistically significant difference in the results of both series.

Myocardial infarction

In spite of very dissimilar clamping times in the three groups of our "coronary sinus" series, the frequency of myocardial infarction was not very different: 4.6% (7/150) in group I, 2.5% (3/117) in II, and 4.5% (1/22) in III.
Moreover, incidence of myocardial infarction in the two series was not significantly different statistically: 3.8% (11/289) and 4% (36/969), for the "coronary sinus" series and the "aortic root" series respectively.

Mortality rate related with myocardial damage

All cases of death that could be related to any myocardial damage (even though there was no electrocardiographical "q" wave or enzymatic increase) such as ventricular arrhythmias, AV conduction disturbances, irreversible low cardiac output, were included.
The results of both series were similar: 4.8% (14/289) in the "coronary sinus" series and 4% (39/969) in the other.
There is no statistically significant difference in the results of both series.

Comments

Infusion of cardioplegic solution via the coronary sinus seems to be an adequate technique for good myocardial preservation during ischemic arrest of the heart. Indeed, our investigations indicate no difference in our two series for hemodynamic improvement after bypass, low cardiac output, myocardial infarction or mortality rate related with myocardial damage.
Besides, in group III of our "coronary sinus" series, protection seems to be very effective despite a very long clamping time of the aorta ($\overline{138.8}$ mn). A low incidence of myocardial infarction was noted: 4.5% and mortality rate related to myocardial damage was satisfactory: 13.6%, in view of the severity of the preoperative functional condition and the high proportion of emergencies.

We believe that this technique of myocardial preservation is the procedure of choice in many circumstances:
– in all cases with aortic insufficiency,
– in all cases with particularly long surgical procedures such as multiple valve replacements, single valve replacement associated with multiple aorto-coronary bypasses, or
– surgery of the aorta.
In all these cases, coronary sinus infusion permits subsequent infusions of cardioplegic solution without risk of air embolism, and without interruption of the surgeon's work.

Authors' address:
Professor C. Rioux
Chirurgie Thoracique et Vasculaire
Centre Hospitalier et Universitaire de Rennes
Hôpital Pontchaillou
35033 Rennes Cedex
France

Pulsatile cardioplegia retroinfusion

O. N. Okike, D. Phillips, C. Hsi, J. M. Gore, T. J. Vander Salm, W. A. Mojica, and J. A. Alpert

Departments of Cardiothoracic Surgery, Cardiology and Radiology, University of Massachusetts Medical Center, Worcester, Massachusetts, U.S.A.

The concept of cardioplegia delivery through the coronary sinus as a mode of myocardial protection during heart surgery is relatively new. Nevertheless, this retrograde perfusion technique has been shown to provide excellent protection for ischemic myocardium (3, 5). In some reports (1, 2), retrograde coronary sinus cardioplegia has been shown to provide superior myocardial protection than antegrade cardioplegia. The observation (4) that continuous retograde coronary sinus cardioplegia causes injury to the microvasculature and induces moderate extracellular edema led us to explore the use of pulsatile cardioplegia retroinfusion. Our hypothesis is that although uninterrupted cardioplegia infusion into the coronary sinus provides provides excellent protection of the ischemic myocardium during periods of hyperkalemic arrest, this mode of cardioplegia delivery leads to a build-up of excessive pressures in the cardiac venous system and thereby causes extravasation of fluid and damage to the microvasculature. Pulsatile delivery of cardioplegia on the other hand can provide excellent myocardial protection without causing extracellular edema or damage to the microvasculature.

We therefore compared intermittent antegrade, continuous non-pulsatile coronary sinus cardioplegia and continuous pulsatile coronary sinus cardioplegia in greyhounds using re-

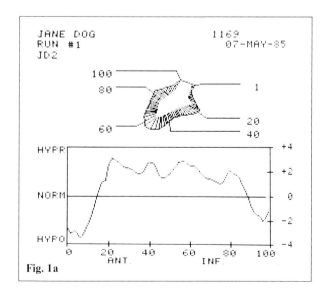

Fig. 1a

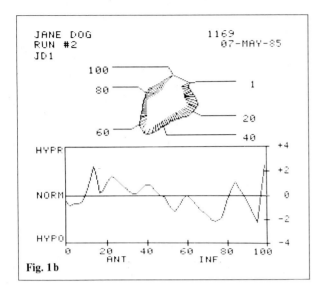

Fig. 1. Digital substraction angiogram of LV function before (1a) and after (1b) myocardial protection with antegrade cardioplegia during 2 hours of hyperkalemic arrest of hypertrophic left ventricle and occlusion of the LAD. There is impairment in the motion of the anterior wall of the left ventricle.

gional wall motion analysis, ejection fractions, myocardial ATP levels and myocardial ultrastructure as indices of myocardial protection.

Materials and methods

Healthy greyhounds weighing 25–40 kg were anesthesized with intravenous sodium pentobarbital (30 mg/kg body weight) endotracheally intubated and ventilated. Aortic, left ventricular and capillary wedge pressures were monitored on a Hewlett Packard 8 Chan-

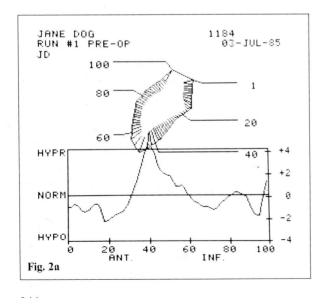

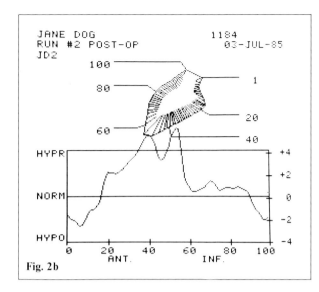

JANE DOG   1184
RUN #2 POST-OP   03-JUL-85
JD2

Fig. 2b

Fig. 2. Digital subtraction angiogram of LV function before (2a) and after (2b) myocardial protection with pulsatile coronary sinus cardioplegia during 2 hours of hyperkalemic arrest of hypertrophic left ventricle and occlusion of the LAD. Anterior wall motion is not impaired.

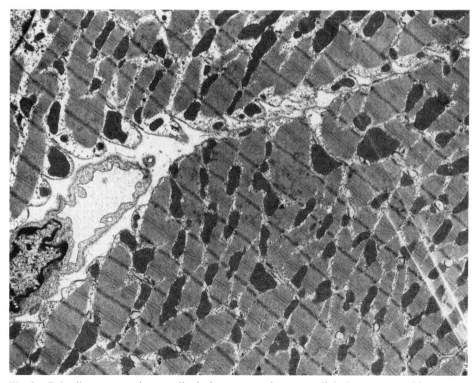

Fig. 3a. Pulsatile coronary sinus cardioplegia preserves the myocardial ultrastructure without extracellular edema.

nel Model No. 77558B Recorder. Following baseline determination of global and regional left ventricular function with digital subtraction angiographic techniques, thoracotomy was performed and total hypothermic (25 °C) cardiopulmonary bypass was established using a Shiley pediatric oxygenator. The LAD and first obtuse marginal branches of the circumflex coronary arteries were exposed.

Delivery of blood cardioplegia

The dogs were divided into three groups following aortic cross-clamping and occlusion of the LAD:

Group   I: Five dogs received cold (8 °C) blood cardioplegia at 500 cc every 20 minutes after initial 1000 cc bolus.

Group II: Five dogs received continuous non-pulsatile blood cardioplegia through the coronary sinus at 25 cc/min after initial 1000 cc given over 20 minutes.

Group III: In 10 dogs a special autoinflatable balloon-tipped retroperfusion catheter was introduced through the free wall of the right atrium into the coronary sinus and connected to a new USCI retroperfusion Pump Model EC-1 (USCI, a division of CR Bard, Inc.). Pulsatile cold (8 °C) blood cardioplegia was infused at 25 cc/min after initial 1000 cc given over 20 minutes.

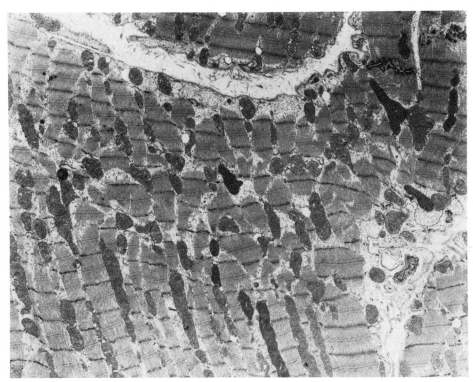

Fig. 3b. Non-pulsatile coronary sinus cardioplegia preserves the myocardial ultrastructure but shows moderate extracellular edema.

248

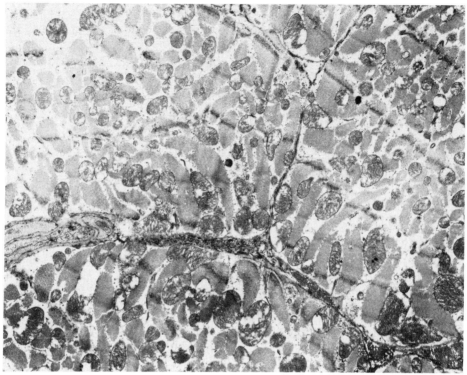

Fig. 3c. Antegrade cardioplegia provides inadequate protection of the myocardial ultrastructure. There is no extracellular edema.
(Original magnifications × 10.000)

Myocardial biopsies of the anterior wall of the left ventricle were taken with Thru-Cut biopsy needle (Travenol) at three time periods: a) before cardiopulmonary bypass, b) after 2 hours of cross-clamping and c) 1 hour after rewarming.

Results

After two hours of ischemia, the motion of the anterior wall of the left ventricle was markedly reduced in the dogs that received antegrade cardioplegia (Figure 1). In contrast pulsatile and non-pulsatile coronary sinus cardioplegia preserved the wall motion of the anterior wall of the left ventricle (Figure 2).

Similarly, myocardial ATP stores were better preserved during pulsatile and non-pulsatile coronary sinus cardioplegia than during antegrade cardioplegia infusion ($p < 0.05$).

Pulsatile coronary sinus cardioplegia showed excellent preservation of myocardial ultrastructure and almost normal extracellular space (Figure 3a). Continuous non-pulsatile cardioplegia, on the other hand, showed mild to moderate extracellular edema even though the myocardial ultrastructure was well preserved (Figure 3b). Antegrade cardioplegia caused moderate to severe ischemic injury of the myocardium (Figure 3c). There was a minimal extracellular edema. The mean pressure during the continuous coronary sinus perfusion was 25 mm Hg. In contrast pulsatile coronary sinus cardioplegia produced a peak pressure of 10 mm Hg and a mean pressure of 7 mm Hg.

Discussion

Comparison of intermittent antegrade, continuous non-pulsatile and continuous pulsatile coronary sinus cardioplegia has confirmed important differences in these modes of myocardial preservation. Pulsatile coronary sinus blood cardioplegia provided the best protection in terms of myocardial ultrastructure and virtual absence of extracellular edema.

References

1. Fabiani JN, Relland J, Carpentier A (1984) Myocardial Protection Via the Coronary Sinus in Cardiac Surgery: Comparative Evaluation of Two Techniques. In: Mohl W, Wolner E, Golgar D (eds) The Coronary Sinus. Steinkopff Verlag, Darmstadt, pp 305–311
2. Gundry S, Kirsch M (1984) A Comparison of Retrograde Cardioplegia Versus Antegrade Cardioplegia in the Presence of Coronary Artery Obstruction. Ann Thorac Surg 38: 124
3. Menasché P, Kural S, Fauchet J (1982) Retrograde Coronary Sinus Perfusion: A Safe Alternative for Ensuring Cardioplegic Delivery in Aortic Valve Surgery. Ann Thorac Surg 34: 647
4. Shaper J, Walter P, Scheld H, Hehrlien F (1985) The Effects of Retrograde Perfusion of Cardioplegia Solution in Cardiac Operations. J Thorac Cardiovasc Surg 90: 882
5. Solorzano J, Taitelbaum G, Chine RCJ (1978) Retrograde Coronary Sinus Perfusion for Myocardial Protection during Cardiopulmonary Bypass. Ann Thorac Surg 25: 201

Authors' address:
O. N. Okike, M.D.
Department of Cardiothoracic Surgery
University of Massachusetts Medical Center
Worcester, MA 01605
U.S.A.

Arterialization of the coronary sinus and retroinfusion

Synchronized retroperfusion.
Developments and current concepts

S. Meerbaum

Senior Research Scientist, Cedars Sinai Medical Center, Los Angeles, California (U.S.A.)

Introduction

The new developments in the area of synchronized retroperfusion (SRP) pertain to the recent start of selected clinical trials (5, 7, 15). We must await definitive reports on these to evaluate the extent to which past experimental studies provided an adequate basis for extrapolation to the clinical setting. In the meantime, it appears desirable to consolidate the essential conclusions from the experimental research and to further pursue the resolution of outstanding questions which may have a bearing on defining optimal operational criteria as well as limitations of the synchronized retroperfusion technique. It is in this spirit that the following older and more recent researches will be recalled. References will be kept to a minimum.

Concept rationale

Work begun in the early 1970s convinced us that the appropriate direction in the area of coronary venous retroperfusion must be a fundamental attack on the frequently reported problem of extended interruption of coronary venous drainage leading to vascular trauma, myocardial edema, hemorrhages and complications which limited application of this fundamentally attractive technique. Our earliest experimental studies in the dog had used a direct non-phased shunt from an arterial blood source to a catheter whose tip was placed deep in the great cardiac vein near its bifurcation with the anterior interventricular veins. After carrying out retroperfusion during about 90 minutes of LAD coronary artery occlusion, we studied the coronary veins and the myocardium. In almost all cases, there was ample evidence of retroperfusion-induced damage, even though the periods of treatment were about 1 hour. We therefore settled on an ECG-synchronized retroperfusion system in which the arterial blood was pumped into the great cardiac vein only in diastole and the objective was to also facilitate coronary venous drainage around the catheter during systole. We first examined this system in open chest preparations, and then proceeded to devise the single lumen autoinflatable balloon catheter which we subsequently used with synchronized retroperfusion (SRP) in a large number of closed chest dog studies.

Open chest dog studies

The initial open chest method used a simple single lumen catheter whose tip was positioned or wedged in the great cardiac vein (12). While retroperfusion pumping was definitively limited to diastole, it was not clear whether the retroinfused blood was occasionally and to some extent also shunted directly to the coronary sinus. During LAD coronary artery ligation, our measurements with myocardial gauges, local ECG probes, pressure and flow from distal to the LAD occlusion, all indicated significant but only partial effectiveness of this temporary retroperfusion treatment. We concluded that the method delivered arterial blood to the jeopardized zone and provided benefits in terms of regional contraction and reduction of ischemic injury. The observed variability of the results was of concern, and was attributed to the coronary venous shunts and inadequate catheterization with insufficient control of the catheter tip positioning or wedging within the great cardiac vein. Importantly, our study after periods equivalent to the earlier nonphased retroperfusion method indicated that limitation of retrograde pumping to diastole along with facilitation of systolic coronary venous drainage greatly reduced the incidence of apparent vascular and myocardial damage. The synchronized system thus promised safer retroperfusion applications. Parenthetically, some of our open chest preparations featured a Roller or Finger displacement pump in series with the pulsatile phased bladder pump to allow fixing a given retroperfusion flow rate.

Closed chest studies

At a time when almost all our laboratory research studies were modified to employ closed chest preparations and newly validated noninvasive measurements, we began employing the single lumen autoinflatable balloon SRP catheter in conjunction with the ECG-synchronized pump (6). The protocols were extended to allow LAD coronary artery occlusions up to 6 hours, which were occasionally followed by extended reperfusion. SRP was generally applied ½ to 1 hour postocclusion because we first wished to evaluate the treatment of acutely yet largely reversibly injured ischemic myocardium. Subsequent limited study of a 3 hour great cardiac vein SRP intervention started 3 hours after LAD occlusion, and then followed by 2 days reperfusion after the 6 hours LAD occlusion, revealed few if any benefits, suggesting that SRP treatment must be initiated early if it is to be successful. Attempts to apply coronary sinus SRP during left circumflex coronary artery occlusions led to highly variable results, and almost all of the subsequent development work concentrated on SRP treatment of LAD-subserved territory. Although the diastolic coronary venous catheter balloon occlusion and systolic collapse now proved safe and reliable, variability in SRP results persisted, presumably because of the unavoidable effects of anatomic coronary veno-venous shunting and its functional consequences depending on factors such as the retrogradely applied pressures and flows.

Nonetheless, a series of encouraging SRP results accumulated in our and other laboratories. SRP was shown to significantly increase myocardial perfusion during LAD occlusion (1). Enhancement of this perfusion up to 50% of control levels was deemed feasible, but there remains controversy about the methodology and observations. One might recall that the significance of SRP-enhanced myocardial perfusion is, of course, related to the underlying ischemic underperfusion, e.g. a small supplemental perfusion may indeed be important and even sufficient in some cases to maintain myocardial viability. Studies of function with sonomicrometry (8) and particularly with quantitative two-dimensional echocardiography (16) proved that SRP leads to significant improvement in ischemic zone cardiac function, with a more moderate enhancement of global left ventricular function. Moreover, these improvements were shown to occur within minutes of the SRP intervention (4, 16). Other studies concentrated on evidence of vascular or myocardial edema and damage to blood cells, and this experimental work in dogs indicated safety (4). Our overall conclusion is that a 6 hour SRP support in acute yet reversible ischemia is both safe and efficacious.

More recently, and after reviewing the SRP benefits as well as potential limitations, we became convinced that two further types of endeavor were indicated. On the one hand, there remained unanswered questions regarding SRP mechanisms, its optimal use and limitations of the synchronized retroperfusion method. It seemed, and still does, that further research is needed to clarify how precisely SRP achieves its effectiveness and over what range of conditions the method may achieve optimal performance. On the other hand, we observed in the canine model instances of apparently unavoidable SRP insufficiency due to anatomic and physiologic factors, which seems to call for supplementation. Thus, various modified synchronized retroperfusion and retroinfusion techniques, such as moderate retrograde hypothermic and drug retroinfusion, were aimed in such cases at reliably extending the SRP effects. As we contemplated SRP applications, we also felt the need for more data on SRP in relation to antegrade reperfusion.

Study of SRP mechanisms

Thus, our first recent moves have been back to the "drawing board", performing in vitro and in vivo studies to assess factors and determine practical criteria of retrograde coronary venous infusions. Available data are being submitted and should be published in the near future (2, 3). We corroborated in a dog study that even under optimal conditions much of the great cardiac vein retroinfusate (50% or more) will be simply shunted to the coronary sinus and the right side of the heart. Premixed radionuclide microspheres in the retroinfused blood, once delivered, were shown to be permanently entrapped in the myocardial microcirculation. The microsphere measurements elucidated some of the factors which must be considered in retroinfusion effectiveness. For example, the actual degree of retrograde delivery (i.e. whether myocardial perfusion in the jeopardized ischemic zone can be increased by 5% or to 50% or normal levels) depends crucially upon the extent, size and flow resistance of the pre-existing coronary veno-venous shunts. When the latter are large, retroperfusion effects may be severely compromised. The placement of the retroperfusion catheter is also crucial; when the catheter tip is in the coronary sinus close to its ostium, performance during LAD obstruction will be much less than when the catheter tip is advanced as far as is possible into the great cardiac vein. The catheter position is to be, in general, in as close proximity as is practicable to the myocardial territory distal to the coronary artery occlusion. The studies also showed that coronary venous retroinfusion effectiveness depends greatly on the pressure potential from the coronary veins to the zone distal to the coronary artery occlusion. Thus, when the myocardial ischemia is moderate, e.g. with end diastolic blood pressure distal to the coronary occlusion of the order of 30 mm Hg, canine study revealed very small effects of retroperfusion.

On the other hand, these effects and benefits were very pronounced when the diastolic coronary artery pressure was of the order of 10 mm Hg, as was the case in many of the dogs after LAD occlusion.

In terms of the beneficial effects of coronary venous retroperfusion and SRP, the recent in vitro and in vivo studies using radionuclide microspheres (3) clearly indicated that retroperfusion provides a highly preferential delivery to jeopardized acutely ischemic myocardium, whereas antegrade treatment tends to deliver more to the nonischemic rather than to the ischemic region. Furthermore, our recent data from closed chest dog studies provide strong evidence of a preferential retrograde delivery to the endocardium, the endo-to-epi ratio being 1.79 ± 0.21 during LAD coronary artery occlusion. It is well to remember that in the presence of pronounced acute ischemia following coronary artery occlusion, the endo-epi ratio with antegradely injected microspheres can be in the range of 0.1 to 0.5. Thus, while mentioned in previous papers, the renewed studies clearly reveal the uniquely selective features of retroperfusion. Further studies in our laboratory using digital angiography and retrograde monastral blue dye injections (2) have shown that great cardiac vein SRP delivers its diastolic flow pulses in a forceful cumulative fashion to the myocardial microcirculation, and even across capillaries into the coronary arterial bed distal to the LAD occlusion. We have also demonstrated that a significantly enhanced myocardial washout is associated with the use of great cardiac vein SRP during LAD coronary artery occlusion. These current measurements point toward further development of the SRP methodology to maximize its effectiveness.

Supplement SRP

A somewhat separate series of retroperfusion investigations were also carried out when it became clear that SRP alone may occasionally not be sufficiently effective. We studied hypothermic retroperfusion (9, 11) and also cardioactive drug retroinfusion (14) and found that further improvement of regional cardiac function and infarct salvage were possible, even in most severely jeopardized myocardial zones which were not sufficiently benefited by normothermic SRP. For thrombotic LAD coronary artery occlusions, we demonstrated in the dog that great cardiac vein retroinfusion of streptokinase allowed retrograde lysis of the LAD thrombus even while SRP provided the desired support and maintained myocardial viability (13). Retroinfusion of procainamide has been shown to be useful in terminating arrhythmias which were refractory to intravenous treatment (10). Clearly, the potential for drug retroinfusion is substantial and encompasses many possible agents. For example, current study in our and other laboratories indicates a promising potential for superoxide dismutase and catalase which have received much recent attention as treatment of myocardial ischemia and reperfusion.

SRP and reperfusion

We also asked the question: can SRP treatment of coronary occlusions alleviate the frequently encountered sudden reflow derangements, and thus serve as a useful adjunct of reperfusion? An encouraging answer was obtained in an experimental study of a 3 hour

LAD occlusion followed by 7 days reperfusion (9). Thus, myocardial edema and hemorrhages following sudden reperfusion were prevented by SRP. There were hardly any post-reflow arrhythmias, and function of the ischemic zone remained enhanced early after reperfusion, indicating avoidance or reversal of the undesirable myocardial stunning.

SRP and applications

Currently, SRP is envisioned as a temporary support to bridge periods of ischemic jeopardy which are refractory to other treatment, and are both serious and rapidly advancing toward irreversible myocardial damage. The SRP support could prove very useful for extending viability during hours or days pending definitive surgical or nonsurgical correction of coronary artery obstructions, or else during multiple brief occlusions of complex PTCA or laser procedures aimed at correction of severe coronary stenosis. Regardless of the specific applications envisioned, a few operational generalities might be kept in mind for SRP use:

1. Early venography, and possibly digital subtraction methods, should be applied to assess the specific coronary venous anatomy and the degree of coronary veno-venous shunting, as well as to reveal the placement and operation of the SRP catheter and its balloon at the particular physiologic conditions.
2. Adjustment of SRP flow, catheter tip positioning, and monitoring of the SRP-induced blood pressure within the coronary veins, are among the controls and procedures needed to reach optimal operational setting without exceeding hazardous pressures.
3. Whereas brief obstruction of coronary veins could be tolerated, and the SRP system is to make adjustments for elevated heart rate and disturbances of rhythm, attention must be paid to any persisting malfunctioning of the coronary venous SRP catheter balloon deflation or inflation.
4. For primary right coronary occlusion, SRP treatment may not be effective although moderately hypothermic SRP was shown to benefit most regions of the heart. During primary left circumflex coronary artery occlusion, SRP treatment should be administered as close as possible to the coronary sinus ostium. When LAD occlusion is accompanied by significant left circumflex stenosis, great cardiac vein SRP may be very effective because of the severe drop in blood pressure in the distal LAD.

References

1. Berdeaux A, Farcot JC, Bourdarias JP, Barry M, Bardet J, Guidicelli JF (1981) Effects of diastolic synchronized retroperfusion on regional coronary blood flow in experimental myocardial ischemia. Am J Cardiol 47: 1033–1040
2. Chang B, Drury JK, Fishbein MC, Meerbaum S, Corday E. Ischemic myocardial washout and retrograde blood delivery with synchronized coronary venous retroperfusion. Not yet published
3. Chen Sh, Chang B, Meerbaum S, Drury K, Corday E. Coronary venous retroinfusion in canine hearts: factors affecting myocardial delivery and distribution. Not yet published
4. Drury JK, Yamazaki S, Fishbein MG, Meerbaum S, Corday E (1985) Synchronized diastolic coronary venous retroperfusion: Results of a preclinical safety and efficiency study. JACC 6 (No 2): 328–35

5. Farcot J, Berland J, Cribier A, Letac B, Bourdarias JP (1985) Diastolic synchronized retroperfusion in the coronary sinus during percutaneous transluminal angioplasty: preliminary experience. Circulation 72 (Suppl III): 470 (abstr)
6. Farcot JC, Meerbaum S, Lang TW, Kaplan L, Corday E (1978) Synchronized retroperfusion of coronary veins for circulatory support of jeopardized ischemic myocardium. Am J Cardiol 21: 1191–202
7. Gore JM, Weiner BH, Sloan KM, Benotti JR, Okike N, VanderSalm TJ, Ball SP, Corrao J, Albert JS, Dalen JE (1986) Human experience with synchronized coronary sinus retroperfusion: feasibility and safety. Abstract, JACC
8. Gundry SR (1982) Modification of myocardial ischemia in normal and hypertrophied hearts utilizing diastolic retroperfusion of the coronary veins. J Thorac Cardiovasc Surg 83: 659
9. Haendchen RV, Corday E, Meerbaum S, Povzhitkov M, Rit J, Fishbein MC (1983) Prevention of ischemic injury and early reperfusion derangements by hypothermic retroperfusion. JACC 1 (4): 1067–80
10. Karagueuzian HS, Ohta M, Drury JK, Fishbein MC, Corday E, Meerbaum S, Mandel WJ, Peter T (1984) Coronary venous retroinfusion of procainamide in the management of inducible ventricular tachyarrhythmias in conscious dogs, during chronic myocardial infarction. In: Mohl W, Wolner E, Glogar D (eds): The Coronary Sinus. Steinkopff Verlag, Darmstadt, pp 385–391
11. Meerbaum S, Haendchen RV, Corday E, Povzhitkov M, Fishbein M, Rit J, Lang TW, Uchizama T, Aosaki N, Broffman J (1982) Hypothermic coronary venous phased retroperfusion: A closed chest treatment of acute myocardial ischemia. Circulation 65: 1435–1445
12. Meerbaum S, Lang TW, Osher JV et al (1976) Diastolic retroperfusion of acutely ischemic myocardium. Am J Cardiol 37: 558–98
13. Meerbaum S, Lang TW, Povzhitkov M, Haendchen R, Uchizama T, Broffman J, Corday E (1983) Retrograde lysis of coronary artery thrombus by coronary venous streptokinase administration. J Am Cardiol I: 1262–1267
14. Povzhitkov M, Haendchen RV, Meerbaum S, Fishbein M, Rit J, Corday E (1982) Protective effect of coronary venous prostaglandin El retroperfusion during acute myocardial ischemia. Am J Cardiol 49: 1017
15. Weiner BH, Gore JM, Sloan K, Benotti JR, Gaca JMJ, Okike ON, Vander-Salm TJ, Ball SP, Corroa J, Alpert JS, Dalen JE (1986) Synchronized coronary sinus retroperfusion during LAD angioplasty. Abstract JACC
16. Yamazaki S, Drury JK, Meerbaum S, Corday E (1985) Synchronized coronary venous retroperfusion: prompt improvement of left ventricular function in experimental myocardial ischemia. J Am Coll Cardiol 5: 655–63

Authors' address:
Samuel Meerbaum, Ph.D., F.A.C.C.
5741 El Canon Avenue
Woodland Hills, Ca., 91367
U.S.A.

Effect of coronary sinus (CS) retroperfusion on left ventricular function in experimental ischemia

M. G. Lepilin, R. S. Akchurin, A. A. Shiriajev, J. B. Brand, and S. A. Partigulov

All-Union Cardiological Research Center, Academy of Medical Science, Moscow (U.S.S.R.)

Summary: The effect of coronary sinus and great cardiac vein retroperfusion with arterial blood (20 ± 3 ml/min), glutamic acid (5.0 ± 0.2 mg/kg · min) and insulin (5 U/min) was studied in open-chest dogs 30 min after ligation of the left coronary artery branches and development of acute cardiac failure. A sensor-tipped catheter in the left ventricle and aorta was used. Ten dogs were treated with coronary sinus retroperfusion, 10 dogs served as control.
Six untreated animals died during 120 min of the study. At 30 min after coronary artery ligation severe depression in cardiac and stroke indices as well as in left ventricular $dp/dt_{max.}$ was noted both in control and treated animals: SI 13 ± 6 and 13 ± 5 ml/beat, respectively, CI 1.4 ± 0.6 and 1.3 ± 0.5 l/min, respectively, $dp/dt_{max.LV}$ 728 ± 124 and 620 ± 135 mm Hg · sec, respectively, SV 6 ± 3 and 7 ± 2 ml/beat, respectively. With retroperfusion significant improvement in cardiac performance and contractility was evident. By 90 min retroperfusion (120 min of myocardial ischemia) in treated dogs stroke volume increased to 12 ± 3 ml/beat, stroke index increased to 25 ± 6 ml/beat, cardiac index was 2.4 ± 0.6 l/min, and $dp/dt_{max.LV}$ increased to 1150 ± 50 mm Hg · sec. Some reduction of increased left ventricular end-diastolic pressure was noticed.
Thus, coronary sinus retroperfusion with arterial blood containing glutamic acid and insulin can improve cardiac pump function and contractility in acute cardiac failure.

Coronary venous perfusion with blood was proposed as a means to reduce myocardial ischemia at the end of the 19th century (14). Attempts at permanent surgical coronary sinus (CS) ligation and/or arterialization were only partially effective and accompanied a high incidence of myocardial edema and subsequent injury (8). Therefore interest in this form of myocardial reperfusion was lost for many years. In the 1970s methods of intermittent occlusion or synchronized diastolic retroperfusion of the CS were developed due to the progress in catheterization, perfusion and monitoring technology (1, 10). In experimental studies these methods have been shown to reduce ischemic areas and improve myocardial contractility (16).
The present study was performed to determine whether CS retroperfusion with arterial blood enriched with glutamic acid (GA) and insulin can improve the left ventricular pump function during severe ischemia and acute cardiac failure (ACF).

Methods

Twenty open-chest mongrel dogs weighing 12 to 17 kg were anesthetized with thiopental sodium (20 mg/kg intravenously) after premedication with dehydrobenzperidol (0.5 mg/kg intramuscularly). After tracheal intuabation dogs were ventilated with a volume respirator (PO-5, USSR) to maintain the P_{O_2} art. ⩾ 100 mm Hg, P_{CO_2} art. ⩽ 40 mm Hg.

The pH was maintained at 7.35 to 7.45 by sodium bicarbonate infusion. Supplemental intravenous doses of sodium thiopental were administered when needed to maintain the anesthesia. After thoractomy heparin (4 mg/kg) was administered.

A 7F catheter with pressure and flow sensors (Millar, Houston, Texas) was introduced via the left carotid artery. Pressure sensors were placed in the aorta and left ventricle, a flow velocity sensor was placed in the ascending aorta and calibrated intraoperatively with an electromagnetic flowmeter (Hellige) probe.

The 7F balloon-tipped retroperfusion catheter was introduced under fluoroscopic control through the right internal jugular vein and advanced via the right atrium and coronary sinus into the great cardiac vein. An arterial 8F catheter was inserted into the right femoral artery and attached to the perfusion pump (AIK-5, USSR). An infusion line with GA (5.0 ± 0.2 mg/kg.min) and insulin (5U/min) was connected to the retroperfusion catheter just near the pump outlet. A retroperfusion roller pump delivered the continuous flow directed to the great cardiac vein during distole by balloon inflation with an ECG-synchronized IABP console. The calculated fraction of active diastolic flow was 20 ± 3 ml/min.

After thoracotomy and pericardiotomy the left anterior descending coronary artery and some branches of left and circumflex coronary artery were ligated step-by-step until ACF signs (left ventricular end-diastolic pressure elevation, 20% or more drop in mean arterial pressure, cardiac index lower than 2.0 l/min.m2) were evident. Ten randomized animals underwent CS retroperfusion from 30 min to 120 min of myocardial ischemia. Ten control dogs had no treatment during 120 min after coronary occlusion. Hemodynamic variables were obtained in the baseline pre-occlusion state and after 15, 30, 45, 60, 75, 90, 105, and 120 min of myocardial ischemia. At the end of the study the dogs were sacrificed and pathologic inspection of CS and cardiac vein intima was performed to detect the post-retroperfusion injury.

All data are expressed as mean ± standard deviation. Data obtained during CS retroperfusion were compared with control group data and with pre-retroperfusion variables in ACF state (treatment group). Differences were compared using Student's t-test for paired and unpaired data. The level of significance was set at a probability value of less than 0.05.

Results

Of 20 dogs studied 4 had evidence of ACF after ligation of the distal portion of the left descending coronary artery, 12 had ACF signs after proximal ligation of the left anterior descending (LAD) coronary artery and 4 dogs developed ACF symptoms after proximal ligation of the LAD artery with subsequent ligation of distal branches of the left circumflex coronary artery. Three dogs had ventricular fibrillation episodes within 30 min of coronary occlusion, treated successfully with 1 or 2 direct-current shocks of 20–30 J.

Of 10 control dogs 6 died within 110 min of the study from recurrent ventricular fibrillation or pump failure with circulatory arrest. All dogs treated with CS retroperfusion were sacrificed after 120 min of myocardial ischemia. Pathologic inspection of the cardiac veins intima did not reveal any significant injury caused by catheterization and/or retroperfusion.

260

Hemodynamic variables are summarized in Figs. 1 and 2. No significant differences were seen between the control and treated group in baseline pre-ligation values. After coronary artery ligation the rapid decline in cardiac and stroke indices, mean arterial pressure, left ventricular systolic pressure and dp/dt$_{max.}$ was seen, indicating the contractility failure. Low cardiac performance and contractility resulted in death in 60% of control animals during the study period. CS retroperfusion was associated with significant improvement in cardiac and stroke indices, a significant rise of left ventricular systolic pressure was observed when compared with control group and pre-occlusion data. Simultaneously some drop in left ventricular end-diastolic pressure and a small but statistically significant rise in dp/dt$_{max.}$ LV were seen. Left ventricular performance and contractility values did not restore to pre-ligation baseline levels but stable improvement during 90 min of CS retroperfusion was registered. Heart rate changes were not significant, presumably due to large fluctuations during ACF (a-v conduction defects, ventricular or supraventricular tachycardia etc.).

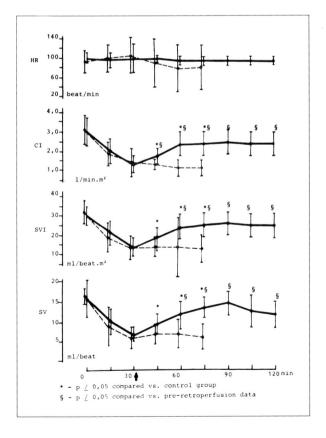

Fig. 1. Left ventricular function during CS retroperfusion (n = 20); hemodynamic parameters. HR: heart rate; CI: cardiac index; SVI: stroke index; SV: stroke volume.

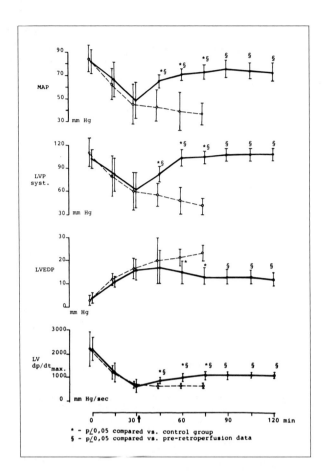

Fig. 2. Further hemodynamic parameters of left ventricular function during CS retroperfusion (n = 20). MAP: mean arterial pressure; LVP syst.: Left ventricular systolic pressure; LVEDP: left ventricular enddiastolic pressure; LV dp/dt$_{max.}$: maximal rate of left ventricular pressure rise.

Discussion

Recent experimental studies have demonstrated that synchronized diastolic cardiac vein retroperfusion delivers blood flow to the capillary network in the ischemic zone subserved from the occluded LAD coronary artery and is capable of reducing the acute infarction size with improved regional contractility (2–7, 12). As a rule no changes in integral cardiac pump function have been observed, presumably due to the use of local ischemia models incapable of inducing cardiac failure.

Experimental and clinical studies of metabolic myocardial preservation techniques in total heart hyperfusion and/or hypoxia revealed the improvement in myocardial metabolism and function after intracoronary infusion of physiologically active metabolic substances, glutamic acid (GA) and insulin (9, 11, 15). In postoperative patients with ACF we observed some improvement in left ventricular function during intravenous infusion of 1% GA solution (13). Due to rapid GA elimination from the intravascular compartment after intravenous infusion the cardiac GA effect was transient (15–20 min).

262

In the present study we investigated the combined effect of retrograde reperfusion of ischemic myocardium and metabolic protection with glutamic acid and insulin administered directly into the coronary capillary network. The model used was created to achieve the significant depression of integral left ventricular contractility and performance. Hemodynamic measurements revealed that cardiac veins retroperfusion with blood containing GA and insulin can improve left ventricular pump function and contractility during ACF caused by coronary arteries ligation. The degree of improvement was comparable with survival and its duration was 90 min.

However, before considering a clinical trial in ACF patients or postoperative low cardiac output patients, reperfusion and metabolic components of the effect obtained must be separated and long-term retroperfusion effects must be studied.

Conclusions

1. Coronary sinus retroperfusion with arterial blood containing glutamic acid and insulin improved left ventricular pump function and contractility after 30 min of acute cardiac failure caused by the ligation of left coronary artery branches.
2. Improved hemodynamic parameters were stable during 90 min of retroperfusion.
3. Coronary sinus retroperfusion with blood, glutamic acid and insulin can presumably prevent the immediate circulatory arrest caused by the extensive myocardial ichemia.

References

1. Arealis EG, Moulopoulos SD, Kolff WJ (1977) Attempts to increase blood supply to an acutely ischemic area of myocardium by intermittent occlusion of the coronary sinus (preliminary results). Med Res Eng 12: 4–7
2. Berdeaux A, Farcot JC, Bourdarias JP, Barry M, Bardet J, Guidicelli JF (1980) Effect of diastolic synchronized retroperfusion on regional coronary blood flow in experimental myocardial ischemia. Am J Cardiol 47: 1064–1070
3. Farcot JC, Berdeaux A, Giudicelli JF, Vilaine JP, Bourdarias JP (1983) Diastolic synchronized retroperfusion versus reperfusion: effects on regional left ventricular function and myocardial blood flow during acute coronary occlusion in dogs. Am J Cardiol 51: 1414–1421
4. Geary GG, Sputh GT, Suehiro GT, Jerman C, Siu B, McNamara JJ (1982) Quantitative assessment of infarct size reduction by coronary venous retroperfusion in baboons. Am J Cardiol 50: 1424–1430
5. Gundry SR (1982) Modification of myocardial ischemia in normal and hypertrophied hearts utilizing diastolic retroperfusion of the coronary veins. J Thorac Cardiovasc Surg 83: 659–669
6. Haendchen RV, Corday E, Meerbaum S, Povzhitkov M, Rit J, Fishbein MC (1983) Prevention of ischemic injury and early reperfusion derangements by hypotermic retroperfusion. J Am Coll Cardiol 1: 1067–1080
7. Hochberg MS, Austen WG (1980) Selective retrograde coronary venous perfusion. Ann Thorac Surg 29: 578–588
8. Kay EB, Suzaki A (1975) Coronary venous retroperfusion for myocardial revascularization. Ann Thorac Surg 19: 327–330
9. Kirkendol PL, Perason JE, Robie N (1980) The cardiac and vascular effect of sodium glutamate. Clin Exper Pharm Physiol 7: 617–625
10. Meerbaum S, Lang T, Osher JV (1976) Diastolic retroperfusion of acutely ischemic myocardium. Am J Cardiol 37: 588–598

11. Merin RG (1970) The relationship between myocardial function and glucose metabolism in the halotane-depressed heart. II. The effect of insulin. Anesthesiology 33: 396–400
12. Mohl W, Glogar D, Mayr H, Losert U, Heimisch N, Wolner E (1982) Effect of intermittent coronary sinus occlusion (ICSO) on tissue parameters after ligation of LAD. Thorac Cardiovasc Surg 30: 18
13. Pisarenko OI, Lepilin MG, Ivanov WE (1986) L-glutamic acid effect on the cardiac function in patients with postoperative cardiac failure
14. Pratt FH (1898) The nutrition of the heart through the vessels of Thebesius and the coronary veins. Am J Physiol 1: 85–103
15. Rau EE, Shine KI, Gervais A, Douglas AM, Amos EC (1979) Enhanced mechanical recovery of anoxic and ischemic myocardium by amino acid reperfusion. Am J. Physiol 236: 4873–4879
16. Smith GT, Geary GG, Blanchard W, McNamara JJ (1981) Reduction in infarct size by synchronized selective coronary venous retroperfusion of arterialized blood. Am J Cardiol 48: 1064–1070

Authors' address:
M. G. Lepilin
All-Union Cardiological Research Center
Academy of Medical Science
Moscow
U.S.S.R.

Effectiveness and safety of low pressure coronary venous arterialization treatment of acute myocardial ischemia

J. J. Moll, N. Hatori, A. Miyazaki, S. Meerbaum, M. Fishbein, E. Corday, and J. K. Drury

The Division of Cardiology, Department of Medicine, Cedars-Sinai Medical Center, and the University of California School of Medicine, Los Angeles, California (U.S.A.)

Summary: To compare the effectivenesss and safety of several modes of surgical arterialization of the coronary veins for treatment of acute coronary occlusion, studies were performed in 30 open chest dogs with five hour LAD occlusion. The dogs were randomly divided into four groups: group I served as control and had no intervention after the LAD occlusion; group II dogs were treated with high pressure coronary venous retroperfusion via a cephalic vein aorto-great cardiac vein anastomosis, along with obstruction of the normal coronary venous drainage; group III was similar to group II except that retroperfusion was applied at a lower flow rate through a mammary artery-to-great cardiac vein anastomosis; group IV was also similar to group II except that partial coronary sinus drainage was permitted resulting in relatively low pressure coronary venous retroperfusion. Mammary and venous graft flows in this study ranged from 60–230 ml/min. Significantly less myocardial hemorrhage was noted in groups III and IV in which mean anterior interventricular coronary vein pressure did not exceed 60 mm Hg as compared to group II in which the coronary venous pressure was greater than 60 mm Hg. Myocardial necrosis as percent of the risk area was 90 ± 4% in group I, 29 ± 26% in group II, 28 ± 18% in group III and 21 ± 10% in group IV.
Thus, surgical retroperfusion in dogs with 5 hour LAD occlusion significantly decreased infarct size, regardless of the particular mode of retroperfusion. However marked interstitial hemorrhage, which could influence the eventual result of the treatment, was absent only in those dogs in which a low coronary venous pressure was maintained during retroperfusion.

Introduction

Surgically achieved arterialization of the coronary venous system has been considered as a treatment for chronic myocardial ischemia since the pioneering efforts of Pratt (7), Beck (2), and Moll (6), however despite substantial clinical and experimental research, the role of this therapy for the treatment of coronary artery disease remains uncertain. The initial clinical application in 1948 of the Beck global coronary venous arterialization (3) was associated with a significant operative mortality and was not considered sufficiently safe and effective because of development of myocardial edema and hemorrhages attributed to high (near systemic) coronary venous pressures. Although interest in coronary venous arterialization subsequently diminished with the development of coronary artery bypass graft surgery (CABG), surgical retroperfusion remains potentially useful when the effectiveness of CABG is questionable as in patients with diffuse coronary arteriosclerosis

Financial support for this study was provided by the W. M. Keck Foundation, the Ahmanson Foundation and the Medallion Group of Cedars-Sinai Medical Center, Los Angeles, California; and grants 17651-10 and 14644-10 from the National Heart, Lung and Blood Institute of the National Institutes of Health, Bethesda, Maryland (U.S.A.)

and poor vascular run-off. Moreover there has recently been a renewed interest in retroperfusion due to the development of synchronized diastolic retroperfusion as well as retrograde infusion of pharmacologic agents. Improvements in surgical retroperfusion techniques have also been proposed, such as an aorta-to-regional coronary vein bypass (1).

It is known that the safety and effectiveness of the retroperfusion treatment is related to the pressure developed within the coronary veins. We therefore deliberately modified the surgical retroperfusion method to provide significantly lower coronary venous pressures by: 1) leaving a partially open communication between the regional coronary vein and the coronary sinus (in essence creating an arterio-venous fistula) or else; 2) anastomosing the internal mammary artery to the great cardiac vein. Since the aorta-coronary vein anastomosis was performed at a site well within the regional coronary vein, we predicted that such a modified retroperfusion system would be safe yet effective, providing adequate retrograde delivery of oxygenated blood to the myocardial microvasculature for the protection of jeopardized acutely ischemic myocardium.

Methods

Mongrel dogs weighing 21–45 kg were anesthetized with intramuscular morphine (1 mg/kg) and intravenous sodium pentobarbital (10 mg/kg), followed by ethrane anesthesia. Respiration was maintained through a cuffed endotracheal tube, and ventilation was with a mixture of room air, oxygen and 3% ethrane (by volume) using a constant volume respirator (Harvard, Waltham). Catheters were placed in the cardiac vein, the thoracic aorta and the left ventricle for pressure monitoring, and in the femoral vein for fluid and drug administration. A Swan-Ganz catheter was placed in the pulmonary artery for pressure and cardiac output measurement. Pressure and electrocardiographic tracings were recorded on a multichannel recorder (Gould Instruments or Electronics for Medicine). Pavulon 0.25 mg/kg (pancuronium bromide 2 mg/ml) was administered intravenously, and thoracotomy in the left fifth intercostal space was performed. The lungs were retracted and the heart was suspended in a pericardial cradle. For the anastomosis to the coronary vein, a cephalic vein was removed from the lower part of the left front leg, or else the dog's internal mammary artery was dissected free for subsequent anastomosis. The LAD coronary artery was dissected from the adjacent tissue at a site proximal to the first diagonal branch and regional acute ischemia in the anterior wall of the left ventricle was instituted by LAD ligation. To prevent bleeding during creation of the anastomosis, two 4.0 sutures on small tourniquets were placed around the great cardiac vein both proximal and distal to the intended site of the vein graft or internal mammary artery anastomosis. The graft was anastomosed in the beating heart with a 7.0 prolene suture to the great cardiac vein at its bifurcation into the two anterior interventricular veins. Flow through the graft was measured by an electromagnetic flow probe and flowmeter (Micron Instruments RC 1000) 2 minutes after LAD occlusion and thereafter every hour throughout the 5 hour experiment.

Dogs were randomly divided into four groups:

Group I (n = 8) Control group with untreated 5 hour LAD occlusion.

Group II (n = 8) 5 hour coronary artery occlusion with retroperfusion via a cephalic vein graft anastomosis, with retrograde flow started 1 min post LAD occlusion. The great cardiac vein was ligated distal to the site of the anastomosis to prevent direct shunting of arterial blood to the coronary sinus. This method caused an increase in the coronary venous pressure.

Group III (n = 7) 5 hour coronary artery occlusion with coronary venous retroperfusion by internal mammary artery anastomosis to the great cardiac vein. Distal to the site of anastomosis, the great cardiac vein was again ligated to prevent an arterio-venous fistula. Treatment was started 1 min post LAD occlusion.

Group IV (n = 7) 5 hour coronary artery occlusion with retroperfusion via a cephalic vein graft anastomosis, started 1 min post LAD occlusion. In this group, the great cardiac vein was only partially occluded distal to the site of anastomosis, allowing some direct shunting toward the coronary sinus and reducing the mean coronary venous pressure below 60 mm Hg.

Before sacrificing the dogs, the arterio-coronary venous bypass was clamped and 10 mCi of technetium 99m human albumin microspheres (mean diameter 20 μ, 3M company) were injected into the left atrium for assessment of the zone of myocardial hypoperfusion. The anesthetized dogs were sacrificed by intravenous injection of 1 mEq/kg potassium chloride. The free wall of the right ventricle, atria and great vessels were removed from the left ventricle, and the left ventricle was cut parallel to the atrioventricular groove into 4 mm thick slices. To assess the extent of myocardial necrosis (infarct size) all slices were incubated at room temperature in a 1% solution of triphenyltetrazolium chloride for 20 minutes, which stained the normal myocardium bright red and rendered the infarcted area yellow. Infarct size (IS) was expressed as percent of the cross-sectional area of the left ventricle. To assess the extent of the hypoperfused zone of the left ventricle, all slices were autoradiographed by placing them on X-ray film (Cronex 4 Dupont or Kodak XRP-1) in a Spectroline cassette (Spectronics Corp.) with two medium speed intensifying screens. The areas without blood flow were "cold" whereas the areas with blood flow were "hot". Soft X-ray exposures (25 kVp, 100 mAs) were made to delineate more accurately the perimeters of the slices, and were superimposed on the autoradiographs. In this manner the otherwise invisible inner and outer arcs, the borders of the "cold areas", could be visualized. The outlines of both areas were traced onto plastic sheets and measured by planimetry. The risk zone was then calculated as percent of the total cross sectional area of the whole left ventricle. In each dog, the percent of the area at risk that evolved to necrosis was calculated by determining the infarct zone to risk zone ratio and multiplying by 100.

Results

All groups of dogs studied were comparable in terms of pre-intervention heart rate, arterial pressure and cardiac output. There was also no statistical difference in risk zones as determined by autoradiography at the end of the experiment. Prior to the coronary artery occlusion, mean heart rate was 135 ± 27 beats/min in the control group (group I) not significantly different from groups II, III and IV in which it was 150 ± 10, 136 ± 14 and 130 ± 30 respectively. The mean arterial systolic pressure was 97 ± 15 mm Hg in the control group, and 110 ± 6, 97 ± 11 and 95 ± 15 in group II, III and IV. The mean cardiac output before intervention was 2.51 ± 0.85 (L/min) in the control group, 2.48 ± 0.31 in group II, 2.78 ± 0.84 in group III and 2.70 ± 0.63 in group IV. The

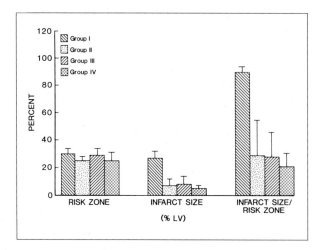

Fig. 1. Comparison of risk zones, infarct size as percent of left ventricle and infarct size as percent of risk zone in dogs of group I, II, III and IV. Note the significant reduction in infarct size of all the retroperfused dogs as compared to the untreated control occlusion dogs.

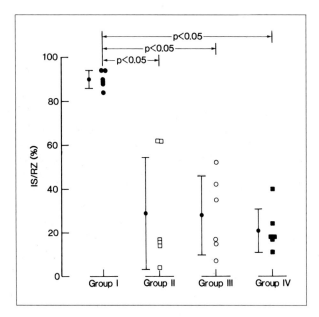

Fig. 2. Comparison of mean values and of variability of infarct size as percent of the risk zone in dogs of control group I, higher coronary venous pressure group II, mammary artery anastomosis group III, and low coronary venous pressure group IV.

mean ischemic risk zone was $30 \pm 4\%$ of the left ventricle in the control group. In the groups of dogs treated by retroperfusion it was 26 ± 4, 29 ± 5 and 25 ± 6 in group II, III and IV respectively.

As shown in Figures 1 and 2, the degree of hypoperfused risk zone evolving to necrosis was $90 \pm 4\%$ (ranging from 84 to 94%) in group I (control), 29 ± 26 (range 4 to 62%) in group II, 28 ± 18 (range 7 to 52%) in group III, and 21 ± 10 (range 11 to 40%) in group IV. The extent of risk zone evolving to necrosis was significantly less in all the retroperfusion treated groups than in the controls ($p < 0.05$). There was no statistically significant difference in infarct size of the treated dogs, suggesting that the retroperfusion induced decrease in necrosis in this acute 5 hour study did not depend on the level of regional coronary venous pressure. However macroscopic hemorrhage was encountered in the majority of hearts in the high pressure group (group II) whereas only relatively minor hemorrhage was noted in the mammary artery group (group III) and in the deliberately low pressure cephalic vein retroperfusion group (group IV).

The hemorrhage was primarily located in the subepicardium and mid myocardium of the left ventricle. Subendocardial hemorrhage was not seen in the treated dogs, nor was any hemorrhage noted in the control dogs.

Discussion

The purpose of this study was to determine the safest and most effective surgical coronary venous retroperfusion technique. We have shown that 5 hour retroperfusions of ischemic myocardium by various surgical techniques were equally effective in terms of myocardial salvage, however hemorrhagic complications were significantly more pronounced with high pressure retroperfusion. It was interesting to note that the hemorrhages were located in the mid myocardium and subepicardium and not in the subendocardium, presumably due to protection of the subendocardial micro circulation from the high venous pressure. Another observation was that the myocardial necrosis in the treated animals was predominantly localized in the mid-myocardial and subepicardial regions of the left ventricle, with sparing of the subendocardium. This is contrary to the usual pattern of necrosis in the absence of treatment, which has been shown to propagate from the subendocardial regions toward the epicardium. Our finding would suggest preferential delivery of the retroperfusate to the endocardium, which is consistent with previously described investigations of retrograde delivery using radiolabelled microspheres.

The mammary artery anastomosis carried less blood into the ligated coronary vein than the cephalic vein graft, resulting in coronary venous pressures less than 60 mm Hg, similar to those obtained with cephalic vein anastomosis combined with a partial coronary venous obstruction.

There remains substantial controversy concerning the efficacy of chronic surgical retroperfusion. Zajtchuk (8) found in his experimental study that six to eight months after mammary artery anastomosis to the anterior interventricular vein, there was intimal fibrosis and luminal stenosis of the retroperfused coronary veins in all dogs. In contrast, Hochberg (4) found that 3 to 5 months after interposing a saphenous vein graft between the aorta and the coronary veins in dogs (mean graft flow approximately 50 ml/min), transmural flow in the ischemic region was partially restored without evidence of venous sclerosis, thrombosis, interstitial edema or hemorrhage. Marco (5) reported a reduction in transmural myocardial infarction with LAD ligation and mammary artery anterior vein anastomosis, compared to LAD ligation alone. However, there was occlusion of the anastomosis by the sixth week in all animals. Since there was no sign of acute or chronic thrombosis, he concluded that occlusion was due to venous obliteration with fibrous tissue.

From these previous studies one might conclude that the difference in late results was primarily due to differences in surgical technique, including site and type of graft anastomosis. Based on our previous experience with chronic animal studies and anastomosis models which allowed control of the coronary venous pressure, we decided to reassess optimization of the surgical retroperfusion method by focusing on the generated coronary venous pressure. We also wanted to determine if the mammary artery carries sufficient blood to achieve adequate myocardial salvage and yet maintain safe coronary venous pressures. From our data it appears that the mammary artery does provide adequate arterial blood retroperfusion for treatment of the LAD subserved acutely ischemic zone, while maintaining a "safe" coronary venous pressure of less than 60 mm Hg. Cephalic vein anastomosis with partial coronary venous occlusion is also an acceptable coronary venous retroperfusion technique.

References

1. Andreadis P, Natsikas N, Arealis E, Lazardies DP (1974) The aortocoronary venous anastomosis in experimental acute myocardial ischemia. Vasc Surg 8: 45
2. Beck DS, Leighninger DC (1954) Scientific basis for the surgical treatment of coronary artery disease. JAMA 159: 1264
3. Beck DS (1948) Revascularization of the heart. Ann Surg 128: 854
4. Hochberg MS, Roberts WC, Morrow AG, Austen WG (1979) Selective arterialization of the coronary venous system: Encouraging long-term flow evaluation utilizing radioactive microspheres. J Thor Cardiovasc Surg 77: 1
5. Marco JD, Hahn JW, Barner HB, Jellinek M, Blair OM, Standeven JW, Kaiser GC (1977) Coronary venous arterialization: Acute hemodynamic, metabolic and chronic anatomical observations. Ann Thor Surg 23: 449
6. Moll JW, Dzieatkoviak AJ, Edelman M, Iljin W, Ratajczyk-Pakalska E, Stengert K (1975) Arterialization of the coronary veins in diffuse coronary arteriosclerosis. J Cardiovasc Surg 16: 520
7. Pratt FH (1898): Nutrition of the heart through the vessels of Thebesius and coronary veins. Am J Physiol I: 86
8. Zajtchuk R, Heydorn WH, Miller JG, Strevey TE, Treasure RL (1976) Revascularization of the heart through the coronary veins. Ann Thor Surg 21: 318

Author's address:
J. Kevin Drury, M.D.,
Cedars-Sinai Medical Center,
Halper Research Building,
8700 Beverly Boulevard,
Los Angeles,
California 90048,
U.S.A.

Synchronized coronary sinus retroperfusion during acute regional ischemia

R. W. Smalling, R. Ekas, Mary Tiberi, Patricia Felli, and R. Ochs

Center for Cardiovascular and Imaging Research, University of Texas Medical School at Houston, Texas (U.S.A.)

Synchronized coronary sinus retroperfusion (SRP) has been shown in dog models to improve regional myocardial blood flow, metabolism and, in some cases, function during periods of ischemia (1, 3, 4, 5, 7). Pressure-controlled intermittent coronary sinus occlusion has been shown to significantly decrease myocardial infarct size (6) as has SRP (2). These studies have been encouraging, however, all have dealt with severe prolonged ischemia.

With the evolution of coronary angioplasty it would be desirable to have a method for temporary support of the left ventricle during angioplasty of difficult, multiple or proximal (left main) coronary occlusions. In an attempt to test the applicability of SRP in this situation, we developed a canine model to test the hypothesis that: synchronized coronary sinus retroperfusion will support left ventricular function during brief periods of regional myocardial ischemia similar to that seen during percutaneous coronary angioplasty.

Methods

Six conditioned mongrel dogs were aseptically instrumented during general anesthesia with the following: left ventricular micromanometer and pressure catheter, circumflex coronary cuff occluder, pressure catheter and flow probe; coronary sinus pressure catheter; left anterior descending cuff occluder and flow probe; ascending aortic pressure catheter; left atrial pressure catheter; right atrial pacing wires; and sonomicrometer crystals in the left anterior descending, circumflex and border zone regions mid-wall in the circumferential plane. These animals were allowed to recover from surgery for approximately 7–14 days. The animals were then returned to the laboratory where they were lightly anesthetized with fentanyl and systemically heparinized. A coronary sinus SRP catheter was placed percutaneously via the right external jugular vein. An arterial supply catheter was placed via cut-down into the right femoral artery and attached to the SRP pump similar to that described by Drury et al. (2). The SRP catheter position was then verified by contrast injection during fluoroscopy. Measurements were made of the following parameters in the control state prior to coronary sinus retroperfusion: ECG; aortic, left ventricular, circumflex coronary, left atrial and coronary sinus pressure; and segmental shortening in the left anterior descending, border zone and circumflex regions. The animals were paced atrially at a rate approximately 20% above the resting heart rate.

271

Measurements were repeated during a three minute occlusion of the circumflex or left anterior descending coronary artery. After coronary artery occlusion, the animals were allowed to recover for 10 minutes or until hemodynamics and coronary flow stabilized. Repeat measurements were then made during occlusion of the remaining artery. After a 10 minute recovery period, synchronized coronary sinus retroperfusion was initiated with flow levels of 75–150 cc/min depending on catheter stability. Measurements during coronary occlusion were then repeated during SRP. Thus, the brief coronary occlusions in the experimental state occurred after SRP had been established for 5–15 minutes. After completion of the experiments, the catheters were withdrawn, the artery repaired and the animal was allowed to recover for 7 days prior to the next set of experiments.

Data analysis

All measurements are presented as the mean ± standard deviation. Due to the small number of samples, mean coronary sinus pressure is reported only as mean. Percent shortening was calculated as:

$$\frac{\text{End Diastolic Segment Length} - \text{End Ejection Segment Length}}{\text{End Diastolic Segment Length}} \times 100$$

Results

Preliminary results of these experiments are presented in Tables 1 and 2. The experimental model was fraught with several problems including frequent thrombosis of the proxi-

Table 1. Regional function during brief left anterior descending occlusions with and without synchronized coronary sinus retroperfusion in five chronically instrumented dogs.

	Baseline		2 minute LAD occlusion	
	Control	SRP	Control	SRP
Heart rate (Beats/min)	123±13	117± 8	122±13	118± 9
Mean aortic pressure (mmHg)	109±16	110±20	102±15	104±22
Mean coronary sinus pressure (mmHg)	9	33	8	31
Percent shortening				
LAD region	12±2	13±3	−3±12	−3±13
Border zone	13±7	10±5	10± 5	6± 5
Circumflex region	8±3	8±3	10± 4	11± 4

LAD – left anterior descending; Mean ± SD.

272

Table 2. Regional function during brief circumflex coronary occlusions with and without synchronized coronary sinus retroperfusion in five chronically instrumented dogs.

	Baseline		2 minute circumflex occlusion	
	Control	SRP	Control	SRP
Heart rate (Beats/min)	114±11	113±11	131±26	128±16
Mean aortic pressure (mmHg)	106± 8	104± 9	102±12	94±11
Mean coronary sinus pressure (mmHg)	9	33	8	31
Percent shortening				
LAD region	8±3	9±5	17±4	15±5
Border zone	10±6	10±5	13±6	11±6
Circumflex region	7±3	8±3	−5±2	−4±2

NAD = Left anterior descending; Mean ± SD.

mal coronary sinus at the site of the chronically implanted coronary sinus catheter. The second problem with the experiments was the difficulty in achieving acceptable flow rates due to SRP catheter instability within the coronary sinus. As depicted in Tables 1 and 2, there was little improvement in regional function in the five dogs studied during brief coronary occlusions. The mean coronary sinus pressure achieved was fairly low during these experiments although coronary sinus pressure could not be reliably measured in each dog due to the problems mentioned above.

In one animal with a patent coronary sinus, as depicted by Figure 1, during a six minute left anterior descending coronary (LAD) occlusion regional function deteriorated significantly with pan-systolic bulging occurring at three minutes. SRP was initiated at three minutes and continued for a total occlusion time of six minutes. At the end of six minutes of left anterior descending ischemia, the pan-systolic bulging had reversed and at end ejection, the segment length was essentially the same as that at end diastole. Contraction of the ischemic segment occurred late after end ejection, but did not contribute to global function. In a separate dog, as shown by Figure 2, initial dysfunction in the left anterior descending region during LAD occlusion was obliterated by one hour of SRP during which time several 3 minute occlusions occurred in both the anterior descending and posterior circulations. After prolonged pumping, occlusion of the left anterior descending coronary artery with or without SRP produced no significant changes in regional function suggesting that collateral channels had been recruited.

Summary

The results in this paper are extremely preliminary due to the problems discussed including coronary sinus thrombosis and inability to achieve adequate coronary sinus flow rates with available SRP catheters. Nonetheless, the following observations may be made: 1)

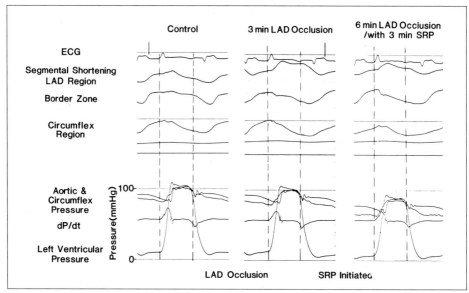

Fig. 1. Improvement in regional function during regional ischemia by synchronized coronary sinus retroperfusion. At 3 minutes of left anterior descending occlusion pan-systolic paradoxical motion of the LAD segments occurred. Three minutes after institution of SRP segmental function is slightly improved.

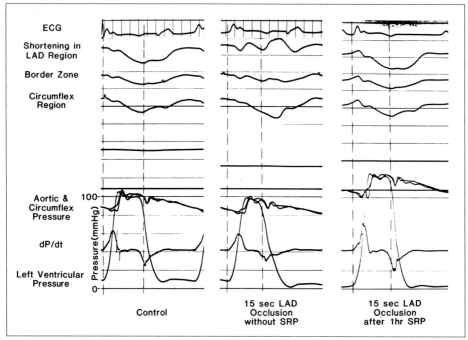

Fig. 2. Correction of contraction abnormalities during regional ischemia after prolonged application of SRP.

274

Efficacy of SRP may depend on the flow rate and/or diastolic coronary sinus pressure achieved; 2) Chronic instrumentation of the coronary sinus at the anterior heart border resulted in partial or total thrombosis in five of six animals studied and may have adversely affected results with anterior ischemia during SRP; 3) Maintenance of regional function was variable but did occur in some animals during SRP and regional ischemia; 4) After prolonged SRP some animals failed to demonstrate a decline in regional function during occlusions with or without SRP suggesting recruitment of collaterals; 5) Hemodynamics and electrical stability appeared to be significantly enhanced with SRP during brief occlusions in that several animals demonstrated ventricular tachycardia and ventricular fibrillation after release of three minute coronary occlusions. In the same animals, these arrhythmias were not observed during SRP.

It is suggested, therefore, that synchronized coronary sinus retroperfusion may be beneficial during acute ischemic syndromes such as with coronary angioplasty. The optimal conditions for application of this technique including maximal allowable flow rates, pressures and duration of pumping remain to be described.

References

1. Berdeaux A, Farcot J-C, Barry M et al (1981) Effects of Diastolic Synchronized Retroperfusion on Regional Coronary Blood Flow in Experimental Myocardial Ischemia. Am J Cardiol 47: 1033–1040
2. Drury JK, Yamazaki S, Fishbein MC et al (1985) Synchronized Diastolic Coronary Venous Retroperfusion: Results of a Preclinical Safety and Efficacy Study. J Am Coll Cardiol 6 (2): 328–335
3. Farcot JC, Meerbaum S, Lang T-W et al (1978) Synchronized Retroperfusion of Coronary Veins for Circulatory Support of Jeopardized Ischemic Myocardium. Am J Cardiol 41: 1191–1201
4. Gundry SR (1982) Modification of Myocardial Ischemia in Normal and Hypertrophied Hearts Utilizing Diastolic Retroperfusion of the Coronary Veins. J Thorac Cardiovasc Surg 83: 659–669
5. Meerbaum S, Lang T-W, Osher JV et al (1976) Diastolic Retroperfusion of Acutely Ischemic Myocardium. Am J Cardiol 37: 588–598
6. Mohl W, Glogar DH, Mayr H et al (1984) Reduction of Infarct Size Induced by Pressure-Controlled Intermittent Coronary Sinus Occlusion. Am J Cardiol 53: 923–928
7. Yamazaki S, Drury JK, Meerbaum S et al (1985) Synchronized Coronary Venous Retroperfusion: Prompt Improvement of Left Ventricular Function in Experimental Myocardial Ischemia. J Am Coll Cardiol 5: 655–663

Authors' address:
Richard W. Smalling, M.D., Ph.D.
Center for Cardiovascular and Imaging Research
University of Texas Medical School at Houston
6431 Fannin/MSB 1.246
Houston, Texas 77030
U.S.A.

On the time course of systolic myocardial wall thickening during coronary artery occlusion and reperfusion in the absence and presence of synchronized diastolic coronary venous retroperfusion in anesthetized pigs

L. Berk, I. O. L. Schmeets, L. M. A. Sassen, R. J. Rensen, R. H. van Bremen, J. M. Hartog, P. W. Serruys, and P. D. Verdouw

The Laboratory for Experimental Cardiology, Thoraxcenter, Erasmus University Rotterdam, Rotterdam (The Netherlands)

Introduction

Synchronized diastolic coronary venous retroperfusion (SRP) partially restores regional myocardial function, when instituted 30 min after occlusion (2). This suggests that SRP can prevent or delay loss of contractile function when started prior or at the time of occlusion. If this proves to be true, SRP could be useful during percutaneous transluminal coronary angioplasty, which involves multiple short-lasting (up to 90 sec) occlusions of a coronary artery. We therefore documented the changes in regional function during coronary artery occlusion and reperfusion in animals with SRP support started at the time of occlusion.

Methods

In pentobarbital-anesthetized pigs (20–45 kg) blood pressures in the descending aorta and left ventricle were recorded from microtipped Millar catheters. After thoracotomy an electromagnetic flow probe was placed around the ascending aorta for the measurement of cardiac output. The left anterior descending coronary artery (LADCA) was prepared free over a length of 0.5–1.0 cm, immediately below the left circumflex branch. Left ventricular wall thickness tracings (5 MHz ultrasound crystal, Krautkramer-Branson, Lewistown, Pa.) were recorded from a section of the myocardium supplied by the LADCA. Because in pigs the left hemiazygous vein empties into the proximal coronary sinus, a ligature was placed around that vein to prevent that retroperfused blood escaped through that route. After removal of air bubbles, the instrument (EC-1, USCI division of C. R. Bard, Inc. Billerica, Mass) (2) was set to pump arterial blood retrogradely into the coronary sinus or directly into the great cardiac vein during diastole at flow rates varying from 30–75 ml · min⁻¹. Heparin (5000–10 000 U) was administered intravenously to prevent clotting.

277

Experimental protocol

After 30 minutes of stabilization, the LADCA was occluded for 20 minutes and subsequently reperfused for two hours. Eight animals served as control, while in 16 animals retroperfusion was started at the time of occlusion and maintained throughout the occlusion period. No antiarrhythmic drugs were administered. In case of ventricular fibrillation, the animals were promptly (within 30–60 sec) defibrillated. Animals in which mean arterial blood pressure fell below 50 mm Hg were excluded from further study.

Results

Retroperfusion via the coronary sinus or great cardiac vein: All hemodynamic changes were independent of the site of retroperfusion. Therefore the data have been pooled. The only difference we observed was in the extent of vessel damage, which was present in some of the animals which were retroperfused via the great cardiac vein.

Ventricular arrhythmias (Table 1): Ventricular fibrillation occurred in 25% of the untreated animals during the occlusion. In two animals, conversion attempts were not successful. A high ectopic activity (> 25 beats $\cdot$ min^{-1}) was observed in all animals during the first 10–15 minutes of reperfusion with a ventricular fibrillation during the first minute.

From the 16 animals with retroperfusion, 4 (25%) had a ventricular fibrillation during coronary artery occlusion. In two cases defibrillation was successful within 30 sec, but two animals had to be excluded because of a failure to do so within 3 minutes. Since two other treated animals had to be excluded because of severe heart failure, reperfusion was started in 12 SRP treated animals. In 11 of the 12 animals ventricular fibrillation occurred during the first five minutes of reperfusion.

Hemodynamics (Table 2): No significant differences were observed in the hemodynamic changes of either group during the 20 min occlusion period. Except for a much higher heart rate in the control animals during the first minutes of reperfusion no differences existed between the two groups.

Table 1. Ventricular arrhythmias during 20 min of coronary artery occlusion and 2 hours of reperfusion in SRP-treated and control animals.

	SRP	Control
Occlusion		
n	16	8
VF	4	2
$\geqslant 5$PVCs $\cdot$ min^{-1}	8	2
Reperfusion		
n	12	6
VF	11	6
$\geqslant 25$PVCs $\cdot$ min^{-1}	9	6

VF – ventricular fibrillation; PVCs – premature ventricular contractions

278

Table 2. Effect of SRP during 20 min of coronary artery occlusion and two hours of reperfusion on cardiovascular performance.

		Baseline	Occlusion[+]		Reperfusion[+]		
			2'	20'	22'	50'	80'
CO	SRP	2.7±0.2	−0.3±0.1	−0.6±0.2	−0.9±0.4	−0.5±0.3	−0.3±0.3
	C	3.0±0.4	−0.3±0.2	−0.2±0.2	−0.9±0.6	−0.2±0.4	−0.1±0.4
HR	SRP	88±7	6±3	8±7	25±12*	2±7	.5±10
	C	88±9	3±1	14±9	74±17	11±4	19±12
SV	SRP	31±1	−6±2	−8±2	−16±3	−7±2	−6±3
	C	34±3	−4±2	−7±4	−23±5	−5±6	−5±6
LVEDP	SRP	10±1	2.9±1.0	4.0±2.1	−0.3±0.9	1.2±1.0	−0.1±0.9
	C	13±1	3.5±0.9	2.4±0.7	−1.9±1.6	3.3±0.9	1.1±1.1
LVdP/dt	SRP	1730 ±210	−450 ±160	−530 ±300	−540 ±400	−380 ±320	−100 ±370
	C	1790 ±240	−370 ±90	−260 ±60	−120 ±150	−160 ±110	−10 ±200
MAP	SRP	76±5	−12±3	−15±6	−34±9	−17±7	−12±8
	C	82±3	−12±3	−13±2	−37±4	−10±2	−14±2
SVR	SRP	30±3	−4±3	1±3	−1±6	−3±4	−1±3
	C	30±4	−3±2	−2±4	0±8	−2±4	−6±4
SWT	SRP	32±3	−27±3	−30±3	−20±4	−23±4	−22±6
	C	30±3	−24±3	−26±4	−26±5	−26±4	−24±5

CO = cardiac output ($1 \cdot min^{-1}$); HR = heart rate (beats $\cdot min^{-1}$; SV = stroke volume (ml); LVEDP = left ventricular end-diastolic pressure (mmHg); LVdP/dt = maximum rate of rise of left ventricular pressure (mmHg $\cdot s^{-1}$); MAP = mean arterial blood pressure (mmHg); SVR = systemic vascular resistance (mmHg $\cdot 1^{-1}$.min); SWT = systolic wall thickening (%); + = all data are expressed as change from baseline (mean ± SEM); * = $p < 0.05$ for treated (T) vs. untreated (C) animals.

Systolic wall thickening (Table 2): Within one minute following LADCA occlusion there was a complete loss of systolic wall thickening as wall thickness at end-diastole decreased and did not change during systole. Only a partial recovery was seen during the two hours of reperfusion. Retroperfusion neither delayed the loss of function during ischemia nor enhanced its recovery during reperfusion.

Discussion

Complete occlusion of the LADCA resulted in decreases in mean arterial blood pressure and cardiac output. The latter was entirely at the expense of a decreased stroke volume as heart rate was not affected. From the determinants of stroke volume, myocardial contractility was most impaired because of a complete loss of contractile function of the ischemic segment during the first minute after coronary artery occlusion. SRP did not modify any of the afore-named changes. Because a prompt improvement in function has been reported when retroperfusion was instituted 30 minutes after occlusion it was expected that in our study a complete loss of systolic function in the ischemic segment could be prevented or at least delayed. The reason why we did not observe any improvement during this earliest period of occlusion can only be speculated upon. We used pigs, a species known for a coronary anatomy similar to that of man, but with a lack of functional collaterals. Reduction of coronary flow to approximately 30% of baseline already results in a complete loss of function (1). This implies that SRP must increase perfusion of the ischemic segment by at least 25–30% of the pre-occlusion flow before any improvement in function should be noticeable. We could not accomplish this despite SRP flow rates from 30–75 $ml \cdot min^{-1}$.

Left atrial injection of radioactive labelled microspheres revealed that entrapment by the myocardium was not increased during SRP. After direct injection of microspheres into the SRP system 95% of microspheres were detected in the lungs which implies that they were unable to reach the arterial bed of the myocardium retrogradely via collaterals or arteriovenous anastomoses.

In summary, we could not demonstrate a delay in loss of function or an enhanced recovery when SRP was instituted at the time of coronary artery occlusion in pigs.

References

1. Verdouw PD, Ten Cate FJ, Schamhardt HC, van der Hoek TM, Bastiaans OL (1980) Segmental myocardial function during progressive coronary flow reduction and its modification by pharmacologic intervention. In: Heiss HW (ed) Advances in Clinical Cardiology. Quantification of Myocardial Ischemia. Gerhard Witzstrock Publishing House, Inc, New York, pp 270–284
2. Yamazaki S, Drury JK, Meerbaum S, Corday E (1985) Synchronized coronary venous retroperfusion: prompt improvement of left ventricular function in experimental myocardial ischemia. J Am Coll Cardiol 5: 655–663

Authors' address:
P. D. Verdouw, Ph.D.
Laboratory for Experimental Cardiology
Thoraxcenter
Erasmus University Rotterdam
P.O. Box 1738
3000 DR Rotterdam
The Netherlands

Clinical evaluation of safety and hemodynamic effects of diastolic coronary venous retroperfusion

J. Berland*, J.-C. Farcot**, A. Cribier*, J.-P. Bourdarias**, and B. Letac*

Summary: The safety and the hemodynamic consequences of a diastolic coronary venous synchronized retroperfusion system (SRP) have been studied in 7 coronary artery disease patients without acute ischemia after routine coronary arteriography. In all the patients the SRP catheter could be inserted in the mid-portion of the coronary sinus (mean time for the procedure 8 minutes). The system was activated during 15 minutes. For a mean arterial blood retroperfused flow of 100 ml/min, no changes in hemodynamic parameters occurred, no ECG modifications were recorded and no patient complained of chest pain. Therefore the evaluation of efficacy of SRP in various acute ischemic clinical settings is warranted.

Introduction

Prior experimental studies suggested that coronary venous retroperfusion may represent a potentially effective treatment of myocardial ischemia (2, 4, 6). Before starting a clinical trial of the efficacy of the previously described ECG synchronized catheter pump system (3), we studied in 7 CAD patients (at the end of a coronary angiography procedure), the feasibility and ease of coronary sinus catheter insertion, as well as system logistics and hemodynamics effects of synchronized arterial blood shunting from the femoral artery to the coronary sinus.

Method

Patient description

Seven male patients complaining of angina (35 to 68 years) were referred to the cardiac catheterization laboratory for coronary angiography. Two had had a previous anterior infarction, a third one had suffered an inferior infarct. Their mean left ventricular ejection fraction was 51%. Two patients exhibited severe anterior hypokinesia secondary to a chronic obstruction of the left anterior descending coronary artery (LAD). Four patients had triple vessel disease, 1 double vessel disease, and two had single LAD disease.

Synchronized retroperfusion technique

At the end of the angiographic procedure and after informed consent was obtained from the patient, the right anterial jugular vein was punctured and a 10 French length dual slit

---

 * Service des Soins Intensifs Cardiologiques et des Explorations Hemodynamics Cardiovasculaires, Centre Hospitalier et Universitaire, Hôpital Charles-Nicolle, Rouen, and
** Service de Cardiologie, Hôpital Ambroise Paré, Boulogne (France)

sheath (*) was introduced over a guide wire. Then the synchronized retroperfusion catheter (**) was inserted through the sheath and passed over the guide wire. After removal of
the wire, the catheter was advanced under fluoroscopic control and positioned with its tip
in the mid portion of the coronary sinus. Afterwards, and 8F sheath was placed in the left
femoral artery to withdraw the arterial blood retroperfusate and this cannula was connected the coronary sinus balloon catheter via a pulsatile gas activated diastolic synchronized retroperfusion pumping unit (3). This system propels arterial blood during
diastole through the coronary sinus catheter.

The auto inflatable balloon of the catheter is activated directly from the central lumen of
the catheter through several holes, and ensures unidirectional diastolic retrograde infusion of the blood toward the ischemic zone. Just before the onset of systole, a sudden
stoppage and even slight reversal of the arterial blood flow due to the pulsatile pump
operation, causes a rapid and total collapse of the balloon in the coronary sinus, allowing
normal coronary venous drainage.

In vitro and in vivo experimental studies (1, 3) indicated that the pumping balloon system converts a simple arteriovenous shunt flow into an augmented pulsed shunt flow,
with maximal retrograde coronary venous flow in diastole and trivial negative flow in
systole.

The mean flow rate was assessed in this study by using a previously calibrated doppler
flow meter placed around the retroperfusion line.

Protocol and measurements

After the retroperfusion system was fully set up but before it was activated, a 5F micromanometer tip catheter (Millar instruments) was positioned into the left ventricle through
the right femoral artery sheath to assess LV pressure and dP/dt, and a 7F Swan Ganz
Catheter was placed in the pulmonary artery to measure pulmonary pressure as well as
cardiac output.

The arterial blood pressure was measured through a side port in the femoral sheath, connected to a fluid filled transducer.

The ECG leads ($D_1 V_F V_5$) were continuously monitored during the procedure. Approximately twenty minutes the end of coronary arteriography, a complete set of hemodynamic parameters were recorded on a multi-channel Siemens recorder. Then the retroperfusion system was activated for 15 minutes, and measurements were repeated at 5, 10 and
15 minutes during pumping as well as five minutes after the pump was turned off. To record an in situ retroperfused coronary venous angiogram, five minutes after starting the
synchronized retroperfusion pump, 3 ml of 76% Renografin was injected directly into the
pumping circuit. The venogram was recorded on a 35 mm film at 50 frames/second over
a period of 6 to 10 seconds. The patients were repeatedly asked to indicate whether they
felt any chest pain or discomfort.

At the end of the procedure, the coronary sinus catheter was pulled out from the right internal jugular over the guide wire. After removal of the sheath, a simple compression of
the vein prevented bleeding.

---

 * USCI, Billerica MA UA
** Plastimed Soc F95320 Saint Leu La Foret France

Twenty-four hours subsequent to the acute study a 2D echocardiogram was recorded in multiple views to visualize the pericardium and assess left ventricular contractility. In each of the patients, a modified apical four chamber view was recorded, aimed specifically to visualize the first few centimeters of the coronary sinus.

All changes in hemodynamic parameters were studied by an analysis of variance.

Results

Safety of the procedure

In all the seven patients we succeeded without difficulty in positioning the coronary sinus catheter in the middle portion of the coronary sinus. The mean time to completion of this catheterization was 8 minutes. In two patients the catheter diameter was 8 French and in 5 patients 7 French.

No patients complained of angina or exhibited ECG changes.

The coronary venous angiogram clearly showed both the diastolic retrograde flow pattern as well as the contrast wash-out in systole. An example of this veno angiogram (Fig. 1) in a patient with complete chronic obstruction of the left anterior descending artery indicated retrograde penetration of the contrast material deep into the intraventricular vein.

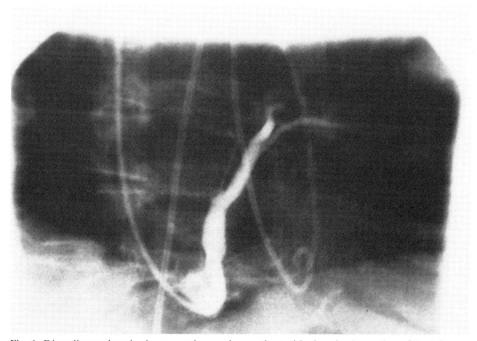

Fig. 1. Diastolic synchronized veno-angiogram in a patient with chronic obstruction of the left anterior descending artery showing retrograde penetration of the contrast material into the interventricular vein.

283

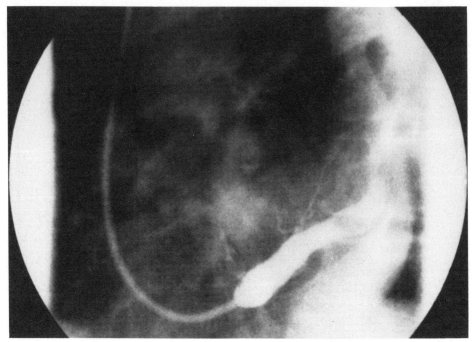

Fig. 2. Veno-angiogram in a patient without LAD obstruction. The retroperfused contrast agent did not reach the anterior venous system.

In patients without total LAD obstruction the retroperfused contrast agent did not reach the anterior venous system (Fig. 2).

At the end of the procedure it was necessary to first remove the sheath before pulling out the balloon catheter from the jugular vein and after compression no local hematoma was noted. 24 hours later neither a pericardial effusion nor a decrease in left ventricular contractility were seen upon echocardiographic examination. The first few centimeters of the coronary sinus visualized in each of the patients showed no abnormality.

Hemodynamic parameters

No changes in the various hemodynamic parameters were observed during the retroperfusion period (Fig. 3). The mean heart rate remained stable (around 70 beat/min), as well as the cardiac index; the mean aortic pressure and the positive first derivative of left ventricular pressure were all stable. In two patients with low cardiac index (below 2 liters/minute) no deterioration in the hemodynamic status was observed.

The individual retroperfusion flow rate data are listed in Figure 4. The mean flow was 106 ml/min ± 17 30 seconds after the retroperfusion was started, and decreased slightly to 96 ml/m ± 23 after 15 minutes of pumping (NS). The two patients with the 8 French catheter exhibited the highest flow rate (120 ml/min 140 ml/min). In two patients the flow rate decreased by 20 ml/min at 25 minutes, without changes in aortic blood pressure.

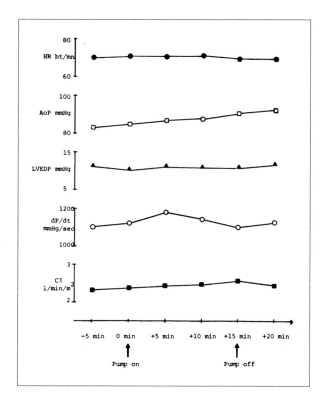

Fig. 3. Mean values of the hemodynamic parameters during the retroperfusion period. hr: heart rate, AoP: mean aortic pressure, LVEDP: Left ventricular and diastolic pressure, dp/dt max: positive pic of the first derivative of left ventricular pressure, CI: cardiac index. No changes were significant.

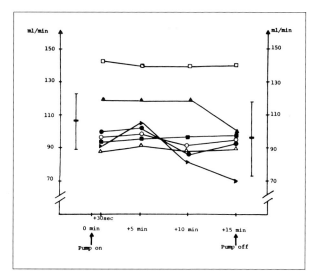

Fig. 4. Individual values of retroperfusion flow during the protocol. An 8 French retroperfusion catheter was used in patients □ and ▲, and a 7 French catheter for the others. The mean flow values (± SD) after 30 seconds and 15 minutes retroperfusion are also drawn. No changes were significant.

Discussion

This limited study demonstrated the apparent feasibility and safety of the new diastolic synchronized retroperfusion system in patients with coronary artery disease and absence of acute myocardial ischemia. Because the system has not as yet been used in a clinical setting, it was first necessary to show the lack of adverse consequences of the procedures before applying this new device in critically ischemic patients. It was not attempted in this phase to place the tip of the catheter deep in the coronary sinus. Despite the approximated mid coronary sinus position, interventricular anterior venous retrograde opacification was noted in one patient with chronic obstruction of the LAD, suggesting that an absence of antegrade flow is a factor in obtaining a satisfactory retroperfusion flow. The mean flow with a 7 F catheter (90 ml/min) was higher than during the experimental studies (50 to 60 ml/min) (1). This increase in flow may be related to the lower heart rate of this clinical study (70 beat/min) as compared to the experimental mean heart rate (140 beat/min). This is allowed a prolonged retroperfusion diastolic time and lowered the pressure in the venous system for a higher flow.

The lack of deleterious hemodynamic consequences during repeated systolic occlusion of the coronary sinus is in agreement with Faxon (5) who observed no change in heart rate and left ventricle pressure for 20 seconds coronary sinus occlusion in 22 patients.

In conclusion, the safety and feasibility of a diastolic synchronized retroperfusion system has been demonstrated in seven LAD patients without acute ischemia.

It is believed possible to commence studies of diastolic synchronized retroperfusion in various clinical ischemic settings, for example as a percutaneous support of transluminal coronary angioplasty, unstable angina or myocardial infarction.

References

1. Berdeaux A, Farcot JC, Bourdarias JP, Barry M, Bardet J, Giudicellia JF (1980) Effects of Diastolic Synchronized Retroperfusion on Regional Coronary Blood Flow in Experimental Myocardial Ischemia. Am J Cardiol 47: 1033–1040
2. Farcot JC, Meerbaum S, Lang TW, Kaplan L, Corday E (1978) Synchronized Retroperfusion of Coronary Veins for Circulatory Support of Jeopardized Ischemic Myocardium. Am J Cardiol 41: 1191–1201
3. Farcot JC, Barry M, Bourdarias JP, Bardet J, Giudicelli JF (1981) New catheter-pump system for diastolic synchronized retroperfusion. Med Prog Technol 8: 19–37
4. Farcot JC, Berdaux A, Giudicelli JF, Vilaine JP, Bourdarias JP (1983) Diastolic Synchronized Retroperfusion Versus Reperfusion: Effects on Regional Left Ventricular Function and Myocardial Blood Flow During Acute Coronary Occlusion in Dogs. Am J Cardiol 51: 1414–1421
5. Faxon DP, Jacobs AK, McSweeney SM, Coats WD, Kellett MA, Ryan TJ (1984) Coronary Sinus Assessment of Left Ventricular Pressure in Man. In Mohl W, Wolner E, Glogar D (eds) The Coronary Sinus. Steinkopff Verlag, Darmstadt, pp 424–429
6. Meerbaum S, PhD, Lang TW, Osher JV, Hashimoto Keiichi, Lewis GW, Feldstein C, Corday E (1976) Diastolic Retroperfusion of Acutely Ischemic Myocardium. Am J Cardiol 37: 588–598

Authors' address:
J.-C. Farcot, M.D.
Service de Cardiologie
Hôpital Ambroise Paré
9. Avenue Charles-de-Gaulle
92100 Boulogne
France

Recent experience with synchronized coronary sinus retroperfusion

J. M. Gore, Bonnie H. Weiner, O. N. Okike, J. R. Benotti, Kathy M. Sloan,
T. J. Vandersalm, J. M. J. Gaca, S. P. Ball, Jeanne M. Corrao, J. S. Alpert,
and J. E. Dalen

Divisions of Cardiovascular Medicine and Cardiothoracic Surgery, University of
Massachusetts Medical School, Worcester, Massachusetts (U.S.A.)

A nonsurgical approach to maintain cardiac viability through coronary sinus retroperfusion was reported from the laboratory of E. Corday (5) in 1976. This system provides retrograde perfusion of arterialized blood, synchronized to the cardiac cycle during diastole, while permitting normal physiologic coronary venous drainage during systole. The method is intended as a temporary treatment for acute myocardial ischemia.

Extensive animal studies have been performed demonstrating improvement in cardiac function and salvage of jeopardized myocardium with the use of synchronized retroperfusion of the coronary venous system for support of acutely ischemic myocardium (2, 6). To date, the intervention has only been applied to experimental animals for up to a maximum of six hours (1).

The retroperfusion system is comprised of four major components. The supply catheter delivers arterialized blood to the pump. The pump chamber assembly includes a piston driven chamber which propels the arterialized blood into the coronary sinus by mechanized displacement. The monitor console permits ECG synchronization of blood delivery and regulation of the amount of flow. The coronary sinus catheter with an autoinflatable balloon permits intermittent occlusion of the coronary sinus to allow retrograde flow without needing a separate inflation vehicle (gas).

Prior to human clinical trials, we undertook a study of the feasibility and safety of this new synchronized coronary sinus retroperfusion system for periods up to 24 hours (3). We studied animals for periods up to 24 hours (range 3 to 24 h). There was no significant change in coronary sinus pressure for periods up to 24 hours. In addition, right heart pressures, arterial pressure and heart rate remained relatively constant. Coronary sinus pressure appears to be directly related to retroperfusion flow: the greater the flow, the higher the peak systolic coronary sinus pressure. With cessation of retroperfusion, there is an immediate return to baseline pressure in the coronary sinus.

There is evidence of minor damage to blood cells at higher flow rates (greater than 100 cc/min), but it is not any different than has been reported by others (1). Blood cell damage may be due to the instrumentation of the animals, not the actual device. Gross and microscopic examination of the coronary sinus, coronary veins and right atrium do not reveal any evidence of significant damage from prolonged retroperfusion.

Prompted by these encouraging animal results, we initiated a Phase I trial to evaluate the feasibility and safety of this intervention.

Patients with unstable angina unresponsive to maximum medical therapy, including intravenous nitroglycerin, beta blockers, calcium channel blockers and morphine, who were felt to be at high risk for a major cardiac event were studied. Unstable angina was defined as multiple episodes of ischemic pain lasting more than five minutes but less than 30 minutes associated with ECG changes. The ECG changes were at least 1.5 mm of ST segment depression, in two contiguous precordial leads, which improved with relief of symptoms. The patient could not have any of the predetermined exclusion criteria and had to be able to give informed consent as approved by the Committee on the Protection of Human Subjects in Research at the University of Massachusetts Medical Center.

Retroperfusion was performed at the bedside in the coronary care unit. After the patients were prepped and draped, introducers were placed in the femoral artery and internal jugular vein. Through the femoral artery introducer an 8 French arterial supply catheter (USCI, Billerica MA) was placed in the distal descending aorta. A 7 French auto-inflatable retroperfusion balloon catheter (USCI, Billerica MA) was inserted through the introducer in the neck. The catheter was advanced into the right atrium. The catheter was then advanced to the tricuspid valve and slowly rotated posteriorly until the tip engaged the ostium of the coronary sinus. The catheter is then advanced into the coronary sinus and the position is verified by obtaining a coronary sinus blood saturation and by the hand injection of contrast material to outline the great cardiac vein and surrounding structures. The catheter is then advanced with a guide wire if necessary, into the great cardiac vein. The patients are then heparinized and maintained at an activated clotting time 2 to 2–½ times control.

Retroperfusion is initiated at a flow rate of 0.5 cc/kg/min of total body weight. The flow rate is increased every 10 minutes until there is relief of symptoms of ischemia or until the maximum flow rate of 2.2 cc/kg/min (or 150 cc/min the maximum output of the system) is achieved. The patients have continuous ECG, arterial blood pressure, pulse and pulmonary artery pressure monitored. Coronary arteriography is performed within 24 hours of the institution of retroperfusion. At this time, a decision is made whether the patient is a candidate for angioplasty or coronary artery bypass surgery.

Our clinical experience to date has indicated that retroperfusion can be performed at the bedside. It takes a little more than 1/2 hour from preparation of the patient to institution of therapy. In most patients the coronary sinus can be cannulated in under 1 minute, however, in some individuals, there appears to be a valve or some other anatomic variant overlying the orifice of the sinus and more time is required to enter the coronary sinus. To date, in the patients we have studied, a flow rate of 0.75 cc/kg/min has been adequate to control angina symptoms. Once an adequate flow rate is obtained there are attempts of decreasing flow requirements over time, which has been successful in some patients, in other patients, attempts at weaning result in recurrence of symptoms.

There has been no indication of any untoward effects from retroperfusion. In addition to careful monitoring of the hemodynamic parameters previously delineated, patients have not reported any discomfort or annoyance due to the system. Hematologic testing reveals no adverse effects to red blood cells or platelets.

Several clinical variables have been followed in an attempt to gain some information on the clinical efficacy of retroperfusion. Patients have been used as their own controls. The frequency of angina attacks, ECG parameters, pain medication requirements and hemodynamic parameters have all indicated a significant clinical improvement for patients while on retroperfusion (4).

288

Our preliminary experience with synchronized coronary sinus retroperfusion indicates that it is a feasible, safe, and clinical effective intervention. It appears that this intervention may increase the time window during which definitive therapy can be applied in an unstable patient. It may also greatly increase the likelihood of more complete recovery from a variety of acute myocardial ischemic events. The rediscovery of the coronary sinus as a potential route for myocardial perfusion may represent a new era for interventional cardiology.

References

1. Drury JK, Yamazaki, S, Fishbein MC, Meerbaum, S, Corday E (1985) Synchronized diastolic coronary venous retroperfusion: Results of a preclinical safety and efficacy study. JACC 6: 328
2. Farcot JC, Meerbaum S, Lang T, Kaplan L, Corday E (1978) Synchronized retroperfusion of coronary veins for circulatory support of jeopardized ischemic myocardium. Am J Cardiol 21: 1191
3. Gore JM, Weiner BH, Sloan KM, Cuenoud HF (1985) The safety of synchronized coronary sinus retroperfusion (SCSR) for up to 24 hours. Chest (abstr) 88: 73
4. Gore JM, Weiner BH, Sloan KM, Benotti JR, Okike ON, Vandersalm TJ, Ball SP, Corrao JM, Alpert JS, Dalen JE (1986) Human experience with synchronized coronary sinus retroperfusion (SCSR) feasibility and safety. JACC (abstr)
5. Meerbaum S, Lang T, Osher JV et al (1976) Diastolic retroperfusion of acutely ischemic myocardium. Am J Cardiol 37: 588
6. Zalewski A, Goldberg S, Slysh S, Maroko P (1985) Myocardial protection via coronary sinus interventions: Superior effects of arteriolization compared with intermittent occlusion. Circulation 71: 1215

Authors' address:
J. M. Gore, M.D.
Division of Cardiovascular Medicine
University of Massachusetts Medical School
55 Lake Avenue North
Worcester, Massachusetts 01605
U.S.A.

The role of synchronized coronary sinus retroperfusion during LAD angioplasty

Bonnie H. Weiner, J. M. Gore, Kathy M. Sloan, J. R. Benotti, J. M. J. Gaca, O. N. Okike, T. J. Vandersalm, S. P. Ball, Jeanne M. Correo, J. S. Alpert, and J. E. Dalen

Divisions of Cardiovascular Medicine and Cardiothoracic Surgery, University of Massachusetts Medical School Worcester (U.S.A.)

Coronary sinus retroperfusion (CSRP) has been shown to effectively support acutely ischemic myocardium in animals (2, 4, 6). A current system consisting of an autoinflatable balloon catheter inserted into the coronary sinus, an arterial supply catheter, a piston driven pump chamber, and monitor console for synchronization, has been shown to be both safe and effective in animals for up to 6 hours (1). Our experience has confirmed its safety for periods of up to 24 hours (3).

The animal studies of this technique have involved acute occlusion of a previously normal coronary artery. This situation rarely occurs in man, in a setting where CSRP can be readily applied. On the other hand, during percutaneous transluminal coronary angioplasty (PTCA), balloon inflations are in most instances limited by the appearance in the patient of the signs and symptoms of acute myocardial ischemia. It is not known whether longer inflation times (up to several minutes) might play a role in addressing two of the major difficulties facing PTCA today; i.e. re-stenosis and the development of occlusive dissections. We therefore undertook a study to determine whether CSRP had a beneficial effect during PTCA. We have initially studied patients undergoing LAD PTCA, as from our early animal experience we felt the effect might be more evident.

Patients undergoing LAD angioplasty with evidence of ECG changes associated with ischemia were invited to participate. Informed consent as approved by the committee on the Protection of Human Subjects in Research at the University of Massachusetts Medical Center was obtained.

The patients were brought to the cardiac catheterization laboratories where both groins and the area of the right internal jugular vein were prepared and draped in a standard sterile fashion. Following local anesthesia, introducers were inserted into both femoral arteries, either one or both femoral veins or the internal jugular vein, depending on the intended approach to the coronary sinus. A 7 F pacing Cournand catheter (U.S.C.I. Billerica, MA) was then inserted via the left femoral vein. The 7F autoinflatable coronary sinus catheter (U.S.C.I., Billerica, MA) was then inserted via either the right internal jugular or right femoral vein. The catheter was positioned in the coronary sinus. Its position was verified fluoroscopically and by hand injection of radiographic contrast media. The tip was then advanced to the great cardiac vein, over a guide wire if necessary. The patients then received 10,000u intravenous heparin for anticoagulation. Further heparin was determined by the length of the angioplasty procedure. A continuous infusion of heparin was not utilized.

The PTCA then proceeded with angiography of the affected vessel, crossing of the stenosis with the appropriate dilation system, and two inflations were then performed. During these inflations, in addition to continuous ECG recording, transtenotic gradient, pulmonary artery pressure, and symptoms were recorded. The patients were allowed to return to their baseline state between inflations.

Following the second inflation, CSRP was initiated by inserting an 8F arterial supply catheter (U.S.C.I., Billerica, MA) via the right femoral arterial introducer, which was then connected to the inflow side of the pumping device. After purging the system of all air, the outflow was connected to the coronary sinus catheter (U.S.C.I., Billerica MA) and retroperfusion initiated. Flow was increased to a maximum of 1.5 ml/kg/min and maintained at that level for 10 minutes prior to continuing the procedure.

Two further inflations were performed, monitoring the same parameters as above. The first of these was maintained until symptoms dictated release or 90 seconds had elapsed. The second was maintained again until symptoms made deflation necessary or the balloon had been inflated for 3 minutes. The patient was then weaned from the retroperfusion device and the 50 ml of blood contained in the system returned by flushing with heparinized saline from the connection to the arterial catheter. The pump was then disconnected and the catheters were left in place. In the event of acute coronary occlusion, CSRP could again be rapidly instituted.

Ten minutes following cessation of CSRP, 2 additional inflations were performed in the same manner as the initial inflations. All catheters were removed following determination of a successful outcome from the PTCA and final angiography.

Preliminary review of our experience in these patients suggests that although there is some training effect with respect to symptoms, CSRP delayed the appearance of symptoms and that this effect was even more marked with the second inflation during CSRP, perhaps related to a time delay necessary for the development of the effectiveness of retroperfusion. Similarly there may be an incomplete washout effect observed during the first post CSRP inflation. Similar findings are seen when inflation time alone, time to initial and comparable ECG changes, and a measure of the rate of development of ECG changes are evaluated.

There were no changes in pulmonary artery pressure or transtenotic gradients attributable to CSRP. No complications related to this procedure have occurred and the prolongation of the procedure has been approximately 30 minutes. If this device were to be used as a clinical tool, rather than as part of a research protocol as described, it would not prolong a routine PTCA procedure significantly as the time necessary for catheter insertion and institution of CSRP was rarely more than 5 minutes.

This initial experience with CSRP during LAD angioplasty suggests several avenues for further investigation. First the expansion of its application to patients undergoing angioplasty of other vessels, i.e. left circumflex and particularly right coronary arteries. Its effectiveness in protecting the right heart and the inferior wall of the left ventricle have yet to be definitely established. There is, however, suggestive evidence from our experience that this is possible.

The use of CSRP in patients with multivessel disease would also be of interest as these are frequently longer procedures and therefore more difficult for the patients. Attenuation of symptoms would be particularly beneficial in that setting. The application of this procedure might also provide the mechanism for approaching left main stenoses in a much safer manner. If the myocardium distal to such lesions can be effectively supported, the risks not only during balloon inflation, but also in the event of complications would be greatly reduced.

It is not currently known whether longer inflation times have a role to play in reducing the incidence of re-stenosis. To date inflation times of several minutes could only be achieved in patients who do not develop significant symptoms during occlusion, a small percentage of the PTCA patients. This may now be possible to evaluate with the protection of the myocardium by CSRP. Similarly, additional time for safely attempting to re-open occlusive dissections and the ability to use longer inflations to accomplish this may now be possible. Current experience with CSRP is limited, however preliminary data are very encouraging and allow for guarded but enthusiastic speculuation about its future roles in interventional cardiology.

References

1. Drury JK, Yamazaki S, Fishbein MC, Meerbaum S, Corday E (1985) Synchronized diastolic coronary venous retroperfusion: Results of a preclinical safety and efficacy study. JACC 6: 328
2. Farcot JC, Meerbaum S, Lang T, Kaplan L, Corday E (1978) Synchronised retroperfusion of coronary veins for circulatory support of jeopardized ischemic myocardium. Am J Cardiol 21: 1191
3. Gore JM, Weiner BH, Sloan KM, Cuenoud HF (1985) The safety of synchronized coronary sinus retroperfusion (SCSR) for up to 24 hours. Chest (Abstr) 88: 73
4. Meerbaum S, Lang T, Osher JV et al (1976) Diastolic retroperfusion of acutely ischemic myocardium. Am J Cardiol 37: 588
5. Weiner BH, Gore JH, Sloan KH, Benotti JR, Gaca JHJ, Okike ON, Vander Salm TS, Ball SP, Corrao J, Alpert JS, Dalen SE. Synchronized coronary sinus retroperfusion (SCSR) during LAD angioplasty. JACC (in press)
6. Zalewski A, Goldberg S, Slysh S, Maroko P (1985) Myocardial protection via coronary sinus interventions: Superior effects of arteriolization compared with intermittent occlusion. Circulation 71: 1215

Authors' address:
Bonnie H. Weiner, M.D.
Division of Cardiovascular Medicine
University of Massachusetts Medical School
Worcester, MA 01605
U.S.A.

Coronary venous retroinjection: the role of pressure gradients during selective distribution to ischemic myocardium

M. Meesmann, H. S. Karagueuzian, T. Ino, A. McCullen, W. J. Mandel, and T. Peter

Division of Cardiology, Cedars-Sinai Medical Center, Department of Medicine, UCLA School of Medicine, Los Angeles, California (U.S.A.)

Coronary venous retroinjection is associated with preferential drug delivery to ischemic myocardium (1, 2). The mechanism of this distribution, however, is not defined. We therefore sought to delineate distribution patterns of coronary venous retroinjections under various conditions of myocardial perfusion pressure using Monastral blue dye as a marker. In 22 open chest dogs dye injections were made via a balloon catheter in the distal great cardiac vein with systolic pressures in the anterior interventricular vein (AIV) reaching 60 to 85 mm Hg. The dye injections were made according to 3 protocols. In protocol I the aortic pressure was normal (systolic 90 to 130 mm Hg) and no myocardial staining occurred despite retrograde filling of the AIV (n = 11). In protocol II (normal aortic pressure) the left anterior descending coronary artery (LAD) was occluded leading to a clearly defined cyanotic area. Dye injections, made one minute after onset of ischemia, resulted in selective staining of the ischemic area in 15 out of 18 dogs. In protocol III the dye injections were made during ischemic hypotension (systolic pressures less than 55 mm Hg). This resulted in complete staining of the myocardium drained by the AIV (n = 5). Post mortem examination of left ventricular slices showed that staining, if present, was transmural.

In six dogs simultaneous pressures recordings were obtained from the AIV, the LAD (distal to occlusion), the aorta and the left ventricle. During retroinjection the following pressure gradients were observed: from the AIV to the distal LAD (35 to 50 mm Hg) during systole and from the AIV to the left ventricular chamber (8 to 30 mm Hg) during diastole. There was no diastolic gradient between the AIV and distal LAD. Pressure gradients in the normal myocardium within the AIV territory were reduced in amplitude but remained arteriovenous in direction (i.e. arterial pressure > venous pressure).

We conclude: 1) the pattern of retrograde coronary venous distribution is influenced by myocardial perfusion pressure with higher pressures in the arterial side preventing coronary venous retrograde delivery 2) the systolic and/or diastolic pressure gradients might form the basis for selective retrograde flow to ischemic myocardium.

Supported in part by Cedars-Sinai ECHO fund. Dr. Meesmann is recipient of research grant Me 799 of the Deutsche Forschungsgemeinschaft, West Germany. Dr. Karagueuzian is recipient of Research Career Development Award HL 01293-03, National Heart, Lung, and Blood Institute, Bethesda, M.D., U.S.A.

The extravascular resistance of the ischemic myocardium, in particular the subendocardium (3), presumably limits retrodistribution during systole. Further studies are needed to determine the relative importance of these pressure gradients.

References

1. Cibulski A, Markov A, Lehan P, Galyean J, Smith R, Flowers W, Hellems H (1974) Retrograde radioisotope myocardial perfusion pattern in dogs. Circulation 47: 1033–40
2. Karagueuzian HS, Ohta M, Drury JK, Fishbein MC, Meerbaum S, Corday E, Mandel WJ, Peter T (1986) Coronary venous retroinfusion of procainamide: a new approach for the management of spontaneous and inducible sustained ventricular tachycardia during myocardial infarction. J Am Coll Cardiol 7: 551–63
3. Sabbah H, Stein P (1982) Effect of acute regional ischemia on pressure in the subepicardium and subendocardium. Am J Physiol 242: H240–H244

Authors' address:
Hrayr S. Karagueuzian, Ph.D.
Cedars-Sinai Medical Center
Div. of Cardiology, Room 5314
8700 Beverly Blvd
Los Angeles, CA 90048
U.S.A.

Comparative electrophysiological effects of coronary venous versus systemic intravenous procainamide on acutely ischemic myocardium

M. Meesmann, H. S. Karagueuzian, T. Ino, A. McCullen, W. J. Mandel, and T. Peter

Division of Cardiology, Cedars-Sinai Medical Center, Department of Medicine, UCLA School of Medicine, Los Angeles, California (U.S.A.)

Great cardiac vein retroinjection of procainamide (GCV-P) has shown greater efficacy than the systemic intravenous route in the treatment of ventricular tachycardias associated with experimental myocardial infarction after permanent occlusion of the left anterior descending coronary artery (3). Increased drug delivery to ischemic myocardium was suggested to be the underlying mechanism. Little, however, is known about the local electrophysiological effects associated with this new mode of drug delivery. We therefore compared the actions of GCV-P (5 mg/kg) to intravenous procainamide (IV-P) (5 mg/kg) on ischemic myocardium in 5 open chest dogs 3 to 7 minutes after complete occlusion of the left anterior descending coronary artery. In each dog both modes of injections were applied in a randomized fashion and compared to each other at corresponding times. Ninety minutes were allowed for recovery and drug washout between the two measurements. Monophasic action potentials were recorded from the ischemic epicardium with contact electrodes at pacing cycle lengths of 500, 400 and 300 ms (2).

After GCV-P the epicardial conduction time in the ischemic myocardium was 192% more prolonged than after IV-P ($p < 0.05$). GCV-P was also associated with a significantly greater slowing of the upstroke velocity of monophasic action potentials than IV-P ($90 \pm 11\%$ versus $54 \pm 21\%$, $p < 0.05$), often leading to rate-dependent conduction block in the ischemic myocardium. No conduction block occurred after IV-P. The rightward shift of strength-interval curves was 3 to 5 times more pronounced after GCV-P than after IV-P, progressively leading to complete inexcitability of the ischemic myocardium. In contrast, however, excitability was preserved after IV-P.

We conclude: 1) great cardiac vein retroinjection of procainamide has more pronounced electrophysiological actions on ischemic myocardium than the intravenous administration; 2) this increased action could account for the enhanced efficacy of retroinjection of procainamide in the treatment of ventricular tachycardias in the setting of anterior myocardial infarction (3).

The findings of this study provide further evidence that coronary venous retroinjection leads to enhanced delivery of drugs to ischemic myocardium. Such an effect may be of great benefit in controlling and suppressing otherwise "drug-resistant" ventricular tachy-

Supported in part by Cedars-Sinai ECHO fund. Dr. Meesmann is recipient of research grant Me 799 of the Deutsche Forschungsgemeinschaft, West Germany. Dr. Karagueuzian is recipient of Research Career Development Award HL 01293-03, National Heart, Lung, and Blood Institute, Bethesda, MD, U.S.A.

cardias (1). Because of the pronounced electrophysiological effects associated with retroinjection of procainamide, low doses should be tested initially to avoid the danger of arrhythmia aggravation (3).

References

1. Duffy CE, Swiryn S, Bauernfeind RA, Strasberg B, Palileo E, Rosen KM (1983) Inducible sustained ventricular tachycardia refractory to individual class I drugs: effects of adding a second class I drug. Am Heart J 106: 450–8
2. Franz MR, Flaherty JT, Platia EV, Bulkley BH, Weisfeldt ML (1984) Localization of regional myocardial ischemia by recording of monophasic action potentials. Circulation 69: 593–604
3. Karagueuzian HS, Ohta M, Drury JK, Fishbein MC, Meerbaum S, Corday E, Mandel WJ, Peter T (1986) Coronary venous retroinfusion of procainamide: a new approach for the management of spontaneous and inducible sustained ventricular tachycardia during myocardial infarction. J Am Coll Cardiol 7: 551–63

Authors' address
Hrayr S, Karagueuzian, Ph.D.
Cedars-Sinai Medical Center
Div. of Cardiology, Room 5314
8700 Beverly Blvd
Los Angeles, CA 90048
U.S.A.

Coronary venous retroinfusion of procainamide and verapamil: for the management of spontaneous sustained ventricular tachycardia during myocardial infarction. Comparative study with the systemic intravenous route

H. S. Karagueuzian, M. Ohta, Malte Meesman, T. Ino, J. K. Drury,
M. C. Fishbein, S. Meerbaum, E. Corday, W. J. Mandel, and T. Peter
With the technical assistance of A. McCullen

The Division of Cardiology and Anatomic Pathology, Department of Medicine and Pathology, Cedars-Sinai Medical Center, UCLA School of Medicine, Los Angeles, California (U.S.A.)

Introduction

Drug therapy of ventricular tachycardia in the setting of ischemic heart disease is often unsatisfactory as these arrhythmias manifest refractoriness to either individual or combined antiarrhythmic drug therapy both in clinical and experimental settings (1, 4, 6, 10, 14, 18, 20). Patients manifesting resistance to antiarrhythmic drug therapy may have deficient and/or inadequate myocardial distribution of the drug, especially in and around severely ischemic zones. Alternatively resistance to drug therapy may be a characteristic of the drug itself, relatively independent of drug concentration. In the present study, a conscious canine model of anterior myocardial infarction caused by the left anterior descending coronary artery (LAD) occlusion with spontaneous ventricular tachycardia (11) was used to determine whether regional retrograde coronary venous infusion of procainamide or verapamil would provide effective antiarrhythmic therapy (2, 3). The great cardiac vein was selected because it predominantly drains the left anterior descending coronary artery perfusion zone (17). The effectiveness of coronary venous drug retroinfusion is compared to conventional intravenous therapy.

Methods

Surgical procedures

Sixteen closed chest mongrel dogs of either sex weighing between 22–26 kg were premedicated with intramuscular morphine sulphate (1 mg/kg) and anesthetized with intravenous sodium pentobarbital (30–35 mg/kg). The left anterior descending coronary artery

Presented in part to the 34th Annual Meetings of the American College of Cardiology in Anaheim, California, March 1985 and to the International Symposium on Ventricular Tachycardia, Vittel France May, 1986.
Supported in part by ECHO Research Fund of Cedars-Sinai Medical Center. H. S. Karagueuzian is recipient of Research Career Development Award No. HL 01293-03, National Heart Lung Blood Institute, Bethesda, MD

was occluded in the closed chest just proximal to its first diagonal branch by inflating the balloon of a Fogarty, Arterial Embolectomy Catheter (Edwards Laboratories, Inc.), inserted through the left carotid artery. Complete occlusion was confirmed fluoroscopically by noting absence of flow distal to the inflated balloon after injection of a small amount of contrast medium (Renografin-76) proximal to the balloon (12). A 7F autoinflatable balloon catheter (5, 13) was inserted through the left internal jugular vein into the coronary sinus and advanced to the great cardiac vein where it bifurcates into the anterior intraventricular coronary veins. During retrovenous drug injection through the tip of this catheter, the balloon automatically inflates, thus preventing direct backward shunting from the regional coronary veins into the right atrium. The drug is delivered retrogradely via the great coronary vein to the specific myocardial region supplied by the left anterior descending coronary artery.

Two Tygon Catheters (3.17 mm o.d., 1.58 mm i.d.) were inserted, one through the right carotid artery to record ascending aortic blood pressure and the other through the right internal jugular vein for systemic intravenous drug injection. The dogs were then returned to their cages for recovery and subsequently studied in the conscious, mildly sedated (intramuscular morphine 1 mg/kg) state, 24 hours after left anterior descending coronary artery occlusion. Surface electrograms, arterial blood pressure and intracardiac recordings were amplified using an Electronics for Medicine DR 16 system, and recorded on magnetic tape (Bell and Howell data tape CPR 4010) for subsequent selective retrieval (paper speed 50 to 100 mm/sec).

Experimental protocol

The efficacy of procainamide (13 dogs) or verapamil (3 dogs) by a given mode were tested by administering incremental bolus doses of procainamide (3 to 5 mg/kg up to 35 mg/kg) and 0.05 up to 0.15 mg/kg for verapamil. The order of intravenous or great cardiac vein mode of drug injection was randomized. Only one drug was tested in a given dog. After testing by a particular mode and prior to the alternate route of drug study, baseline spontaneous ventricular tachycardia was present in each dog. To determine the effects of coronary venous administration of a non active control substance on the tachycardia, saline was retroinfused during baseline ventricular tachycardia.

For the coronary venous retroinfusion, the drugs were diluted in 5 ml normal saline and warmed at 37 °C and were then administered over a 5 second period, immediately followed by a 5 seconds retrograde 5 ml saline flush at 37 °C. Thus, for each retroinfusion the coronary vein remained occluded for a total of 10 seconds.

Histopathologic examinations

Just prior to sacrifice, 5 ml of Monastral blue and Monastral red dye (Dupont) were injected to delineate grossly the areas of myocardial procainamide distribution. When red dye was injected into the great cardiac vein, blue dye was simultaneously injected into the left ventricle, in an attempt to delineate the areas of both retrograde and antegrade myocardial perfusion. Areas of myocardial necrosis were evaluated by planimetry after gross staining of the myocardium by the triphenyl tetrazolium chloride technique (9). For his-

300

tologic evaluation, six micron thick sections were stained with hematoxylin and Eosin (H and E), or with toluidine blue.

Results

Effects of systemic intravenous procainamide

Figure 1 illustrates the effect of intravenous procainamide in a representative dog with spontaneous ventricular tachycardia. In ten of the thirteen dogs studied, incremental doses of systemic intravenous procainamide up to 35 mg/kg were ineffective in suppressing the tachycardias. In 3 dogs, intravenous procainamide at a mean dose of 30 ± 3 mg/kg promptly suppressed the tachycardias and restored normal sinus rhythm with a mean rate of 132.5 ± 17 beats/min for a period of 3 to 7 min (mean of 4.2 ± 2.1 min), thereafter, ventricular ectopic activity re-emerged gradually and developed within 3 hours

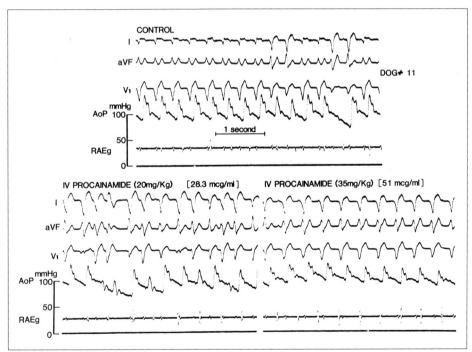

Fig. 1. Inefficacy of systemic intravenous procainamide administration to suppress spontaneously occurring ventricular tachycardia in a conscious dog one day after permanent left anterior descending coronary artery occlusion. Top panel shows ventricular tachycardia at a rate of 192 beats/min during control condition. After intravenous administration of 20 mg/kg of procainamide, causing a peak plasma level of 28.3 μg/ml of procainamide, tachycardia was not suppressed (lower left panel). Additional 15 mg/kg of procainamide injection (total of 35 mg/kg) caused a peak plasma level of 51 μg/ml of procainamide (lower right panel); tachycardia was still not suppressed, but its rate was reduced to 162 beats/min. (From Karagueuzian et al. (13), J Am Coll Cardiol Volume 7, 1986.)

301

to a tachycardia with originally observed rate and QRS configuration. In the ten dogs in which normal sinus rhythm could not be restored despite a total cumulative dose of 35 mg/kg, there was a significant ($P < 0.05$) reduction in the rate of the tachycardia without significant change in aortic blood pressure.

Effects of great cardiac vein procainamide retroinfusion

Figure 2 illustrates in one dog the efficacy of great cardiac vein procainamide retroinfusion in terminating spontaneous ventricular tachycardia. This mode of procainamide delivery was effective in eleven of the thirteen dogs studied in suppressing the tachycardias, with prompt restoration of normal sinus rhythm. This retroinfusion effect was statistically significant when compared to the systemic intravenous route of procainamide treatment ($P < 0.01$). The mean rate of re-established normal sinus rhythm was

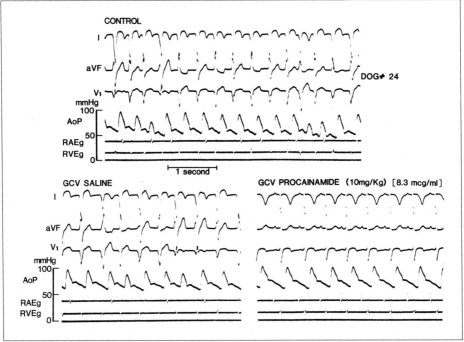

Fig. 2. Comparative effects of great cardiac vein retroinfusion of normal saline and procainamide in a conscious dog with spontaneously occurring ventricular tachycardia one day after permanent occlusion of the left anterior descending coronary artery. This figure is organized in the same fashion as in Fig. 1, with the addition of right ventricular bipolar electrogram (RVEg) on the bottom of each panel. The top panel is a control run of ventricular tachycardia. Retroinfusion of 10 ml of normal saline through the great cardiac vein (GCV) (lower left panel), had no detectable effect on tachycardia. In contrast, however retroinfusion of 10 mg/kg of procainamide through the GCV (lower right panel), promptly terminated the tachycardia with the resumption of normal sinus rhythm. This was associated with a peak plasma level of 8.3 µg/ml. (From Karagueuzian et al. (13), J Am Coll Cardiol Volume 7, 1986.)

121.5 ± 13.1 beats/min (range 95–135 beats/min) and lasted 11.3 ± 3.2 min (range 3–18 minutes), which was comparable to the duration of systemic procainamide administration ($P < 0.1$). Thereafter ventricular ectopic beats re-emerged progressively, and after 3–4 hours tachycardia similar in rate and QRS morphology to that noted prior to procainamide retroinfusion, re-emerged. In the two dogs in which a cumulative retrograde dose of 35 mg/kg procainamide was ineffective, a reduction in tachycardia rate was noted from 215 to 182 and from 197 to 166 beats/min respectively. Systolic blood pressure did not change after a mean dose of 19.6 ± 8.8 mg/kg procainamide retroinfusion, however, a small but significant ($P < 0.05$) elevation in diastolic blood pressure was noted.

Effect of normal saline infusion on ventricular tachycardia

Coronary venous retroinfusion of normal saline had no effect on either spontaneously occurring ventricular tachycardia or on aortic blood pressure (Figure 2).

Effects of verapamil

In three additional dogs, the effects of great cardiac vein and systemic intravenous administration of a cumulative dose of (0.15 mg/kg) verapamil was tested. In all three dogs great cardiac vein retroinfusion of verapamil successfully converted ventricular tachycardia to normal sinus rhythm, whereas systemic intravenous verapamil was without effect. The aortic blood pressure after systemic intravenous administration of verapamil was much more profoundly reduced than after great cardiac vein retroinfusion of similar doses of verapamil.

Myocardial dye distribution after great cardiac vein and systemic intravenous administrations

Most of the dye retroinfused through the coronary vein distributed over the anterior wall of the left ventricle into regions supplied by the occluded artery. Various degrees of staining were consistently seen in all preparations within the general zone of the infarction including the subepicardial and subendocardial regions overlying the infarcted zone (n = 6). The least amount of dye after coronary venous retroinfusion was seen in the posterior septum and the posterior papillary muscle. The demarcation between the anterior and posterior wall distribution was variable; in some cases it was sharply delineated and in others it was less distinct. In contrast, areas of dye distribution after left ventricular injection were mostly confined to the posterior wall of the left ventricle, with no or very little staining in the anterior wall, including the zone of infarction. Myocardial zones bordering the infarct appeared to be within the territory of both left ventricular and coronary venous routes of drug delivery (zone of overlap) as both dyes were present in these zones. Mean myocardial infarct size estimated by planimetry was 23.5 ± 52 per cent of the left ventricle (range 18.5–35.6 percent).

Discussion

The major finding of the present study is that great cardiac vein procainamide and vera-pamil retroinfusion is significantly more effective than systemic intravenous administration in suppressing spontaneous sustained ventricular tachycardia in a conscious canine model of myocardial infarction. These findings of procainamide were similar to the canine tachycardia model of chronic myocardial infarction, in which programmed electrical stimulation induces sustained ventricular tachycardia caused by a re-entrant mechanism (13).

The electrophysiological mechanisms underlying spontaneously occurring ventricular tachycardia one day after permanent left anterior descending coronary artery occlusion seem to be more complex than originally anticipated. Both re-entrant and automatic mechanisms (triggered or abnormal or both) have been implicated in the genesis of these late phase tachycardias, with ectopy arising at both epicardial and endocardial sites overlying the infarcted left anterior wall (7, 8, 19). We do not know the precise electro-physiological mechanism(s) responsible for tachycardia conversion to normal sinus rhythm by either procainamide or verapamil. The elevation of myocardial excitability threshold with prolongation of refractoriness in ischemic myocardial sites as shown by Michelson and associates (16) may well be (at least in part) important operative mechanisms. Drug-induced decrease in myocardial excitability has been shown to be associated with effective arrhythmia suppression one day after coronary artery occlusion (12). It is possible that procainamide at certain critical myocardial sites can suppress an arrhythmia generating mechanism (re-entry, and/or automaticity) by virtue of appreciable decrease in myocardial excitability along with a prolongation of myocardial refractoriness. On the other hand, the ability of verapamil to terminate both abnormal and/or triggered automatic mechanisms (7) at critical ischemic myocardial sites otherwise not accessible by systemic intravenous route may be the mechanism responsible for the greater efficacy of great cardiac vein verapamil compared to systemic intravenous route. Further studies are needed to resolve these issues.

Clinical implications

Retrograde coronary sinus delivery of hypothermic cardioplegic solutions has been used to protect myocardium during aortic valve surgery (15). The use of the coronary sinus and the great cardiac vein as an alternate and possibly effective route for antiarrhythmic drug delivery has not as yet been tested in man. In light of the present experimental observations, it seems plausible that some patients with "drug refractory" ventricular tachyarrhythmias may be considered as suitable candidates in emergency situations in the intensive care setting. However, both dosage regimen and safety issues for this new retrograde delivery route need to be carefully evaluated.

Acknowledgements

We kindly acknowledge Ms. Carol Ginyard and Rose Isidro for typing this manuscript and Ms. Brenda Williams for editing the manuscript.

References

1. Bagwell EE, Wale T, Drayer DE, Reindenberg MM, Pruett JK (1976) Correlation of the electrophysiological and antiarrhythmic properties of the N-acetyl metabolite of procainamide with plasma and tissue drug concentrations in the dog. J Pharmacol Exp Ther 197: 38–48
2. Berdeaux A, Farcot JC, Bourdarias JP, Barry M, Bardet J, Guidicelli JF (1981) Effects of diastolic synchronized retroperfusion on regional coronary blood flow in experimental myocardial ischemia. Am J Cardiol 46: 1033–1040
3. Cilbulski AA, Markov A, Lehan PH, Galyean JR, Smith RO, Flowers WM Jr, Hellums HK (1974) Retrograde radioisotope myocardial perfusion patterns in dogs. Circulation 50: 159–166
4. Davis J, Glassman R, Wit A (1982) Method for evaluating the effects of antiarrhythmic drugs on ventricular tachycardias with different electrophysiologic characteristics and different mechanisms in the infarcted canine heart. Am J Cardiol 49: 1176–83
5. Drury JK, Yamazaki S, Fishbein MC, Meerbaum S, Corday E (1985) Synchronized diastolic coronary venous retroperfusion: results of a preclinical safety and efficacy study. J Am Coll Cardiol 6: 328–335
6. Duffy CE, Swiryn S, Bauernfiend RA, Strasberg B, Palileo E, Rosen KM (1983) Inducible sustained ventricular tachycardia refractory to individual class I drugs: Effects of adding a second class I drug. Am Heart J 106: 450–458
7. El-Sherif N, Gough WB, Zeiler RH, Mehra R (1983) Triggered ventricular rhythms in 1-day-old myocardial infarction in the dog. Circ Res 52: 566–79
8. El-Sherif N, Mehra M, Gough WB, Zeiler RH (1982) Ventricular activation patterns of spontaneous and induced ventricular rhythms in canine one-day-old myocardial infarction. Evidence for focal and reentrant mechanisms. Circ Res 51: 152–66
9. Fishbein MC, Rit JYU, Lando U, Kanmatsuse K, Mercier JC, Ganz W (1980) The relationship of vascular injury and myocardial hemorrhage to necrosis after reperfusion. Circulation 62: 1124–1129
10. Graboys TB, Lown B, Podrid PJ, DeSilva R (1982) Long-term survival of patients with malignant ventricular arrhythmia treated with antiarrhythmic drugs. Am J Cardiol, 50: 437–443
11. Karagueuzian HS, Fenoglio JJ Jr, Weiss MB, Wit AL (1979) Protracted ventricular tachycardia induced by premature stimulation of the canine heart after coronary artery occlusion and reperfusion. Circ Res 44: 833–846
12. Karagueuzian HS, Fujimoto T, Katoh T, Peter T, McCullen A, Mandel WJ (1982) Suppression of ventricular arrhythmias by propafenone, a new antiarrhythmic agent, during acute myocardial infarction in the conscious dog. A comparative study with lidocaine. Circulation 66: 1190–1198
13. Karagueuzian HS, Ohta M, Drury JK, Fishbein MC, Meerbaum S, Corday E, Mandel WJ, Peter T (1986) Coronary venous retroinfusion of procainamide: A new approach for the management of spontaneous and inducible sustained ventricular tachycardia during myocardial infarction. J Am Coll Cardiol 7: 551–563
14. Mason JW, Winkle RA (1978) Electrode-catheter arrhythmia induction in the selection and assessment of antiarrhythmic drug therapy for recurrent ventricular tachycardia. Circulation 58: 971–985
15. Menasché P, Kural S, Fauchet M, Lavergne A, Commin P, Bercot M, Touchot B, Georgiopoulos G, Piwnica A (1982) Retrograde coronary sinus perfusion: A safe alternative for ensuring cardioplegic delivery in aortic valve surgery. Ann Thorac Surg 34: 647–657
16. Michelson EL, Spear JF, Moore EN (1981) Effects of procainamide on strength-interval relation in normal and chronically infarcted canine myocardium. Am J Cardiol 47: 1223–1232
17. Roberts RL, Nakazawa HK, Klocke FJ (1976) Origin of great cardiac vein and coronary sinus drainage within the left ventricle. Am J Physiol 230: 486–492
18. Ross DL, Sze DY, Keefe DL, Swerdlow CD, Echt DS, Griffin JC, Winkle RA, Mason JW (1982) Antiarrhythmic drug combinations in the treatment of ventricular tachycardia. Efficacy and electrophysiologic effects. Circulation 66: 1205–1210
19. Scherlag BJ, El-Sherif N, Hope R, Lazzara R (1974) Characterization and localization of ventricular arrhythmias resulting from myocardial ischemia and infarction. Circ Res 35: 372–83

20. Waxman HL, Buxton AE, Sadowski LM, Josephson ME (1982) The response to procainamide during electrophysiologic study for sustained ventricular tachyarrhythmias predicts the response to other medications. Circulation 67: 30–37

Authors' address:
Hrayr S. Karagueuzian, Ph.D.
Cedars-Sinai Medical Center
8700 Beverly Boulevard
Division of Cardiology, Room 5314
Los Angeles, CA 90048
U.S.A.

Workshop on synchronized retroperfusion

J. M. Gore and B. H. Weiner

Division of Cardiovascular Medicine University of Massachusetts Medical School, Worcester (U.S.A.)

To begin the workshop, a videotape was presented to review the basic concepts of coronary sinus retroperfusion and the implementation of the procedure in an animal.

Following a schematic of the coronary sinus retroperfusion system showing the pump console that allows for ECG timing and pump control, we showed the SRP catheter being inserted through an introducer placed in the internal jugular vein. The catheter is positioned in the coronary sinus approximately 4 to 5 centimeters into the great cardiac vein. The catheter has side holes near the tip surrounded by an autoinflatable balloon as well as an end hole, where the arterialized blood is ejected in a retrograde fashion. The side holes of the catheter allow for the inflation and deflation of the balloon, using the patient's own arterialized blood. Thus, no other agent such as helium, is required to inflate and deflate the balloon, which is one of the advantages of the sysem. We have been able to place this catheter into the coronary sinus from both the femoral vein and internal jugular vein approach.

The connection of the catheters and the pump console involves the following: inlet tubing, made of polyurethane, is connected to a femoral artery supply catheter. This takes the arterialized blood and delivers it to the pump, of which the two major components, are the main pump chamber and a blood reservoir. The latter smooths out the delivery of blood so that there is less trauma to the cells and minimal hemolysis. From here, arterialized blood, in a synchronized fashion, is delivered through another polyurethane tube to the SRP catheter located in the coronary sinus. The arterial supply catheter used, an 8 French 35 cm polyurethane catheter with side and end holes, aspirates blood from an artery. In this case, we used the femoral artery and placed the catheter just beyond the bifurcation of the central aorta. An animal retroperfusion catheter was then presented. The balloon, located near the tip, has about a 1 cc volume. The human catheter balloon is much larger with a volume of about 3–4 cc and a larger diameter when fully inflated.

The pump console has a cathode ray tube, which allows for continuous electrocardiographic monitoring, and options for measuring other parameters, including arterial pressure. We also have the capability of monitoring pump timing and cycling. In the future, we will be able to measure continuous coronary sinus pressure. The controls for the pump are divided into four panels. The top panel controls the flow, allowing us to adjust SRP flow from 25 to 150 cc per minute. We usually begin at low flow rates. There is some data in the literature that indicates that institution at high flow rates may cause some arrhythmias. We usually commence at 25 cc per minute and increase gradually over 5 minutes until we achieve the target flow rate, or there is relief of symptoms. The other two main controls of the console are the pump delay and the pump run time. The system can be synchronized off the electrocardiogram, arterial pressure, or internal triggers. The machine triggering is based on the R wave. A specific delay is set after perception of the R wave before commencing retroperfusion. A fixed amount of the cardiac cycle, usually 30–40%, is actual retroperfusion time, during which retroperfusion of arterialized blood occurs. When perfusion stops, the balloon deflates and allows for the egress of blood out of the coronary sinus.

An example of an animal instrumented for SRP was then shown. Through cutdowns, introducers are inserted into the femoral artery and internal jugular vein. In humans, these introducers are placed percutaneously. The SRP catheter is placed through the internal jugular vein into the right atrium. The key to catheter placement is to "bounce" it off the tricuspid valve. The catheter frequently ends up in the inferior vena cava, especially when the introducer is placed too deeply and ends up in the right atrium. Having found the tricuspid valve, the catheter is rotated slowly in a counter-clockwise manner and it will find its way into the coronary sinus. We inject hypaque (Winthrop) to show the outline of the coronary sinus. We look for good filling of the coronary venous system, in addition to adequate washout of contrast material through the right atrium.

The ECG and arterial pressure are monitored prior to instituting SRP. Retroperfusion is started by attaching the femoral artery catheter. The stopcock of this catheter is opened, allowing the arterialized blood to displace the heparinized saline in the tubing and pump chamber. Arterialized blood fills the pumping reservoir and the pump chamber and the blood comes out through the other side and flows towards the coronary sinus catheter. When there is free flow of blood from the outlet tubing, it is connected to the SRP catheter, and the system is then activated. To create ischemia, we use a 2.0 mm angioplasty dilatation catheter, left fully inflated, positioned in the proximal LAD. In our own work we have not found instantaneous reversal of electrocardiographic ischemic changes. It usually takes about 10–20 minutes. It has been our experience in humans also, that it takes a few minutes before we see positive ECG changes as a result of SRP.

To briefly review the system itself, it essentially has four components. First, the arterial supply catheter provides the arterialized blood. We hope that in the future the system will be simplified to exclude the arterial supply catheter; we are working on a venous oxygenator, which would enable us to use oxygenated venous blood. Secondly, there is the pump chamber assembly, a piston driven chamber, which actively propels the blood into the coronary sinus. This occurs through mechanized displacement, and it is calibrated so that flow can be set off the main console. In fact, it is calibrated relative to the catheter length. Thirdly, the monitor console permits ECG synchronization, or arterial blood pressure synchronization, and regulation of the amount of blood. The fourth component is a single lumen coronary sinus balloon catheter, which is autoinflatable.

With regard to the anatomy, there is a close relationship between the venous and arterial systems of the heart. There is a rich network of arteriovenous anastomoses. The coronary sinus empties into the right atrium in a posterior orientation. The proximal position of the SRP catheter is in the great cardiac vein before it courses anteriorly. This position generally provides good occlusion of the sinus during inflation with excellent filling of the anterior intraventricular vein, and because of the veno-veno we see good filling of the entire coronary venous system. Even when the catheter is positioned quite far into the coronary venous system there is good filling of the right ventricular and inferior venous channels.

The ostium of the human coronary sinus is found in the right atrium and is a fairly large structure. The valvular structure near the orifice occasionally causes the bulk of the balloon to hang up as the catheter is being inserted. This becomes an important point since sometimes a guide wire is required to get beyond this valve and properly place the catheter in the coronary sinus. When inserting the SRP catheter in humans, the tip may buckle when it approaches the coronary sinus. As in animals, the catheter will go down the inferior vena cava if it is not in the correct orientation. A guide wire is used for this particular insertion as shown.

Using contrast medium, one can actually see the balloon inflate while it is being positioned. A change can be seen in the catheter motion and orientation as it enters the sinus. A guide wire exiting from the tip of the catheter allows the catheter to be advanced further out into the great cardiac vein. The catheter may come back slightly during forceful injections. We have found, for instance using the internal jugular approach, that a guide wire is not required to advance further out of the coronary sinus. However, when injecting contrast you have to be careful that you do not inject too forcefully otherwise the catheter may be forced out of the coronary sinus.

It is not always easy to cannulate the coronary sinus. To orient in terms of catheter size, the right heart catheter is a 7 French catheter, as is the shaft of the SRP catheter. In its inflated configuration the balloon itself is several times the size of the catheter. It is not uncommon to be inferior to the coronary sinus, in a sort of pocket. One of the easiest approaches is to come down the right atrium, to generate a small turn in the tip of the catheter and then rotate posteriorly. Most of the insertions are done in the LAO projection, just to orient anterial and posterial, and are done very quickly with very little manipulation. Once it is in the coronary sinus, the catheter is very easily advanced to the optimal position.

Discussion

Farcot:
We have catheterized over 50 or 60 human coronary sinus and obviously what you said is right. First of all it is important to try to have the right shaped catheter. Secondly, one should get as close as possible to the ostium, and then use a little stearable wire. One can then advance the catheter very easily. I would also like to point out that there is, of course, a learning curve too. From now on, all our students, our residents, ought to be able to insert the catheter very easily. You mentioned that you try to get through without the supply. Four years ago I published almost the whole system in "Medical Progress Through Technology", an engineering publication, and reported that in ten patients we pushed the catheter from the femoral vein up to the area of the kidney drainage. If you sample blood at this level you will see that PO_2 concentration is close to arterial concentration, so we can really think about sharing a system like you show, having blood coming from the area of the kidney drainage, and be able to retroperfuse venous blood with very high oxygen content.

Weiner:
As you said, I think the critical issue is having a very high oxygen content. One of our unstable angina patients became hypoxic during the course of his clinical illness, during which time we had more difficulty with retroperfusion because we were in fact retroperfusing him with venous blood (unoxygenated arterial blood) functionally. Since one of the potential applications for a system like this is in patients who cannot have an intra-aortic

balloon inserted because of peripheral vascular disease, for example, or to make this a much more simple, stream-lined system, that would require only one catheter, to be able to obtain oxygenated venous blood would be a real advantage.

Farcot:
I would like to comment that we still have to prove that oxygen is a key issue.

Gore:
Dr. Peter Maroko's group has published a paper, and we've done some work ourselves with venous retroperfusion. With low oxygen saturations, the beneficial effects of retro-perfusion are lost and there is no infarct-sparing effect as there is with arterialized blood. It seems that oxygenation is a key component of whatever makes the system works.
I agree with Dr. Farcot that there is a learning curve with coronary sinus catheterization. I have found that it is not more difficult to place this catheter than it is to place a pulmonary artery catheter.

Kenner:
What is the range of blood flows which you inject into the coronary sinus?

Weiner:
The pump is calibrated from 25 to 150 ml per minute. In order to inflate and deflate the balloon, a flow rate somewhere between 25 and 50 cc/minute is required. The peak flow achievable with the current pump is 150 ml/min.

Gore:
I stress that we are only using an augmented flow of 100 cc/minute, so that it really has no effect on right sided pressures. We were concerned that SRP might affect thermodilu-tion derived cardiac output but this was not the case. Thus, the amount of extra blood that we are adding to the right side of the heart is really negligible.

Toggart:
How do you determine your optimal flow rate since you are not measuring pressure in the coronary sinus?

Weiner:
In terms of our initial protocols we were limited by the guidelines set by regulatory boards and have determined flow rates on the basis of ml/kg body weight/min (based on our animal experience). Given the range of the existing pump, we have been pumping at rates of approximately 1.5 ml/kg/min.

Gore:
We have done a series of about 70 animals and found a range of flows that seem to give the optimal benefit of SRP. Based on these results, we have determined the flows used in the human studies. In an angioplasty protocol, we have a fixed flow rate that we use and in the unstable angina protocol we start off at the lowest flow rate and increase it until re-lief of symptoms, aiming toward the target flow rate that we know, at least in animals, on a cc/kg/min basis, gave us the best results.

Weisel:
How does this system compare with balloon pumping?

Meerbaum:
The evidence of the effectiveness of intra-aortic balloon pumping on coronary flow is not definitive.

Weisel:
Well, it is different. In the case of a patient with coronary artery dissection as a result of angioplasty, I would put an intra-aortic balloon pump in, unless I had access to the operating room right away. Is your system as good as this? You must have addressed this with your review board.

Gore:
Essentially, we are in the process of evaluating the role of the system for patients with unstable angina as compared to the intra-aortic balloon. The advantage is that we have a system that can be implemented fairly easily at the bedside, at least comparable to the intra-aortic balloon.

Weisel:
It is a little more difficult, since there are two catheters, and fluoroscopy is not required to insert a balloon.

Gore:
We hope that this system increases supply, whereas the balloon works more on decreasing demand. In unstable angina the system may not have that much more benefit than the intra-aortic balloon, except in the delivery of antiarrhythmic agents, vasodilators or thrombolytic agents to where they have to work. The procedure is possible in peripheral vascular disease, aortic dissection, aortic insufficiency. In patients with contraindications to the intra-aortic balloon, we can do the procedure. With regard to angioplasty, Dr. Weiner has not had a complication yet, but there is the possibility that we could support a patient if there was an acute thrombosis or an acute dissection. We have not studied the system in acute infarcts, and I am not aware of any study that shows that the balloon is good for limiting the size of acute infarcts.

Smalling:
I think there is no evidence that balloon pumping limits infarct size, other than temporarily supporting the blood pressure. You have to get blood flow to the myocardium for there to be salvage. There is evidence with PICSO and with SRP that there is infarct salvage.
The problem is, at least in my limited experience, the blood pressure does not increase with coronary sinus pumping. I think a combined approach may be needed.

Farcot:
In the American Journal of Cardiology we published an article on microsphere studies in which we proved, first of all, that synchronized retroperfusion exhibited some redistribution of the blood towards the endocardium in the ischemic zone, as well as some support

in the non-ischemic zone. Balloon pumping reduced after-load and improved non-ischemic area perfusion. It has been proven in many experimental studies and in our lab (this has been duplicated very recently by Dr. Meerbaum's group) that microspheres are delivered to the ischemic zone and favorably redistributed toward the endocardium by synchronized retroperfusion. So this is the main difference of these two techniques.

Gore:
I would be interested to know of studies that show that the intra-aortic balloon is useful in limiting infarct size, since I have only found some reports with thrombolytic agents.

Meerbaum:
Despite extensive studies of intra-aortic balloon pumping concerning perfusion, and our retroperfusion experience, together with some work on the combination of the two, I am not aware of any major proven effect of intra-aortic balloon pumping on achieving an increase in the myocardial perfusion.

Toggart:
At this symposium our surgical colleagues have said that pressures within the coronary sinus rise only to about 40 mm Hg during synchronized retroperfusion. Yet I have heard several surgeons comment that during the initial phases of cardioplegia pressures in the coronary sinus rise to 100–140 mm Hg until the heart arrests.

Gore:
As we heard from Dr. Okike from our institution yesterday, it may be related to whether retroperfusion is pulsatile or non-pulsatile. With a non-pulsatile system you are essentially wedging the catheter to accomplish retrograde flow, you have fixed capacitance. As you increase the flow, pressure will build up. We think the pulsatile system is better because it allows for a short interval pressure build-up during which the retroperfusion of cardioplegia occurs, and with the deflation of the balloon there is a prompt decrease in pressure. Just as with PICSO, as soon as you deflate the balloon, the pressure drops and there is drainage out. This prevents a continuous build-up of pressure and is why, in Dr. Okike's experiments, he found no evidence of edema in the coronary venous system.

Gundry:
I think what you say is right, but the main feature is, as surgeons, we totally occlude the coronary sinus at its orifice so that any venous exit from the coronary sinus and venous system is blocked completely, whereas in almost all these catheter systems the balloon is well down into the great cardiac vein, so that, even if you continuously perfuse this through systole and diastole there is such extensive venous run-off through the other portion that is open that you never can achieve huge pressures. I think that is the main difference.

Weiner:
I think the other point is the difference between a beating heart and a non-beating heart, and the physiology of those two. Those are two entirely different preparations, the surgical approach is much more of a closed system, just by the way in which the methods are currently applied.

312

Hugenholtz:
Returning to the effects of lytic therapy in acute infarction, I think that there is over-whelming evidence that if we are in time with the proper lytic agents and/or further re-duce this obstruction, antegrade flow, in terms of likelihood to succeed as a strategy, would be a much better treatment of myocardial infarction than anything else presented so far.

Gore:
I agree with you. We have studied over a hundred patients now as part of the TIMI trial, and I am aware of the GISSI study that shows that there may be a decrease in mortality.

Hugenholtz:
With regard to unstable angina, from a clinician's viewpoint, it would be much easier to go straight to PTCA. Properly, carried out, with PTCA one can bring mortality down to a few percent, and reinfarction the same.

Farcot:
What percentage of your patients, 100 patients with unstable angina, can you catheterize right away?

Hugenholtz:
Over 50% improve from therapy without talking about recanalization as a first approach. There, presumably, the physiology is mainly one of increased vasomotor tone etc., and the combination of nitroglycerin and beta blockers will be successful. In the remaining 50%, we have found that PTCA performed within the first twenty-four hours is nearly al-ways sufficient. But, we are talking about global strategies, and rather than give the im-pression that this might be a major and early strategy, it should be reserved for the very complex case.
There is a philosophical question to be answered: traditionally we should work through the animal model toward a clinical situation, yet the points that have been made are ex-tremely difficult to reproduce in the animal laboratory. The dilemma we are having, is at what point do you decide to do an experiment on the human when you know that the equivalent situation in the animal cannot be found or recreated? This is an extremely dif-ficult point, not necessarily because of the health controls, and public outcry against ex-perimentation, but because I, as a scientist, would still like to definitely confirm a "hunch".

Harken:
It seems to me that one thing is obvious: We have two techniques that are safe. Whether they delay definitive therapy or not (I believe they do not), and whether you are talking about the court of law or the court of human conscience, we are at a point where we are denying some people relief from suffering, and possibly from death. There are several categories, at least one in global disease, where the peripheral disease is literally unsuita-ble for coronary bypass and the patient is in overwhelming pain, not controlled by our usual techniques. Either PICSO or retrograde perfusion would be morally and ethically justified because the time frame is considerable. Second, there is a whole category of ar-rhythmias. I am not sure how much PICSO would deliver the medication to the point of

need, but surely retrograde perfusion has established that fact. Many patients have unsuitable aortas for inter-aortic balloon counter pulsation. In the past we have cut down on an artery and inserted a catheter into it and then we put a cannula into perform arterial-arterial counter pulsation. Even that reduced infarct size I think, because it reduced the ischemic changes in the electrocardiogram. Then we went to the balloon as you all know. But there are instances where the balloon does not work. Whatever your therapy whether PICSO or retrograde perfusion, you have an ethical obligation to proceed. It is a reasonable calculated risk for you to go ahead and use your techniques on these people. I would accept a pig model as being similar to the human coronary circulation. If, by one of these techniques, you can reduce anaerobic metabolism and correct it to aerobic metabolism, there is sufficient justification to proceed with humans. There are instances where you are justified, so you may consider it as troubling your conscience that you are not proceeding in some of these areas: both moral and legal courts will approve a decision to proceed.

Authors' address:
Joel M. Gore, M.D.
Division of Cardiovascular Medicine
University of Massachusetts Medical School
Department of Medicine
55 Lake Avenue North
Worcester, Massachusetts 01605
U.S.A.

ICSO and PICSO

PICSO (pressure controlled intermittent coronary sinus occlusion) – developments and current concepts

W. Mohl

2nd Surgical Clinic, University of Vienna (Austria)

Introduction

Side by side with synchronized retroperfusion and the retrograde delivery of cardioplegia, PICSO (pressure controlled intermittent coronary sinus occlusion) is one of those alternative methods of protecting ischemic myocardium by a retrograde means which are generally considered as having great potential in becoming viable approaches in cardiac medicine. So far there is much evidence that PICSO is capable of coping with many of the problems associated with the early reperfusion period.

Basic mechanism of PICSO

The rationale of this intervention, developed by Mohl et al., is to elevate the coronary sinus pressure during controlled occlusion of the coronary sinus (3). During this temporary blockade of the coronary sinus a redistribution of venous flow and plasma-dense fluid causes more extensive flow into underperfused zones. This happens in accordance with the rise and fall of certain pressure gradients in the microcirculatory bed (4) (redistribution phase). As the coronary sinus pressure and hence perfusion to ischemic zones gradually rise until a certain plateau of systolic pressure peaks and thus pressure control is reached, mechanic, osmotic and ional forces come to react with the dysfunctioning metabolism of these areas (equilibrium phase).

During the intermittent release of the coronary sinus blockade a rapid change in outflow resistance forces excessive venous loads to drain into the right atrium. Toxic waste accumulated in the course of progressive angina is being washed out (washout period). This phase is followed by a hyperemic response in the coronary artery flow (2).

This cycling of high flow associated with low pressure (during intermittent coronary sinus release) and low flow in the venous vasculature associated with high pressure (during coronary sinus occlusion) appears to reverse the ischemic processes and bring them to a halt. We hypothesize these mechanisms to ultimately prevent cell death and enhance recovery during reperfusion.

PICSO system

PICSO is achieved through a balloon occlusion system, which is driven pneumatically with a pressure-dependent control of the occlusion and release cycles.

A 7F balloon catheter is inserted percutaneously or intraoperatively through the right atrium into the coronary sinus. The coronary sinus pressure is monitored through a central lumen of the catheter. As compared to synchronized retroperfusion, PICSO is a simpler device and more convenient to handle, and we assume that it will ultimately lend itself to use by less experienced hands in community hospitals.

However, PICSO still needs further optimization. In this respect more refined timing of the occlusion/release intervals continues to be the challenge of future research.

Optimization of PICSO

It is important to point out that cycling of the occlusion vs. release intervals is adjusted as indicated by the coronary sinus pressure. Continuous monitoring of the coronary sinus pressure dynamics is thus indispensable if the full benefits of this method are to be exploited.

Another aspect illustrating the necessity of proper cycling of the coronary sinus occlusion and release phases is the fact that washout of toxic metabolites as described above is closely related to coronary sinus pressure elevation during coronary sinus occlusion.

Although plateau CS pressure elevation limits the occlusion period and was hitherto regarded as fairly efficient, a time pattern of PICSO occlusions and releases which, through more exact timing, takes full account of continuously changing parameters such as heart rate or coronary venous flow appears indispensable. This is even more important since rigid regimens of coronary sinus occlusion/release cycles were found to produce either no effect or risked becoming counterproductive. This is due to the fact that an inadequate duration of coronary sinus release appears to be bound to lead to insufficient drainage and hence, to bring about edema formation and a decrease in coronary inflow rather than washout. According to our own studies with short coronary artery occlusions in the setting of reperfusion we found significant variations in coronary sinus pressure dynamics between different stages of coronary artery perfusion. Analysis of the time needed to reach 90% of the CSP plateau level revealed significant differences between normal perfusion, stenosis, coronary artery occlusion and reperfusion. Table 1 demonstrates quite clearly that there is a dependance between CS occlusion/release times and CSP dynamics as much as between CS occlusion/release times and the duration of coronary artery occlusion.

Various authors have focused their studies on the mechanisms and effect of PICSO.

While several authors never adapted CSO to CSP dynamics and therefore failed to produce favourable results, Jacobs et al. tried to use CSP feedback for a study of PICSO during 3 minutes of LAD occlusion and 30 minutes of reperfusion (1, 2, 6).

While Jacobs found PICSO to uniformly blunt reactive hyperemia during reperfusion she at the same time suggested that this be due to mechanical factors rather than to a reduction in the ischemic stimulus. This mechanical blunting of reactive hyperemia corresponds to our conception of the non-adapting ICSO mechanism rather than PICSO.

According to our own studies with short occlusions we found CSP dynamics to differ significantly between coronary artery occlusion and the other stages of reperfusion. This means that a coronary sinus pressure that reaches the plateau before the coronary artery is occluded is not necessarily bound to reach that very plateau during coronary artery occlusion. Moreover, a hyperemic response after release of the coronary artery occlusion

Table 1. Dependance between CS occlusion/release times and CSP dynamics as well as CS occlusion/release times and the duration of coronary artery occlusion.

Pre-coronary artery occlusion		Coronary artery occlusion		Reperfusion	
I	II	I	II	I	II
66.7	51.7	66.7	35.0	76.7	51.7
66.7	66.7	75.0	58.3	83.3	50.0
68.9	40.0	77.8	40.0	77.8	26.7
66.7	46.7	88.9	53.3	66.7	46.7
50.0	25.0	83.3	25.0	75.0	75.0
58.3	66.7	66.7	54.2	75.0	83.0
50.0	30.0	77.8	33.3	88.9	80.0
44.4	46.7	66.7	66.7	77.8	53.3
83.3	50.0	83.3	75.0	83.3	66.7
66.7	66.7	83.3	83.3	83.3	83.3
77.8	40.0	88.9	73.3	77.8	46.7
77.8	73.3	88.9	80.0	88.9	73.3
64.8 ± 12.1	50.3 ± 15.4	78.9 ± 8.7	56.4 ± 19.7	79.5 ± 6.3	61.4 ± 18.1

$p < 0.05$ $p < 0.001$ $p < 0.001$

$p < 0.001$ n.s.

$p < 0.001$

Analysis of T 90%: Time in terms of percentage of the total occlusion time needed for CSP to reach 90% of the plateau.

2 groups: Group I: Occlusion: 6– 9 s
                    Release: 8–11 s
        Group II: Occlusion: 12–15 s
                    Release: 2– 5 s

may produce a prolonged coronary sinus occlusion with the intrinsic risk of becoming counterproductive.

Evidently, this failure to adapt the length of the PICSO cycles to the changes in coronary sinus pressure dynamics does not permit full exploitation of the beneficial effects of PICSO. We are convinced that full exploitation of all the information available on CSP dynamics would help reduce counterproductive effects such as blunting of the hyperemic response.

Another widespread conception we take issue with is the assumption that ischemia is tantamount to perfusion deficit and that the effect of PICSO lies in compensating for this shortage. In our view this in only in part true. It must be clear that PICSO – even in its optimized form – will never make up for this deficit and may only provide relief as to the consequences of ischemia as they manifest themselves in changes in fluid content and the

Table 2. Optimal release times calculated from appropriate correlations between duration of coronary flow and the duration of the release time. Note the trend toward longer release times during ischemia as well as the differences between groups.

	Pre-occlusion	Occlusion	Reperfusion
Dog 1	2.27	2.84	2.89
Dog 2	3.58	3.96	4.04

electrolyte balance in the interstitial and intracellular space through its mechanism of washout of toxic wastes.

Another important parameter for the optimization of PICSO is the response of the flow in the coronary arteries to the cyclic coronary sinus occlusions and releases and hence to the concomitant changes in inflow resistance. Table 2 shows the mean values of release times during normal perfusion, coronary artery occlusion and reperfusion, as calculated from the loss in hyperemic response incurred by a non-adjusted application of CS occlusion and release cycles in two dogs. Release times were found to be subject to considerable variation with a trend toward longer release times during occlusion and reperfusion.

Prediction of infarct size by coronary sinus pressure dynamics

Another recent focus of our research work has been the establishment of a relationship between CSP dynamics and the development of an experimental myocardial infarction. So far preliminary data from our present study (5) suggest that CSP parameters during CS occlusion may be used as valid markers for estimates of the area at risk.

Three groups of dogs (28 in total) with myocardial infarction were investigated: Group I – 5 dogs with 6 hours of coronary artery occlusion, CAO; Group II – 11 dogs with 3 horus of CAO and 3 hours of reperfusion; Group III – 12 dogs with 3 hours of CAO and 3 hours of reperfusion. In each group PICSO was performed throughout the experiment. There were, however, individual variations as to the point of time at which PICSO treatment was initiated. In Group I PICSO was started at 15 min post CAO; in Group II at 30 min post CAO and in Group III at 2.5 hours post CAO and continued throughout reperfusion.

Peak systolic and diastolic coronary sinus pressure during PICSO was measured shortly after the onset of PICSO (A), at 3 hours (B), and at 6 hours after the start of the experiment (C). The following parameters were measured: peak systolic and diastolic CSP and the baseline values of systolic and diastolic CSP upon release. From these quantities the differences between systolic CSP and systolic baseline, and between diastolic CSP and diastolic baseline were computed.

Area at risk and infarct size, assessed upon sacrifice using dye solution and TTC were $28.2 \pm 7.8\%$ of left ventricle and $8.6 \pm 7.2\%$ respectively.

A linear stepwise regression was done to obtain an optimal model in terms of the highest correlation coefficient for both area at risk and infarct size.

A significant relationship was found to exist between area at risk measured post mortem and our 4-component model of CSP measurements, which we assume to be a valid

320

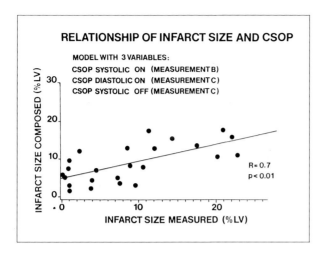

Fig. 1. Comparison of infarct size (% left ventricle) measured and infarct size computed from our 3-component model of coronary sinus pressure (CSP) measurements.

marker for the evolvement of myocardial cell necrosis, the main variables being the measurements taken at the beginning of PICSO.

As to infarct size a less favorable while still significant relationship was established, B and C measurements being the most important variables (Fig. 1).

We conclude that CSP pressure upon coronary sinus occlusion may be a valuable marker for estimating the extent of ischemic injury and evaluating the efficacy of conventional therapies as well as of coronary sinus interventions when applied in settings of acute myocardial injury.

This diagnostic implication, since it links the practical applications of PICSO to basic cardiovascular research, opens up a fascinating new domaine of our PICSO research.

In summary we may say that as with any new therapy, the PICSO technique will, of necessity, be as good or better than current medical or surgical therapy. Towards this end, PICSO will require evaluation against standard therapy or in combination with accepted treatments. It is of the utmost importance that any new method must be shown to be safe. Preliminary experimental and clinical studies have been encouraging in that there has been no evidence of major vascular damage due to PICSO. Investigations into a more refined monitoring of the coronary sinus pressure seem, however, necessary to avoid excessive pressure, prolonged coronary sinus occlusion and inappropriate cycling, which obstructs the full exploitation of the technique's inherent benefits.

References

1. Diltz E, Maines R, Lee J, Underwood T, Mishra A, Vankeyningen C, Nicklas J (1985) Intermittent coronary sinus occlusion does not reduce infarct size or ischemic dysfunction in an occlusion reperfusion model. Circulation 72 (Suppl III): 120
2. Jacobs A, Faxon D, Mohl W, Coats W, Gottsman S, Ryan T (1984) The effect of pressure controlled intermittent coronary sinus occlusion during ischemia. In: Mohl W, Wolner E, Glogar D (eds) The Coronary Sinus. Steinkopff Verlag, Darmstadt, pp 483–489
3. Mohl W (1984) The development and rationale of pressure controlled intermittent coronary sinus occlusion – a new approach to protect ischemic myocardium. WiKliWo 96: 537–548

4. Moser M, Mohl W, Gallasch E, Kenner Th (1984) Optimization of pressure controlled intermittent coronary sinus occlusion intervals by density measurements. In: Mohl W, Wolner E, Glogar D (eds) The Coronary Sinus. Steinkopff Verlag, Darmstadt, pp 529–536
5. Schuster J, Mohl W, Jacobs A, Faxon D, Simon P, Neumann F, Schreiner W (1986) Relationship between coronary sinus pressure dynamics and myocardial infarction (abstr)
6. Zalewski A, Goldberg S, Slysh S, Maroko P (1985) Myocardial protection via coronary sinus interventions: superior effects of arterialization compared with intermittent occlusion. Circulation 71 (Suppl. VI): 1215–1223

Author's address:
Werner Mohl, M.D.
2nd Surgical Clinic
University of Vienna
Spitalgasse 23
1090 Vienna
Austria

Intermittent coronary sinus occlusion in swine

E. Toggart, S. Nellis, and L. Whitesell

University of Wisconsin Hospital and Clinics, Department of Medicine,
Section of Cardiology Madison, Wisconsin (U.S.A.)

Purpose

The purpose of this study was to test the hypothesis that intermittent coronary sinus occlusion improves the metabolic and functional status of ischemic myocardium by retroperfusion, independent of collateral arterial flow.

Methods

An open-chest, in situ, whole blood perfused working swine heart preparation was used for this study. The coronary sinus was cannulated and coronary sinus flow diverted through a solenoid valve which was controlled by an external timing device for intermittent coronary sinus occlusion. Ultrasonic crystal pairs were placed transmurally to measure ischemic and nonischemic bed wall thicknesses. A Millar catheter was inserted into the left ventricle and a polyethylene cannula inserted into the coronary sinus via the hemiazygos vein for pressure measurement. The hemiazygos vein was ligated proximally. Regional myocardial blood flow was measured using 9 micron radio-labeled microspheres injected into a mixing chamber prior to the roller pumps in the coronary perfusion circuit. After baseline measurements the mid left anterior descending was ligated and a small cannula inserted into the distal vessel for pressure measurement and blood sampling.

Hemodynamic measurements including left ventricular and coronary sinus pressure, dp/dt, regional wall motion and samples for oxygen saturation from artery and coronary sinus were obtained at baseline. Microspheres were then injected for the measurement of regional myocardial blood flow. The left anterior descending was ligated. Repeat hemodynamics, blood sampling, and microsphere injection were then performed. The animals were then divided into treatment and control groups. Intermittent coronary sinus occlusion with 15 seconds of occlusion alternating with 5 seconds of release was performed on the treatment group. The solenoid valve was left in the open position for control animals. Data were then recorded at 15 minute intervals for one hour. At one hour a third microsphere injection was performed. Data were analyzed using nonpaired t statistics for comparison of control to treatment groups and paired t statistics for open versus closed within the treatment groups.

Results

Heart rate tended to be higher in the treatment group, although the difference was only significant at the post ligation time point. Peak left ventricular pressure was slightly but statistically significantly lower in the treatment versus control group at 30, 45 and 60 minutes. Despite these differences, global myocardial oxygen consumption calculated from total coronary flow, arterial and coronary sinus saturations was similar for treatment and control animals. Only at 15 minutes post ligation was the treatment group significantly greater than control. With intermittent coronary sinus occlusion both coronary sinus and LAD pressure significantly increased at all time points post ligation (Figs. 1 and 2). During release and in control animals, however, LAD pressure was approximately 12 mm Hg. Ischemic bed wall motion was severely depressed in both control and treatment groups with systolic thinning occurring post ligation (Fig. 3), and remained so for the duration of the study in both groups. Regional myocardial blood flow fell to near zero in endocardial and epicardial segments from the ischemic bed of both control and treatment animals with no change in either group at one hour. Left ventricular dp/dt in both treatment and control groups tended to increase in the treatment group and remained depressed in the control group. However these differences were not statistically significant.

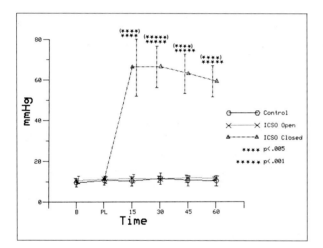

Fig. 1. Mean coronary sinus pressure.

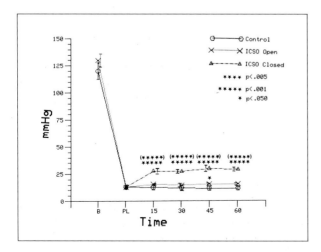

Fig. 2. Mean LAD pressure.

324

Left ventricular end-diastolic pressure rose in both groups post ligation and tended to decrease with time in the treatment group but these differences were not significant. Both end-diastolic and end-systolic ischemic bed thickness fell post ligation in control and treatment groups. While these parameters remained stable in control, a significant increase in thickness occurred in treatment groups comparing post ligation to 60 minutes post ligation. Coronary sinus oxygen saturation tended to be lower in treatment versus control animals however, the differences were significant immediately post ligation and at 45 minutes post ligation. Ischemic bed oxygen saturation remained stable in control animals but fell and remained significantly lower in treatment groups reaching statistical significance at 30, 45 and 60 minutes post ligation (Fig. 4).

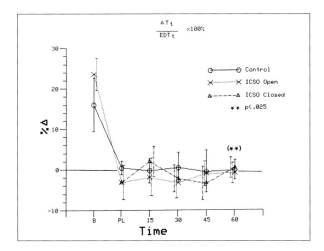

Fig. 3. Thickening of ischemic bed.

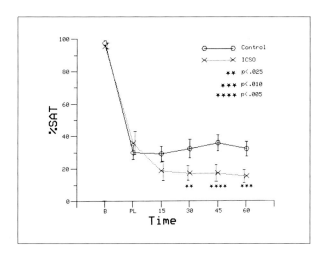

Fig. 4. LAD saturation.

325

Conclusions

1. In an animal model without arterial collaterals (as evidenced by no antegrade flow after LAD occlusion, and low LAD bed pressures during release) intermittent coronary sinus occlusion did not preserve global or regional parameters of mechanical function.
2. Distal coronary pressure, ischemic bed oxygen saturation, and changes in ischemic bed wall thickness are compatible with retroperfusion of the ischemic bed during intermittent coronary sinus occlusion.
3. Increases in end-diastolic and end-systolic wall thickness in the ischemic bed during intermittent coronary sinus occlusion may promote myocardial salvage by decreasing wall tension and thereby decreasing regional myocardial oxygen demand.
4. Lower ischemic bed oxygen saturations with intermittent coronary sinus occlusion are compatible with preservation of myocellular viability despite a lack of preserved mechanical function.

Authors' address:
Edward Toggart, M.D.
University of Wisconsin Hospital and Clinics
600 Highland Avenue
Department of Medicine, Section of Cardiology
Madison, WI 53792
U.S.A.

Hemodynamics of coronary sinus occlusion in the canine heart under an increased sympathetic drive

A. Juhász-Nagy, Violetta Kékesi, and L. Papp

Cardiovascular Surgical Clinic, Semmelweis University, Budapest (Hungary)

Summary: Short-term occlusions of the coronary sinus were performed in open chest dogs narcotized with pentobarbital to explore the coronary hemodynamic effects of this procedure in combination with adrenergic activation. Catecholamines (noradrenalin and adrenaline) were infused into the systemic circulation up to pharmacologic doses (2 μg · kg^{-1} · min^{-1}) to produce strong stimulation. It was found that the basic character of actions exerted by coronary sinus occlusion on arterial inflow and venous outflow (electromagnetic flowmeter) and on myocardial tissue blood flow (heat clearance) remained unchanged despite the great quantitative differences (hemodynamic shifts) between control and stimulated states. It was concluded that coronary sinus interventions may benefit even the sympathetically activated heart.

Ischemic events in the heart are often associated with an increased cardiac sympathetic drive which, especially in an excessive form, may be detrimental for jeopardized cardiac cells. The invention of new and ingenious methods for protecting the jeopardized myocardium via the coronary sinus has created a renewed interest in many relevant problems of coronary hemodynamics. Since little appears to be known about the modification of sinus occlusion-induced responses in hearts activated by adrenergic agents, the purpose of the present study was to assess these actions.

Methods

Seventeen mongrel dogs of either sex (16–28 kg) were studied under pentobarbital (30–35 mg · kg^{-1}) anesthesia. The heart was exposed by a transsternal dissection and cradled in the pericardium. Artificial ventilation was maintained with room air. Intravascular pressures were measured with the aid of Statham gauges (P 23 Db). Coronary blood flow was measured either with a Statham electromagnetic flow probe (SP 2201) fitted on the LAD artery or by using an extracorporeal flow probe (Carolina, Model 601 D) inserted into a large-bore (> 5 mm) closed artificial circuit between the cannulated sinus and a femoral vein. In most cases the coronary sinus was occluded abruptly (usually for 2 min) with a snare occluder placed around its terminal part; in other experiments (sinus outflow determinations) it was blocked in a step-by-step manner by using a screw clamp on the outflow circuit. In 3 dogs myocardial tissue blood flow was recorded with heated copper-constantan thermal probes which were introduced atraumatically into the mid-portion of the left ventricle supplied by the LAD artery. Noradrenalin and adrenaline were infused i.v. to obtain steady state responses. The dose range was 0.25–2.0 μg · kg^{-1} · min^{-1}. For comparison adenosine infusions (100–400 μg · kg^{-1} · min^{-1}) were also tested. Statistically evaluated numerical data are given as mean ± SEM. The significance of results was calculated by using Student's t-test for paired data.

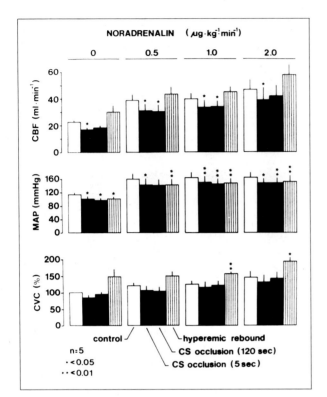

Fig. 1. Hemodynamics of 2 min coronary sinus occlusions. CBF: coronary blood flow (LAD), MAP: mean arterial pressure, CVC: coronary vascular conductance.

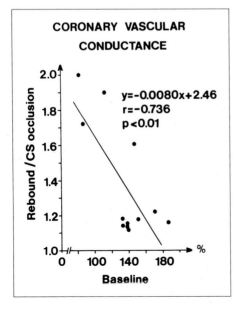

Fig. 2. Relative values of coronary vasodilator responses following sinus release plotted against baseline vascular tone induced by noradrenalin. Significant negative correlation was computed from the two-tailed regression of these responses. Same experiments as in Fig. 1.

Results

Arterial inflow

In five dogs coronary sinus occlusions of 2 min duration were performed during the control state and during noradrenalin infusions. The results as summarized in Fig. 1 showed a moderate steady inflow decrease in the LAD, followed by a short increase (rebound) on release. This hemodynamic pattern was singularly little affected by catecholamine administration. On occluding and releasing the sinus, the variable of coronary vascular conductance (%flow/%pressure) exhibited seemingly less regular changes than flow. Interestingly, the degree of the conductance rebound, i.e. the ratio of postocclusive vasodilation to the value of vascular conductance recorded during sinus occlusion, correlated significantly and inversely with the coronary vasodilation induced by the adrenergic stimulus itself (Fig. 2). This finding suggests the involvement of metabolic autoregulatory capacity of the coronaries during sinus occlusion: experimental proof for this suggestion was provided by eliciting reactive hyperemic responses (Fig. 3).

Venous outflow

The procedure for determining coronary sinus pressure-flow relationships is depicted in Fig. 4. During a gradual occlusion of the outflow tube the values of mean flow and pressure were found to be inversely and linearly related over a sinus pressure of 7–8 mm Hg. Accordingly, the data were arbitrarily normalized for blood flow determined at 10 mm Hg outflow pressure, and this level, as recorded in the control state, was regarded the 100 percent value of outflow. Pressure-flow lines were drawn from least-square regressions between 10 mm Hg and the intercept on the pressure axis, i.e. the occlusion pressure. Catecholamines, without considerably affecting their slopes, forced the lines to make a parallel shift to the right (Fig. 4). In 5 experiments, adrenaline doses of 0.25, 0.5, 1.0, and 2.0 $\mu g \cdot kg^{-1} \cdot min^{-1}$ augmented sinus occlusion pressure (control: 42.7 ± 6.2 mm Hg) by

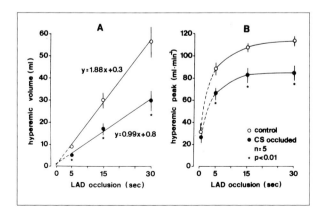

Fig. 3. Reduction of reactive hyperemia in the LAD after coronary sinus occlusion. Same experiments as in Fig. 1.

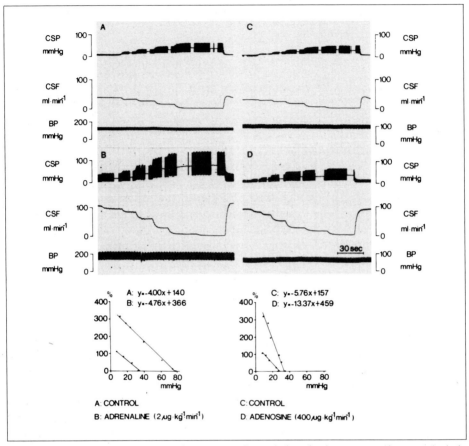

Fig. 4. The method used for determining pressure-flow relations in the coronary sinus: gradual obstruction of the outflow tube. Sinus occlusion pressure (intercept on the pressure axis) was considerably increased by adrenaline (left) but not by adenosine (right) which elicited coronary vasodilation of similar magnitude. CSP: coronary sinus pressure, CSF: coronary sinus flow, BP: blood pressure.

3.5 ± 0.7, 5.9 ± 1.0, 12.9 ± 4.3, and 26.6 ± 5.9 mm Hg, respectively ($p < 0.05$). Noradrenalin (2 dogs) and isoproterenol (2 dogs) elicited similar responses.

Tissue blood flow

The heat clearance technique was utilized to compare, in the same locus, *normal* deep myocardial flow patterns with those occurring during the *collateral-dependent* state 30–60 min after LAD ligation. The dogs were given noradrenalin (1 $\mu g \cdot kg^{-1} \cdot min^{-1}$) as an activator. A typical record (Fig. 5) shows that sinus occlusion elicited a reversed flow pattern after LAD ligation; noradrenalin did not alter the pattern but modified the response. In 3 experiments, on occluding the sinus, tissue blood flow was found to decrease from 100 ± 0 to $71 \pm 5\%$ (control) and from 127 ± 5 to $109 \pm 7\%$ (noradrenalin). After

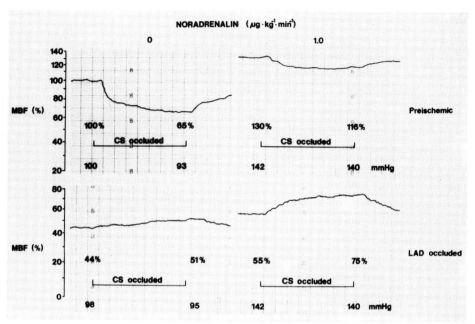

Fig. 5. Responses of myocardial tissue blood flow (heat clearance) before and after LAD occlusion.

LAD ligation the increases were: from 39 ± 4 to $47 \pm 2\%$ (control) and from 44 ± 10 to $57 \pm 12\%$ (noradrenalin), respectively.

Discussion

In most cases coronary sinus occlusion elicited a slight hypotension which was·probably reflex (3, 7); the animals were narcotized with barbiturate to minimize this effect. Nevertheless, a rough estimate of the vascular conductance in the coronary bed revealed a less pronounced fall in this variable than in flow on sinus occlusion. It is probable that compensatory adjustments contributed to the maintenance of myocardial blood supply, at the expense of the autoregulatory reserve, during sinus occlusion. This supposition tallies well with the parallel diminution of reactive hyperemia which follows brief LAD occlusions (Fig. 3). However, an alternative explanation is the mitigating action of coronary sinus occlusion on the hypoxic stimulus itself produced by an arterial inflow stop (2). In general, our observations essentially confirm the results obtained in former excellent studies concerning the dynamics and partition of arterial (1, 4, 5) and venous (6, 8) coronary flow during sinus occlusion. At the same time, our present measurements extend the validity of these findings to the cardiac muscle working under strong sympathetic influences: it seems that in the adrenergically stimulated heart the sinus occlusion-induced pressure-flow relations both in the left arterial and venous coronary bed are shifted to higher ranges but remain unchanged in their character. These observations may have relevance in predicting flow responses to various types of coronary sinus interventions performed under analogous pathologic circumstances.

References

1. Gregg DE, Shipley RE (1947) Studies of the venous drainage of the heart. Am J Physiol 151: 13–25
2. Jacobs AK, Faxon DP, Mohl W, Coats WD, Gottsman SB, Ryan TJ (1984) The effect of pressure controlled intermittent coronary sinus occlusion during ischemia. In: Mohl W, Wolner E, Glogar D (eds) The Coronary Sinus. Steinkopff Verlag, Darmstadt, pp 483–489
3. Juhász-Nagy A, Szentiványi M (1973) Effect of venous coronary reflexes on cardiovascular dynamics. Acta Physiol Hung 43: 287–299
4. Mohl W, Glogar D, Mayr H, Losert U, Sochor H, Pachinger O, Kaindl F, Wolner E (1984) Reduction of infarct size induced by pressure-controlled intermittent coronary sinus occlusion. Am J Cardiol 53: 923–928
5. Muers MF, Sleight P (1972) The reflex cardiovascular depression caused by occlusion of the coronary sinus in the dog. J Physiol (London) 221: 259–282
6. Scharf SM, Bromberger-Barnea B, Permutt S (1971) Distribution of coronary venous flow. J Appl Physiol 30: 657–662
7. Szentiványi M, Juhász-Nagy A (1962) Two types of coronary vasomotor reflexes. Quart J Exp Physiol 47: 289–298
8. Tiedt N, Litwin J, Skolasinska K (1966) The dynamics of the coronary venous pressure in the dog. Pflügers Arch 288: 27–42

Authors' address:
A. Juhász-Nagy
Cardiovascular Surgical Clinic
Semmelweis University
Budapest XII, Városmajor u. 68.1122
Hungary

Pressure controlled intermittent coronary sinus occlusion (PICSO) improves myocardial ischemia in swine

R. J. Capone, F. Fedele, A. Most, and H. Gewirtz

Division of Cardiology, Rhode Island Hospital, Providence, Rhode Island (U.S.A.)

Previous studies demonstrating efficacy of pressure controlled intermittent coronary sinus occlusion (PICSO) have been conducted in animal models during acute coronary occlusion (3, 4) or during coronary occlusion and reperfusion (2). It is, however, not known whether PICSO can favorably affect myocardial ischemic conditions induced by an increase in myocardial oxygen demand. We have therefore employed PICSO in a close-chested model of myocardial ischemia created by placing an intraluminal stenosis into the left anterior descending (LAD) coronary artery and pacing the heart at an accelerated rate. Myocardial metabolism was monitored by following changes in myocardial lactate consumption.

In 10 swine anesthetized with halothane a PICSO catheter was introduced from the right internal jugular vein into the coronary sinus and positioned immediately proximal to the entrance of the azygous vein. A 3 F polyethylene catheter was passed through the distal PICSO lumen into the mid-portion of the anterior interventricular vein (AIV), which drains the area supplied by the LAD. Following instrumentation, the animal was allowed to recover from anesthesia and received light intravenous barbiturate sedation for the remainder of the study. Baseline determinations of myocardial blood flow were made by injection of radioactive-labelled microspheres into the left atrium. Arterial and AIV blood gases and lactate levels were determined. An 80% stenosis was then placed into the LAD from the right carotid artery as previously described (1). The right atrium was paced to 140 beats/minute and repeat metabolic and hemodynamic measurements made at 30, 60, 90, 105, and 120 minutes following LAD stenosis. PICSO was instituted at 30 minutes and continued for 1 hour. Inflation of the PICSO catheter balloon was sustained until the AIV pressure reached approximately 90% of plateau for 3–4 beats (7.5–9 seconds); deflation was maintained for 4 seconds. Five animals were studied without the use of PICSO in order to observe the natural history of lactate dynamics in this preparation.

Lactate consumption was calculated as the product of lactate extraction (arterial – venous) and myocardial blood flow. Statistical analysis was carried out using blocked, one-way ANOVA and Dunnet's test.

With placement of the stenosis, pressure in the distal LAD fell, producing a mean gradient of 47 ± 8 in the PICSO group and a mean of 50 ± 6 mm in the non-PICSO group. Endocardial blood flow fell from a baseline of 1.72 ± 0.47 to 0.89 ± 0.24 ml/min/100 g at 30 minutes in the PICSO group and 2.10 ± 0.27 to 0.88 ± 0.34 ml/min/100 g in the non-PICSO animals. Epicardial blood flow remained normal in both groups. Lactate was consumed at baseline in PICSO animals (33.7 ± 20.0 μmol/min/100 g) and produced during LAD stenosis (-46.7 ± 37.5) $p < 0.01$. During PICSO lactate production was reduced to -13.1 ± 22.6 at 60 minutes and to -7.0 ± 17.6 at 90 minutes, $p < 0.01$. Production remained unchanged following discontinuance of PICSO (−14.9 ± 25.2) at 105 minutes and at 120 minutes (−7.6 ± 19.2).

In the five non-PICSO animals, lactate production following LAD stenosis occurred to a somewhat lesser degree than in the PICSO group (baseline = 55.8 ± 15.1; 30 minutes = −16.1 ± 7.9 μmol/min/100 g). In contrast to the PICSO group, it remained unchanged at subsequent measurements: −7.5 ± 9.7 (60 min), −8.5 ± 13.3 (90 min), −7.0 ± 13.9 (105 min), −3.8 ± 7.0 (120 min). Myocardial oxygen extraction, arterial pressure, left ventricular end-diastolic pressure and arterial blood gases showed no significant changes during the study.

Therefore, this study has shown evidence of a reduction in myocardial lactate production during myocardial ischemia following implementation of PICSO, while in a small group of non-PICSO animals no such change occurred. This finding is consistent with a reduction in myocardial anerobic metabolism and suggests that PICSO favorably affects the balance between myocardial oxygen supply and demand. However, no mechanism for this effect was found.

These studies were performed in swine, an animal without pre-formed collaterals and similar to man in its coronary artery anatomy. Because in swine the azygous vein drains into the coronary sinus, the PICSO catheter balloon was positioned just proximal to its entrance into the coronary sinus; the implementation of PICSO was otherwise similar to studies performed in other animal models.

The study, however, differs from previous work in that a coronary stenosis and atrial pacing were employed to cause ischemia primarily in the subendocardium. The data suggest therefore that PICSO may be of value in relieving ischemia occurring in conditions other than acute myocardial infarction (e.g.; unstable angina pectoris).

References

1. Gewirtz H, Most AS (1981) Production of a Critical Coronary Arterial Stenosis in Closed Chest Laboratory Animals. Am J Cardiol 47: 589–596
2. Guerci AD, Ciuffo AA, Weisfeldt ML (1985) Profound Infarct Size Reduction by Intermittent Coronary Sinus Occlusion (abstr). Circulation 72 (Suppl 3): 64
3. Jacobs AK, Faxon DP, Coats WD, Mohl W, Ryan T (1985) Intermittent Coronary Sinus Occlusion: Effect of infarct Size and Coronary Flow During Reperfusion (abstr). Circulation 72 (Suppl 3): 65
4 Mohl W, Punzengruber C, Moser M, Kenner T, Heimisch W, Haendchen R, Meerbaum S, Maurer G, Corday E (1985) Effects of Pressure-Controlled Intermittent Coronary Sinus Occlusion on Regional Ischemic Myocardial Function. J Am Coll Cardiol 5: 939–947

Authors' address:
Robert J. Capone, M.D.
Division of Cardiology
Rhode Island Hospital
593 Eddy Street
Providence
Rhode Island 02902
U.S.A.

Linear modelling of the coronary circulation during intermittent coronary sinus occlusion in swine

E. Toggart and S. Nellis

University of Wisconsin Hospital and Clinics, Department of Medicine, Section of Cardiology, Madison, Wisconsin (U.S.A.)

Purpose

The purpose of this study was to characterize coronary sinus to ischemic bed pressure transmission during intermittent coronary sinus occlusion.

Methods

The data used for this study were acquired from animals undergoing intermittent coronary sinus occlusion after LAD ligation. The preparation used was an arterial, blood perfused, in situ, working swine heart preparation. A Millar catheter was inserted retrograde to the left ventricle and a cannula placed distal to the LAD ligature for pressure measurement. The coronary sinus was cannulated through the right atrium with coronary sinus flow being directed through a timer controlled solenoid valve and returned to the right atrium. Coronary sinus pressure was measured through a cannula placed into the coronary sinus via the hemiazygos vein. The hemiazygos vein was ligated proximally. Intermittent coronary sinus occlusion was performed using 15 seconds of occlusion and five seconds of release. Coronary flow rates were adjusted to maintain perfusion pressure at LV systolic pressure, correcting for line resistance. Coronary flow was maintained at a constant rate during release and occlusion. Data were recorded at 15 minute intervals after LAD ligation. Statistical analysis comparing release to occluded pressure data was performed using paired t statistics.

Results

There was no significant difference between heart rate or left ventricular end diastolic pressure comparing release to occluded values at all time points. Left ventricular systolic pressure was slightly but statistically significantly less during occlusion compared to release. Coronary sinus (Fig. 1), LAD (Fig. 2), and left main perfusion pressure (Fig. 3) were significantly increased during occlusion compared to release. During occlusion of the coronary sinus, the absolute coronary sinus pressure was significantly greater than the LAD pressure. However during release, the absolute LAD pressure was slightly higher than the coronary sinus. The magnitude of coronary sinus pressure increase during occlusion was significantly greater than the pressure increase which occurred in the left anterior descending or left main coronary artery (Fig. 4). The percent increase in left main perfusion pressure during occlusion remained stable at approximately 15% (Fig. 5).

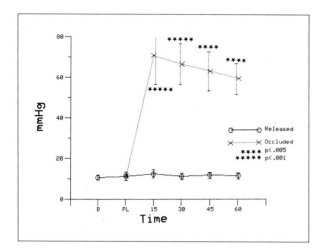

Fig. 1. Coronary sinus pressure.

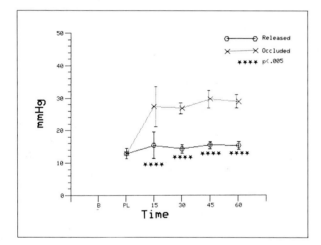

Fig. 2. LAD pressure.

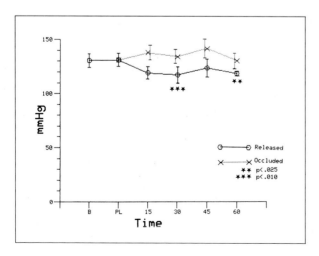

Fig. 3. Coronary perfusion pressure.

336

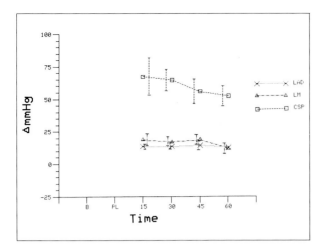

Fig. 4. △ pressure (occluded-released).

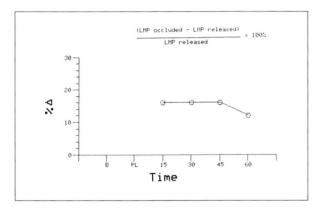

Fig. 5. % Change in LM pressure.

Conclusions

1. The low LAD pressure, comparable to previously reported zero flow pressures, is compatible with minimal arterial-arterial collaterals.
2. Because flow was held constant in the left main, any increase in left main pressure with intermittent coronary sinus occlusion is directly proportional to an increase in resistance. The relatively small increase in left main pressure (resistance) is compatible with a low resistance antegrade noncoronary sinus drainage.
3. If a direct large vein coronary sinus to noncoronary sinus drainage pathway exists, its resistance is high.
4. Because of the lack of a significantly large vein, coronary sinus to noncoronary sinus drainage, retrograde flow into the LAD bed and out through noncoronary sinus drainage must occur. Based on the magnitude of the pressure drop from coronary sinus to

LAD, retrograde resistance from coronary sinus to LAD is approximately equal to antegrade LAD to noncoronary sinus drainage.
5. An alternative explanation of these data is the existence of a nonlinear directionally dependent resistance from coronary sinus to ischemic bed.

Authors' address:
L. Papp
Cardiovascular Surgical Clinic
Semmelweis University
Budapest XII, Városmajor u. 68, 1112
Hungary

The effect of pressure controlled intermittent coronary sinus occlusion during reperfusion

L. Papp, Violetta Kékesi, B. Osváth, A. Juhász-Nagy, and Z. Szabó

Cardiovascular Surgical Clinic, Semmelweis University, Budapest (Hungary)

Summary: The effects of intermittent coronary sinus (CS) occlusion and coronary bypass were measured on the blood supply to an acutely ischemic region of the heart with computer-aided infrared thermography which determines, according to the authors' previous findings, subepicardial distribution of blood flow. Myocardial ischemia was produced by ligating the LAD artery in open chest dogs narcotized with pentobarbital. Three types of experiments were performed on 15 dogs. *A* In the control group untreated ischemia was established. *B* In the second group the local ischemia was influenced by intermittent CS occlusions of different types. *C* Coronary bypass operations were performed on the beating heart 2 h after ligating the LAD branch. It was found that CS occlusion significantly decreased the ischemia-induced local cooling and thus diminished the temperature difference between ischemic and nonischemic myocardial regions. The local blood flow increasing action of CS occlusion was considerably surpassed by the hyperemic effect of a patent coronary artery bypass graft but not by that of a technically deficient graft.

The aim of this study was to examine the thermographic effects of intermittent CS occlusion and coronary bypass on the blood supply to an ischemic region of the dog heart.

Methods

Fifteen dogs of both sexes (12–26 kg) were anesthetized with 30 mg · kg^{-1} of sodium pentobarbital, intubated intratracheally and operated upon under artificial ventilation with room air. Complete transversal thoracotomy was performed in the fourth intercostal space or median sternotomy was taken for coronary bypass operation. Ventricular ischemia was induced by ligating the LAD artery after its first or second branching. The ventricular mass supplied by the occluded artery was determined by premortem injection of Evans-blue into the vessel distal to the ligature: The weight of this muscle (area at risk) was compared to the total ventricular mass.

Arterial blood pressure was continuously measured with a Statham gauge via a cannula introduced into the femoral artery. In some experiments phasic and mean values of blood flow were recorded in the LAD with a Godard-Statham electromagnetic flowmeter (SP 2201). The above variables were registered on a Hellige multiscriptor.

Epicardial distribution of the coronary blood flow was assessed, according to the technique developed at our institute, by means of infrared thermography using an AGA 750 Thermovision camera (4, 5, 6). The sensitivity of the equipment was set to cover a temperature range of 5 °C (0.5 °C for each colour). With the aid of a standard reference heat source the temperature pertaining to a given colour could be detected and calibrated at regular time intervals. The experiments were performed at 23–24 °C room temperature and 50–60% relative humidity.

Computerized data analyses were made according to the procedure developed in our institute and described earlier (4, 5).

Three types of experiments were performed:

A In four control animals untreated local ischemia was established and maintained for 2 hours.

B In a second group the local ischemia was influenced by intermittent CS occlusion of different types: In four dogs which were compared statistically to controls the sinus was alternately occluded and released for 8 and 2 min, respectively. The procedure was also maintained for 2 hours. In another four experiments (not compared to controls) the sinus interventions were varied to collect data about general features and time course of the thermographic events. The CS was obstructed by a snare occluder placed around the terminal part of the sinus.

C Three coronary bypass operations were performed on the beating heart utilizing the mammary artery and the femoral artery graft two hours after LAD ligation.

Student's t-test for unpaired data was used for statistical comparison.

Results

CS occlusion considerably increased heat irradiation from the area at risk, thus decreasing the temperature difference between ischemic and nonischemic zones. On releasing the

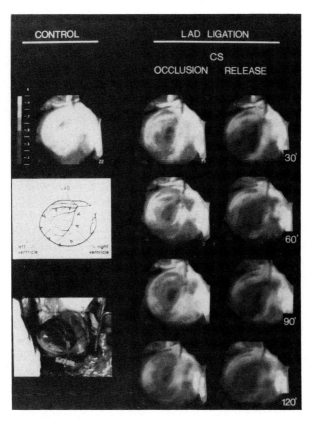

Fig. 1. Thermographic pattern of the CS occluded group. Left panel (Control): thermogram before LAD occlusion (above), schematic drawing (middle) and normal photo after LAD occlusion (below). The ischemic zone is marked with arrows and Evans-blue. Note cardiac mirror image on the thermogram and scheme as compared to the anatomical situation (photo). Right panel: occlusion and release of the CS at various phases of the experiment. Warming during CS occlusion is indicated by lighter shades.

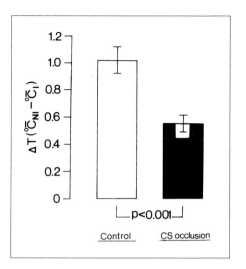

Fig. 2. Summed average (± SEM) of temperature differences between ischemic and non-ischemic areas in controls and in CS occluded group.

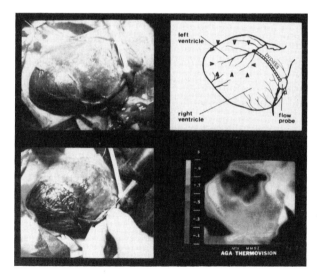

Fig. 3. Technical aspects of coronary artery operation. The graft (on the mid-portion of LAD) is clamped. Normal photo (upper left), schematic drawing (upper right), injection of Evans-blue into the graft (lower left), and thermogram of the latter intervention (lower right).

sinus the difference returned to control ranges. When the procedure was regularly repeated the appearance of this alternate temperature shift could be observed for a period of 2 hours (Fig. 1). In contrast, the control, untreated group exhibited an eveness of temperature difference between the two zones. Average values of temperature differences integrated over the total period of observation were therefore considerably less pronounced in the CS occluded group (Fig. 2). The significantly smaller temperature heterogeneity in the latter group was essentially due to the shrinkage of the cold area during the period of CS occlusion which occupied, according to the experimental protocol, four-fifths of the total

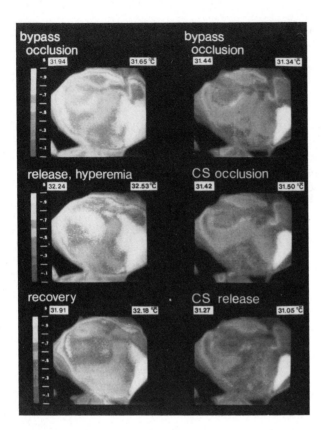

bypass
occlusion

| 31.94 | 31.65 °C |

bypass
occlusion

| 31.44 | 31.34 °C |

release, hyperemia

| 32.24 | 32.53 °C |

CS occlusion

| 31.42 | 31.50 °C |

recovery

| 31.91 | 32.18 °C |

CS release

| 31.27 | 31.05 °C |

Fig. 4. Comparison of effectiveness of coronary bypass (left) and CS occlusion (right). Thermographic changes and their computer-aided evaluation. Figures refer to mean temperature of the total field (left corner) and of the field supplied by the bypass (right corner). CBF values during hyperemia and recovery were 27 and 18 ml min^{-1}, respectively.

time; during CS release the temperature difference was approximately the same in both groups. The area at risk expressed as a proportion of the total ventricular weight was again similar in both groups: 23.4 ± 0.7% (control) and 27.7 ± 1.8% (CS occluded). There was a moderate difference in the behaviour of the arterial blood pressure: at the terminal period this variable was *higher* by 19 ± 11 mm Hg than at the beginning of the experiment in controls, and *lower* by 16 ± 6 mm Hg in the CS group, respectively (p < 0.05). This difference was probably due to reflex (3, 7). Further studies with different relations of clamping and unclamping periods (4 dogs) revealed qualitatively similar actions on epicardial temperature distribution.

Figure 3 is composed of representative photos of an experiment: it depicts the technical aspects of the coronary artery bypass operation. In this animal the excellent patency of bypass was evidenced by the rapid and significant overshot of the local temperature (reactive hyperemic vasodilation) after unclamping the graft (Fig. 4, left). The effect of CS occlusion on local temperature was slight (Fig. 4, right) as compared to the re-establishment of arterial blood supply. However, in another case where a technical problem (kinking of the graft on the very small LAD branch) rendered the bypass only partially patent, both CS occlusion and bypass release elicited a rewarming of similar magnitude. In fact, the

CS intervention was somewhat more effective than the opening of the arterial bypass route.

Discussion

The thermographic method employed in this study can semi-continuously and quantitatively determine the distribution of infrared irradiation from the epicardium. Evidence has been presented that in the exposed heart the mean value of the cardiac surface temperature assessed by the computer-aided thermographic technique is causally related to (5) and empirically dependent on (4) the rate of coronary blood flow, the relation between flow and temperature being approximately linear in the subnormal (ischemic) range of perfusion (4). In the present study it was demonstrated that in an experimental model which closely resembles acute myocardial infarction in man, occlusion of the CS is likely to reduce ischemic heterogeneity of temperature, probably by increasing blood supply to the acutely ischemic ventricular zone. This effect is evidently smaller than that of a patent coronary artery bypass graft, but can be better than of a technically deficient graft. (This raises the possibility that some technique based on the principle of CS occlusion may be of use in the future to extent the time-limits of emergency coronary artery bypass surgery, and even may be a method of choice, when early postoperative thrombosis occurs in the coronary graft.) Amelioration of blood supply to the area at risk can be maintained for hours by intermittent occlusion of the sinus. Direct visualization by thermography of this phenomenon indicated the promptness of the beneficial changes in local perfusion, and supports data that have previously been obtained by using radioactive microspheres (2) and 133 xenon washout curves (1). It was not the purpose of the present study to investigate the actions of sophisticated modalities of CS interventions (e.g. PICSO) on cardiac thermographic images. Since the full time-course of the thermographic method, like that of other techniques which involve the process of temperature exchanges is rather slow (≤ 2 min) as compared to the rapid pressure-flow changes during PICSO, we have tried to establish first the basic, steady state thermographic patterns characterizing the key-step of these interventions: the hindrance of CS outflow. The more refined thermographic signs of the relevant problems remain to be elucidated.

References

1. Ciuffo AA, Guerci AD, Halperin H, Bulkley G, Casale A, Weisfeldt ML (1984) Intermittent obstruction of the coronary sinus following coronary ligation in dogs reduces ischemic necrosis and increases myocardial perfusion. In: Mohl W, Wolner E, Glogar D (eds) The Coronary Sinus. Steinkopff Verlag, Darmstadt, pp 454–464
2. Glogar DH, Mohl W, Mayr H (1984) Pressure controlled intermittent coronary sinus occlusion effects the myocardium at risk and reduces infarct size. In: Mohl W, Wolner E, Glogar D (eds) The Coronary Sinus. Steinkopff Verlag, Darmstadt, pp 445–453
3. Muers MF, Sleight P (1972) The reflex cardiovascular depression caused by occlusion of the coronary sinus in the dog. J Physiol (Lond) 221: 259–282
4. Papp L, Álló G, Kékesi V, Juhász-Nagy A (1985) Correlation between coronary flow and epicardial temperature determined by quantitative infra-red thermography. IRCS Med J 13: 621–622
5. Papp L, Álló G, Szabó Z, Juhász-Nagy A (1985) Natural history of acute regional myocardial ischaemia revealed by infrared thermography in the canine heart. Acta Morph Hung 33: 123–142

6. Papp L, Mezei B, Osváth B, Szabó Z (1982) Thermography in artificially induced coronary circulatory disorders. Acta Chirurg Hung 23: 75–81
7. Szentiványi M, Juhász-Nagy A (1962) Two types of coronary vasomotor reflexes. Quart J Exp Physiol 47: 289–298

Authors' address:
L. Papp
Cardiovascular Surgical Clinic
Semmelweis University
Budapest XII, Városmajor u. 68, 1112
Hungary

344

The effect of pressure controlled intermittent coronary sinus occlusion during reperfusion

A. K. Jacobs, D. P. Faxon, W. D. Coats, W. Mohl, and T. J. Ryan

The Evans Memorial Department of Clinical Research and the Department of Medicine, University Hospital, Boston, Massachusetts (U.S.A.)

It has previously been shown that during experimental myocardial infarction, after sudden occlusion of a coronary artery, a wavefront of necrosis commences in the subendocardium and for several hours proceeds outward to reach the subepicardium (5, 9). It is now well accepted that restoration of arterial flow salvages this ischemic myocardium (2, 7). However, the efficacy of arterial reperfusion is limited by two factors. First, there is a relatively short time interval after which little myocardium can be salvaged (2). Second, there has been concern that arterial reperfusion may lead to cellular processes that extend the area of cell necrosis beyond that which is due to the ischemic insult (3).

Prior studies have demonstrated that pressure-controlled intermittent coronary sinus occlusion (PICSO) reduces experimental infarct size (1, 8). However, with the advent of clinical reperfusion techniques such as thrombolytic therapy and coronary angioplasty, it is important to evaluate PICSO in the setting of reperfusion. Two questions need to be addressed. First, if arterial reperfusion is delayed, will PICSO enhance myocardial salvage if begun during the evolving infarction prior to the onset of reperfusion? Second, if PICSO is started at the time of reperfusion, will it be capable of reducing the injury that occurs during the reperfusion process?

To answer these two questions the effect of PICSO, when begun early after coronary artery occlusion prior to reperfusion as well as its effect when started at the time of reperfusion was examined.

In the first study, we postulated that PICSO performed during ischemia prior to reperfusion would enhance the salvage of myocardium achieved by reperfusion alone, either by delaying cell death or by limiting myocardial necrosis. From a clinical standpoint, this would be analogous to performing PICSO prior to reperfusion while thrombolytic therapy or coronry angioplasty were underway.

In 22 open-chest anesthetized dogs, occlusion of the left anterior descending artery for three hours was followed by three hours of reperfusion. Dogs were randomly assigned to reperfusion alone or reperfusion plus PICSO 30 minutes following coronary artery occlusion. PICSO was performed using a pump inflated coronary sinus balloon catheter during coronary artery occlusion and reperfusion. Risk region was determined by Rhodamine B perfusion and infarct size was measured using triphenyltetrazolium chloride staining.

Infarct size/risk region was $32.7 \pm 4.1\%$ (reperfusion) and $16.7 \pm 4.1\%$ (reperfusion plus PICSO), $p < 0.02$. Coronary blood flow was higher at peak hyperemia (294 ± 31.5 vs. $187 \pm 22.5\%$ above baseline), $p < 0.01$ and throughout reperfusion in the PICSO treated group and infarct size was related to coronary flow following three hours of reperfusion ($r = 0.71$, $p < 0.01$). Heart rate was lower than baseline (125 ± 6.0 bpm) during reperfusion (114 ± 8.7), $p < 0.02$ only in the dogs treated with PICSO.

We conclude that in this canine model, PICSO significantly enhances the salvage of ischemic myocardium achieved by reperfusion alone. The fall in heart rate and the increase in coronary flow during PICSO may reflect preservation of an intact microvasculature.

Since in this first experiment, PICSO was started several hours prior to reperfusion, we cannot distinguish whether PICSO is capable of reducing further cellular damage which occurs during the reperfusion process. One mechanism which has been proposed to account for reperfusion injury, in part, is the accumulation of tissue edema and intracellular fluid which has been demonstrated as early as two minutes following reperfusion in dogs (6).

Although we now know that PICSO is effective in the setting of infarction as well as during infarction and reperfusion, the mechanism of this effect remains largely unknown. It is conceptualized that periodic elevation of coronary sinus pressure results in a redistribution of venous flow to the ischemic zone with washout or drainage of accumulated toxic metabolites and cellular edema occurring following release of coronary sinus obstruction. We postulated that PICSO, by enhancing washout of cellular edema, would potentiate the salvage of ischemic myocardium achieved by reperfusion by reducing part of the damage attributed to the reperfusion process.

We examined this hypothesis in 24 open-chest anesthetized dogs. Occlusion of the left anterior descending artery for three hours was followed by three hours of reperfusion. Dogs were randomly assigned to PICSO plus reperfusion or reperfusion alone. Using a pump inflated balloon-tipped coronary sinus catheter, PICSO was started just prior to reperfusion and continued throughout reperfusion. Coronary blood flow, aortic pressure, and heart rate were recorded continuously.

Although left ventricular mass and percent of the left ventricle at risk of infarction were the same in both groups, infarct size expressed as percent of the myocardium at risk was significantly lower in the group treated with reperfusion plus PICSO (29 ± 5.8) than in the group receiving reperfusion alone (45 ± 2.3), $p < 0.02$. Coronary blood flow and aortic pressure were the same in both groups during reperfusion. However, at peak reperfusion, heart rate was lower with reperfusion plus PICSO (123.8 ± 7.0) vs. reperfusion alone (145.2 ± 7.1), $p < 0.05$.

We conclude that in this experimental model, PICSO performed during reperfusion significantly enhances myocardial salvage. The fall in heart rate at peak reperfusion in the PICSO treated group suggests that PICSO may decrease heart rate by a reflex mechanism which is mediated by vagal afferents (4). This evidence supports the concept of "reperfusion injury" and suggests that PICSO may reduce or prevent that damage which occurs during the reperfusion process.

The above studies document a potential role for PICSO during myocardial infarction in the setting of reperfusion. In the clinical arena, during reperfusion by thrombolysis or coronary angioplasty, PICSO may further enhance myocardial salvage by sparing cells from additional injury.

References

1. Ciuffo AA, Guerci AD, Halperin H, Bulkley G, Casale A, Weisfeldt ML (1984) Intermittent obstruction of the coronary sinus following coronary ligation in dogs reduces ischemic necrosis and increases myocardial perfusion. In: Mohl W, Wolner E, Glogar D (eds) The Coronary Sinus. Steinkopff Verlag, Darmstadt, pp 454–464

2. Ellis SG, Henschke CI, Sandor T, Wynne J, Braunwald E, Kloner (A 81983) Time course of functional and biochemical recovery of myocardium salvaged by reperfusion. J Am Coll Cardiol I (4): 1047–1055
3. Hearse DJ (1977) Reperfusion of the ischemic myocardium. J Mol Cell Cardiol 9: 605–616
4. Juhász-Nagy A, Szabó Z (1984) Hemodynamic pattern of cardiodepression elicitable from reflexogenic areas in left coronary venous system of the dog. In: Mohl W, Wolner E, Glogar D (eds) The Coronary Sinus. Steinkopff Verlag, Darmstadt, pp 231–238
5. Jennings RB (1969) Early phase of myocardial ischemic injury and infarction. Am J Cardiol 24: 753–765
6. Kloner RA, Ganate CE, Whalen DA, Jennings RB (1974) Effect of a transient period of ischemia on myocardial cells. II. Fine structure during the first few minute of reflow. Am J Pathol 74: 399–420
7. Lange R, Kloner RA, Braunwald E (1983) First ultra short acting beta blocker: its effect on size and segmental wall dynamics of reperfused myocardial infarcts in dogs. Am J Cardiol 51: 1759–1767
8. Mohl W, Glogar DH, Myre H, Losert V, Sochor H, Pachinger O, Kaindl F, Wolner E (1984) Reduction of infarct size induced by pressure-controlled intermittent coronary sinus occlusion. Am J Cardiol. 53: 923–928
9. Reimer KA, Lowe JE, Rasmussen MM, Jennings RB (1977) The wavefront phenomenon of ischemic cell death. Myocardial infarct size vs duration of coronary occlusion in dogs. Circulation 56: 786–793

Authors' address:
Alice K. Jacobs, M.D.
Section of Cardiology
University Hospital
75 East Newton Street
Boston, MA 02118
U.S.A.

Effect of PICSO treatment on arrhythmias during early myocardial ischemia

H. Mayr, D. Glogar, W. Mohl, H. Weber, and F. Kaindl

Kardiologische Universitätsklinik and II. Chirurgische Universitätsklinik, Vienna (Austria)

Summary: Pressure controlled intermittent coronary sinus occlusion (PICSO) has shown protective effects during early regional myocardial ischemia. Since coronary artery occlusion (CAO) can cause malignant rhythm disturbances, the aim of the study was to evaluate the effect of PICSO treatment on cardiac arrhythmias.

In eight anesthetized open chest mongrel dogs the LAD was occluded distal to the first diagonal branch. Area at risk was determined by radioactive labelled microspheres. In one group (n = 4) PICSO was started 15 min after CAO as previously described and was continued for 6 hours. The other group (n = 4) served as control. ECG was recorded continuously during the experiment using an Oxford-Medilog recorder and printed on UV paper. Each ECG was evaluated visually at 60 sec intervals according to Lown's classification. The time of observation in the PICSO group was 293 ± 48 min vs. 289 ± 61 min in the control group. The mean Lown value in the PICSO treated group was significantly lower than in the controls (0.37 ± 0.41 vs. 1.31 ± 0.52; p < 0.05). The area at risk was not significantly different between both groups (26.5 ± 10.7% LV vs. 22.0 ± 8.2% LV; n.s.).

It is concluded that PICSO treatment starting 15 min after CAO reduces significantly the quantity and severity of arrhythmias during the first 6 hours of myocardial infarction. This underlines the protective effect of PICSO treatment reported earlier.

Introduction

Pressure controlled intermittent coronary sinus occlusion (PICSO) is a new concept for the treatment of acute myocardial infarction (6, 11–13). It is performed by a closed fluid-filled balloon catheter pump system. The tip of the balloon catheter is introduced into the coronary sinus. Inflation of the balloon leads to a gradual increase of the coronary sinus pressure until a plateau is reached, followed by deflation of the balloon to allow sufficient blood drainage. This procedure has been proven to reduce the area at risk and infarct size during the first 6 hours of acute coronary artery occlusion (12).

Acute coronary artery occlusion can cause severe rhythm disturbances which are responsible for a great number of complications during the first hours of acute myocardial infarction. These arrhythmias are triggered by the increased sympathoadrenergic drive during acute ischemia as well as by focal electrical instability of cell membranes exposed to ischemia. During the course of ischemia the ischemic zone expands gradually from the center of the ischemic bed and the subendocardial regions to the subepicardial myocardium and the edge of the risk zone. This may leave smaller areas of severely ischemic tissue surrounded by either focal necrosis or viable tissue (15–17).

Experimental preparation and protocol

Eight mongrel dogs weighing 20 to 28 kg were anaesthetized with sodium-pentobarbital (30 mg/kg) and ventilated with a 1 : 1 O2/N2O gas mixture using a volume regulated respirator. A throacotomy was performed in the 5th left intercostal space and the heart was suspended in a pericardial cradle. Catheters were placed into a central artery and the left atrium via the atrial appendage for hemodynamic measurements and injection of radioactive labelled microspheres for determination of area at risk (5). A 7 F double-lumen coronary sinus catheter connected to the pump system was inserted through the left jugular vein and guided manually into the orifice of the coronary sinus. The left anterior descending artery was dissected free and ligated permanently distal to the first diagonal branch.

Eight dogs were randomized in 2 groups. Experiments in which primary ventricular fibrillation occurred within the initial 15 minutes of ischemia were excluded from this series (n = 5). Group A received PICSO treatment starting 15 minutes after acute myocardial infarction (n = 4) and group B served as controls (n = 4). Area at risk and infarct size was determined according to a protocol previously described (12). Determination of area at risk was performed prior to the intervention at 15 minutes of coronary artery occlusion with an injection of technetium 99 labelled human albumin microspheres. Infarct size after 6 hours was measured post mortem by incubation in triphenyltetrazolium chloride. For continuous monitoring of the ECG three needle electrodes were placed subcutaneously on the thorax in such a way that the suspended heart represented the center of a triangle. ECG recording was started 15 minutes before acute myocardial ischemia and was continued throughout the experiment. The ECG signal was stored on tape by an Oxford-Medilog recorder. ECGs were printed on UV paper with a speed of 10 mm/sec and evaluated visually in sections of 60 sec according to Lown's classification. The arrhythmia with the highest Lown grade was scored for each respective minute. The overall severity and frequency arrhythmias result for one experiment was expressed as mean Lown value per minute.

Results

The area at risk of necrosis was not significantly different between the PICSO treated animals (group A, 22.0 ± 8.2% of left ventricular mass) and the controls (group B, 26.5% of left ventricular mass, p = n.s. vs. Group A). In contrast, infarct size determined 6 hours after coronary artery occlusion was lower in the PICSO treated group (5.5 ± 9.2% of the left ventricular mass) as compared to controls (22.4 ± 8.4% left ventricular mass, p > 0.05 vs. group A) (Figure 1). Thus, PICSO treatment effectively protected ischemic myocardium with an average of 25% of myocardium at risk infarcted in this series compared to 85% of myocardium at risk in controls.

Long-term ECG recordings were available in all the experiments. The average time of ECG observation was similar between both groups (group A 293 ± 48 minutes and group B 289 ± 61 minutes, p = n.s.). The severity of arrhythmias was significantly higher in the control group than in the PICSO treated group, with an average Lown value (Lown mean 1.31 ± 0.52 in group B vs. 0.37 ± 0.41 in group A, p > 0.05) (Figure 2). The severity of arrhythmias showed a correlation with the area at risk of necrosis and infarct

350

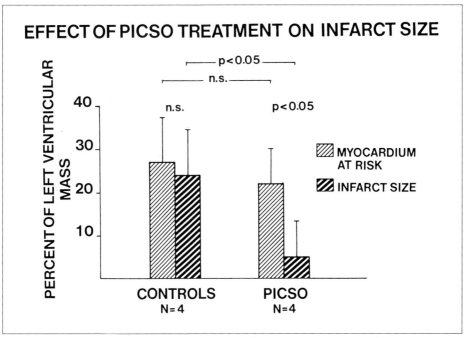

Fig. 1. The columns represent the myocardium at risk (measured 15 minutes after coronary artery occlusion) and infarct size (measured 6 hours after coronary artery occlusion). Values are expressed as a percentage of the left ventricular mass.

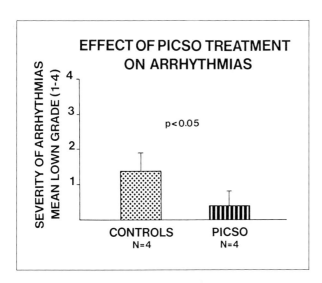

Fig. 2. Mean Lown grade per minute averaged during individual experiments in controls and PICSO treated dogs (mean ± standard deviation).

size (Figure 3). While the eventual size of the infarction was related to the severity and frequency of arrhythmias (mean Lown) that occurred during the course of the acute infarct in both controls and PICSO treated dogs, the myocardium at risk was predictive

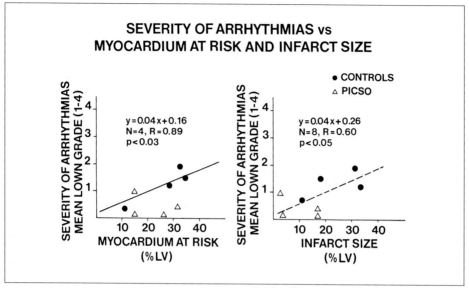

Fig. 3. Left panel: Correlation of severity of arrhythmias to area at risk of necrosis in controls (filled circles) and in PICSO treated dogs (open triangles).

Fig. 4. Right panel: Correlation of severity of arrhythmias to infarct size in controls (filled circles) and PICSO treated dogs (open triangles).

only in the control group. In contrast to the control group hearts even with large areas at risk of necrosis had no higher incidence of malignant arrhythmias if treated with PICSO (Figure 3). There was no evidence of rhythm disturbances triggered by PICSO. There was no increase in mean Lown values following the start of PICSO treatment after 15 minutes of coronary artery occlusion. Also, there were no measurable differencves in mean Lown values if phases of PICSO inflation and PICSO deflation during the initial pump cycles were evaluated separately (13).

Discussion

Our results show that pressure controlled intermittent coronary sinus occlusion (PICSO) started 15 minutes after acute myocardial ischemia and continued for 6 hours is an effective method to reduce infarct size. While 85% of the myocardium at risk became necrotic after 6 hours of coronary artery occlusion in the control group, in PICSO-treated hearts it was only 25%. Despite similar areas at risk of infarction measured 15 minutes after coronary artery occlusion, PICSO treated hearts had a significantly lower incidence and severity of ventricular arrhythmias as compared to to the control group. In our study the mean Lown arrhythmia grade was greater with increasing area at risk and with increasing infarct size in untreated hearts, while such correlation was not seen after PICSO treatment. This may be due to the substantial cardioprotective effects of PICSO leading to a reduction of infarct size as well as to modification of life-threatening arrhythmias.

An easily administered and effective regimen to prevent severe and life-threatening ventricular arrhythmias during acute myocardial infarction would be of considerable clinical value. So far numerous pharmacologic interventions, in particular of different antiarrhythmic agents, have been tested (3, 8–10). Most studies have failed to reach a definite statistical conclusion (1, 4, 14, 18). Several large scale beta-blocking trials for management of acute myocardial infarction have shown some beneficial effets of betablockade on severity of arrhythmias and the frequency of episodes of sudden death (2, 7). The present experimental paper attempts to address the question of management of arrhythmias during acute myocardial infarction from the perspective of infarct size and the use of effective means to reduce the extent of the infarction. PICSO has been shown by several investigators to be of great potential for the management of acute myocardial infarction. Its beneficial effect on arrhythmias is most likely due to its antiischemic properties leading to a preservation of potentially severely damaged tissue. Several theories have been offered to explain the mechanism of PICSO treatment such as washout of edema, protection of cellular metabolism, increased border zone flow, etc., all of which may be of great importance for preservation of tissue viability as well as for maintenance of electrical stability.

In summary, the present study demonstrates that PICSO treatment not only has cardioprotective potential but also reduces effectively the frequency and severity of arrhythmias during the initial hours of acute myocardial infarction.

Acknowledgement

The authors acknowledge the skilful secretarial help of Miss Margit Kuzmics and Gabriele Bambasek in preparing the manuscript. This work was suppoted in part by the Ludwig Boltzmann-Institut für Herzchirurgische Forschung.

References

1. Anderson J, Mason J, Winkle R et al (1978) Clinical electrophysiologic effects of tocainide. Circulation 57: 685–91
2. Beta-Blocker Heart Attack Study Group (1981) The Betablocker heart attack trial. JAMA 246: 2073–2080
3. Campbell R, Achuff S, Pottage A, Murray A, Prescott L, Julian D (1979) Mexiletine in the prophylaxis of ventricular arrhythmias during acute myocardial infarction. J Cardiovasc Pharmacol 1: 43–52
4. Campbell R, Bryson L, Bailey B, Murray A, Julian D (1981) Prophylactic administration of tocainide in acute myocardial infarction. In: Pottage A, Ryden L (eds) Workshop on tocainide. AB Haessle, Goteborg, pp 201–4
5. Campbell R, Hutton I, Elton R, Goodfellow R, Taylor E (1983) Prophylaxis of primary ventricular fibrillation with tocainide in acute myocardial infarction. Br Heart J 49: 557–63
6. Glogar D, Mohl W, Mayr H, Losert U, Sochor H, Wolner E, Kaindl F (1982) Pressure controlled intermittent coronary sinus occlusion reduces myocardial necrosis. Am J Cardiol 49: 1017
7. Hjalmarson A, Herlitz J, Malek I, Ryden L, Vedin A, Waldenstrom A, Wedel H, Elmfeldt D, Holmbert S, Nyberg G, Swedberg K, Waagstein F, Waldenstrom J, Wilhelmsen L, Wilhelmsson C (1981) Effect on mortality of metoprolol in acute myocardial infarction. Lancet 2: 823–827
8. Jones D, Kostuk W, Gunton R (1974) Prophylactic quinidine for the prevention of arrhythmias after acute myocardial infarction. Am J Cardiol 33: 655–60

9. Koch-Weser J, Klein S, Foo-Canto L, Kastor J, DeSanctis R (1969) Antiarrhythmic prophylaxis with procainamide in acute myocardial infarction. N Engl J Med 281: 1253–60
10. Lie K, Wellens H, Van Capelle F, Durrer D (1974) Lidocraine in the prevention of primary ventricular fibrillation. N Engl J Med 291: 1324–6
11. Mayr H, Mohl W, Glogar D, Losert U, Wolner E, Kaindl F (1983) Infarktgrößenbeeinflussung durch druckkontrollierte intermittierende Koronarsinusokklusion (ICSO). Z Kardiol 72 (Suppl 1): 59
12. Mohl W, Glogar D, Mayr H, Losert U, Sochor H, Pachinger O, Kaindl F, Wolner E (1984) Reduction of infarct size induced by PICSO. Am J Cardiol 53: 923–928
13. Moser M, Mohl W, Gallasch E, Kenner T (1984) Optimization of pressure controlled intermittent coronary sinus occlusion intervals by density measurements. In: Mohl W, Wolner E, Glogan D (eds) The Coronary Sinus. Steinkopff Verlag, Darmstadt, pp 529–536
14. Rehnquist N (1981) Comparison of tocainide with lidocaine in AMI. In: Pottage A, Ryden L (eds) Workshop on tocainide. AB Haessle, Goteborg, pp 187–9
15. Reimer K, Jennings R (1979) The "wave front phenomenon" of myocardial ischemic cell death. II. Transmural progression of necrosis within the framework of ischemic bed size (myocardium at risk) and collateral flow. Lab Invest 40: 633–644
16. Reimer K, Jennings R (1981) Energy metabolism in the reversible and irreversible phases of severe myocardial ischemia. Acta Med Scand Suppl 651: 19
17. Reimer K, Lowe J, Rasmussen M, Jennings R (1977) The wavefront phenomenon of ischemic cell death. I. Myocardial size vs duration of coronary occlusion in the dog. Circulation 56: 786–794
18. Ryden L, Arnman K, Conradson T, Hofvendahl S, Mortensen, O, Smedgard P (1980) Prophylaxis of ventricular tachyarrhythmias with intravenous and oral tocainide in patients with and recovering from acute myocardial infarction. Am Heart J 100: 1006–12

Author's address:
H. Mayr, M.D.
Kardiologische Universitäts-Klinik
Garnisonsgasse 13
A-1090 Vienna
Austria

Characterization of the reactive hyperemic response time during intermittent coronary sinus occlusion

Y. Sun and W. Mohl

University of Rhode Island (U.S.A.) and University of Vienna (Austria)

Summary: The coronary sinus occlusion pressure (CSOP) and circumflex coronary blood flow waveforms were analyzed in 12 canine studies conducted with pressure controlled intermittent coronary sinus occlusion (PICSO). The time interval (Tp) to reach the peak of reactive hyperemic response during the release phase of PICSO was characterized. Information extracted from the CSOP waveform was used to predict Tp.

The coronary sinus pressure-flow relations were simulated by use of an analog, resistor-capacitor circuit. The systolic and diastolic envelopes of CSOP were characterized by use of first-order exponential functions. Parameters extracted from the CSOP envelopes included heart rate, systolic/diastolic plateaus and time constants.

The measured Tp showed a mean of 3.4 sec (1.6 to 5.8 sec, SD = 0.9 sec, n = 128). We found weak correlations between individual CSOP parameters and Tp; nevertheless, an estimator (Tp') which optimally combines several parameters resulted in the following relation: Tp' = 0.92 Tp + 0.00 (r = 0.64, p < 0.001).

This study has demonstrated a method to predict the occurrence of reactive hyperemic response during the release phase of PICSO by use of information obtained from the CSOP. The result should prove useful in optimizing the PICSO cycle.

Introduction

The timing of occlusion/release cycle may have critical influence on the performance of pressure controlled intermittent coronary sinus occlusion (PICSO). Moser and colleagues (10) evaluated the washout effect of PICSO by measuring the instantaneous coronary sinus blood density. They found that the amplitude of density variation showed a maximum when a 10/8 sec occlusion/release cycle was employed. Mohl and colleagues (8) indicated that a sufficient release period is necessary for the repayment of flow which lasts for 4 ± 1.5 sec during repetitive occlusion and as long as 14 ± 4 sec during permanent release.

Several investigators have suggested that myocardial protection by PICSO is likely due to a mechanism of washing out edema and toxic substances from the ischemic zone (2, 9). The effects of washout as well as flow repayment are related to the reactive hyperemic coronary flow during the release phase of PICSO. Since the reactive hyperemia can be significantly suppressed by inappropriate PICSO timing, a feedback control algorithm which synchronizes PICSO with respect to the hyperemic response should be useful. Unfortunately, the present-stage knowledge concerning the optimal timing control for PICSO is limited.

Accordingly, in this study the time interval (Tp) to reach the peak reactive hyperemic response during the release phase of PICSO was characterized. In addition, a mathematical model was developed to assist interpretations of the observed coronary sinus occlusion

355

pressure (CSOP) waveforms. An empirical formula was also developed to predict Tp based on information extracted from the CSOP. The purpose of this study was to establish both a mathematical and experimental basis for the implementation of an optimal PICSO system with feedback timing control.

Mathematical model

The pressure-flow relations observed in the coronary sinus during PICSO are simulated by use of an electrical equivalent circuit as shown in Fig. 1. During the occlusion phase, the capacitance C is charged up towards an intramyocardial pressure source (Pim) through the coronary venous resistance (R). The time-varying Pim represents an average transmural pressure which has morphology similar to the left ventricular pressure but with a smaller dynamic magnitude (3, 11). The capacitance C represents the compliance of the coronary sinus. The resistance Ro represents a large distal venous resistance during the occlusion phase (Ro = infinity, for complete occlusion). During the release phase, the capacitance is discharged through a relatively small distal venous resistance Rr. The values of R and C are periodically varied by the contraction of the heart according to

1. $R = Rs; C = Cs$; during systole.
   $R = Rd; C = Cd$; during diastole.

Thus, the systolic and diastolic envelopes of the coronary sinus occlusion pressure (CSOP) waveform may have different time constants: $Ts = Rs\,Cs$ and $Td = Rd\,Cd$, respectively.

Based on the proposed mathematical model, the CSOP systolic envelope (Psi, i = 1, 2, ..., n) can be described by a first-order exponential function (Fig. 2):

2. $Psi = As\,(1 - e^{-tsi/Ts})$

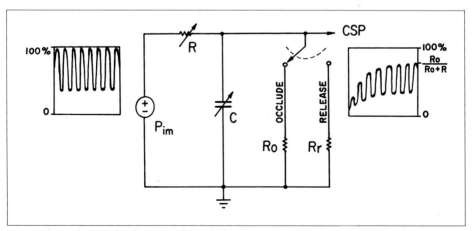

Fig. 1. The equivalent circuit used to simulate the coronary venous circulation during PICSO: Pim = intramyocardial pressure; R = proximal coronary venous resistance; C = coronary sinus capacitance; Ro = distal venous resistance during occlussion; Rr = distal venous resistance during release, where Ro ≫ Rr.

356

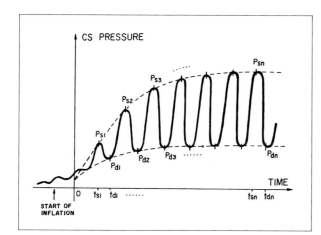

Fig. 2. The systolic envelope (Psl ... Psn) and the diastolic envelope (Pdl ... Pdn) of a CSOP waveform. First-order exponential functions (dashed curves) are fitted to the envelopes.

where As is the systolic plateau and tsi is the time instant that Psi is measured. A "slow rise" phase is usually observed during the first second of measured CSOP waveforms. This phenomenon is likely an artifact caused by a slowly inflated PICSO balloon and, thus, ignored in the present analysis. The beginning of the occlusion interval (i.e. the $t = 0$ reference) is chosen slightly after the instant of balloon inflation.

Given the measurements of CSOP envelopes, there exist two unknown variables, namely As and Ts, in equation 2. Assuming the occlusion period is sufficiently long such that a CSOP plateau is reached, the plateau As is roughly equal to the maximum of Psi, for $i = 1$ to n. To determine the time constant Ts, equation 2 is first linearized according to

3. $1/\ln[(As\text{-}Psi)/As] = (-1/tsi)\ Ts,$

for all i except at the maximum pressure point. Equation 3 represents an over determined system of simultaneous equations. Next, a least-squares estimation is used to determine Ts.

4. $Ts = \dfrac{-\sum\limits_{i} tsi^2}{\sum\limits_{i} tsi \cdot \ln[(As-Psi)/As]}$

The diastolic plateau Ad and time constant Td can be obtained in a similar way. Thus, the systolic and diastolic envelopes of the CSOP waveform are completely represented by use of four parameters: As, Ad, Ts, and Td.

Estimation of the peak hyperemic response time

The parameters extracted from the CSOP were utilized to predict the peak hyperemic response time Tp. This was done by use of five basic parameters: As, Ad, Ts, Td, and HR (heart rate); and nine derived parameters: RRI (R to R wave interval), As/Ad, Ad/As,

Ts/Td, Td/Ts, As/RRI, Ad/RRI, Ts/RRI, and Td/RRI. First, linear regression analysis was performed between each individual parameter and Tp. An intercept and slope was obtained from the regression line. Next, each parameter was normalized by subtracting out the intercept and then divided by the slope. This procedure was to ensure that, when all parameters are linearly combined, the resultant estimator be unbiased. Finally, an empirical formula is obtained to predict Tp based on a linear combination of all 14 normalized parameters. The optimal set of weight coefficients for the linear combination was obtained in a least-square-error sense.

Experimental method

A retrospective analysis was performed on hemodynamic waveforms obtained from 12 open chested dogs. Coronary sinus pressure and circumflex coronary flow were simultaneously recorded on paper during PICSO. The experimental procedures have been described in detail elsewhere (8).

A stylus-type, x-y digitizer (GTCO Corporation, Rockville, MD) was used to identify the CSOP envelopes and the reactive hyperemic response time (Tp). The digitizer has a spatial resolution of 0.025 mm, which is equivalent to a resolution of 1.25 mm Hg in pressure and 0.1 sec in time on the recorded traces. Data from the digitizer were processed by an IBM Personal Computer. A typical recorded CSOP and coronary flow trace is shown on the left of Fig. 3, with the digitized CSOP waveform shown on the right.

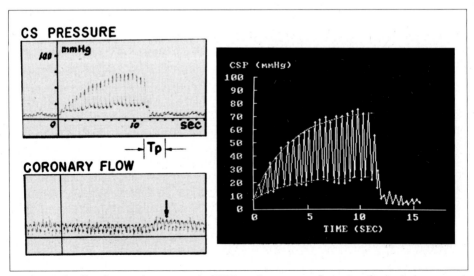

Fig. 3. Left: Simultaneously measured CSOP and coronary flow waveform during a typical PICSO cycle; Right: The systolic and diastolic envelopes of CSOP identified by using an x-y digitizer. The extracted points are connected by line segments just for clarity.

358

The complete course of each experiment was carefully examined. Data acquisitions were selectively performed at times when significant variations occurred on either the CSOP or the reactive hyperemic flow response.

Results

In all, 128 PICSO cycles from the 12 canine studies were analyzed. High correlations were found between the measured CSOP envelopes and the predictions by the first-order exponential model: $r = 0.98 \pm 0.05$ for systolic envelopes; and $r = 0.83 \pm 0.21$ for diastolic envelopes. The plateaus and time constants fitted by the model showed the following result: As = 63 ± 13 mm Hg, Ts = 4.2 ± 1.6 sec for systole; and Ad = 14 ± 4 mm Hg, Td = 3.7 ± 1.7 sec for diastole. There exists a correlation ($r = 0.71$) between Ts and Td. A paired t-test indicated that Ts is significantly higher than Td ($p < 0.001$).

The measurements of time interval (Tp) to reach the peak reactive hyperemia had a mean of 3.4 sec (1.6 to 5.8 sec, SD = 0.9 sec, n = 128). As shown in Figure 4 and Table 1, we found weak correlations between individual parameters and Tp. The three parameters which showed the highest correlation were the normalized diastolic time constant (Td/RRI: $r = -0.32$), normalized systolic time constant (Ts/RRI: $r = -0.21$), and heart

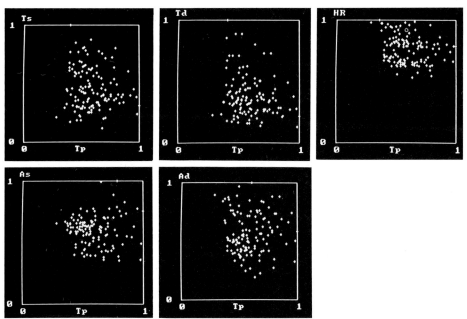

Fig. 4. The five basic parameters plotted versus the peak hyperemic response time (Tp), where Ts and Td = systolic and diastolic time constant, respectively; As and Ad = systolic and diastolic plateau, respectively; HR = heart rate. The maximum amplitudes for all parameters are normalized to unity. Weak correlations were observed between these parameters and Tp.

Table 1. The results of linear regression analyses between individual CSOP parameters and the peak hyperemic time (Tp), where Parameter = a Tp + b; with correlation coefficient r; all p < 0.001.

Parameter	r	a	b
Ts	−0.11	−0.21	4.89
Td	−0.21	−0.39	5.04
As	−0.00	0.05	62.0
Ad	−0.01	−0.04	13.9
HR	−0.21	−4.19	127.2
RRI	0.19	0.02	0.48
Ts/Td	0.14	0.06	0.98
Td/Ts	−0.18	−0.06	1.13
As/Ad	−0.05	−0.07	5.08
Ad/As	0.00	0.0002	0.22
Ts/RRI	−0.21	−0.63	9.77
Td/RRI	−0.32	−0.92	9.84
As/RRI	−0.10	−3.92	131.5
Ad/RRI	−0.09	−1.21	30.8

rate (HR: r = −0.21). By contrast, the prediction (Tp') generated by an optimal linear combination of all parameters showed a significantly increased correlation with respect to the measured Tp. Linear regression analysis resulted in: Tp' = 0.92 Tp + 0.00, with r = 0.64, SEE = 0.9 sec, p < 0.001 (Fig. 5). Tp' was calculated by use of the following empirical formula:

5. Tp' = −0.26 As + 1.6 Ad − 1.6 Ts + 0.82 Td − 0.0081 HR
 + 18 RRI − 0.51 As/Ad − 53 Ad/As + 3.7 Ts/Td − 3.5 Td/Ts
 + 0.065 As/RRI − 0.38 Ad/RRI − 0.10 Ts/RRI + 0.15 Td/RRI + 7.7

where As and Ad in mm Hg; Tp', Ts, Td, and RRI in sec; HR in bpm.

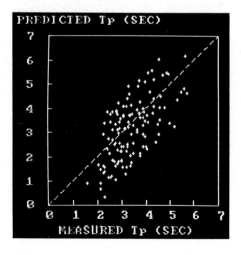

Fig. 5. The predicted peak hyperemic response time (Tp') from equation 4 is plotted versus the measured Tp. Linear regression analysis resulted in: Tp' = 0.92 Tp + 0.00; r = 0.64; n = 128; SEE = 0.9 sec.

Discussion

The coronary sinus occlusion pressure (CSOP) contains valuable diagnostic information: By extracting parameters from CSOP, it is possible to assess the end diastolic left ventricular pressure (3), coronary blood flow (4), and infarct size (1). In this study, a resistor-capacitor circuit analog to the coronary venous circulation was developed to interpret the CSOP waveforms. The systolic and diastolic envelopes of the CSOP were accurately described by first-order exponential functions. The systolic time constant was significantly longer than the diastolic time constant (Ts = 4.2 > Td = 3.7 sec, p < 0.001). This phenomenon can be explained by a significant increase of coronary venous resistance during systole. As a result, the decreased coronary venous blood flow takes a longer period to charge up the coronary sinus capacitance.

The mathematical model also served as a useful tool for parameter extraction. Information from the CSOP waveform was compressed into four parameters, namely, the systolic/diastolic plateau and time constant. These parameters were optimally combined to predict the occurrence of reactive hyperemic flow response during PICSO. We were able to identify an empirical formula which generates an unbiased estimator of the peak hyperemic response time (Tp) with a reasonable correlation.

Although the exact mechanism of myocardial protection by PICSO is still not clear, several studies have shown that a possible criterion for the optimization of PICSO is to maximize the reactive hyperemic flow response during the release phase of PICSO (8, 9, 10). It has also been reported that, when a relatively short release period (2 sec) was employed, PICSO suppressed hyperemia and failed to reduce ischemia (5). We think there is a strong indication from these results that the adjustment of PICSO release period should be keyed to the peak reactive hyperemic response. Moreover, data from this study have shown that the peak hyperemic response time may vary between 1.6 and 5.8 sec (mean = 3.4, SD = 0.9). Thus, it is questionable that the benefit of PICSO can be maximized by choosing a unique, constant occlusion/release cycle.

To access the coronary hyperemic flow response, an open chest surgery is generally required. Otherwise, for nonsurgical procedures, special instrumentations must be employed (6,7). By contrast, the CSOP waveform is easily accessible during PICSO. The algorithm developed in this study allows us to predict the upcoming reactive hyperemia during PICSO by use of information solely extracted from the present CSOP waveform. Since the required computation (equations 4 and 5) can be accomplished on a microcomputer within milliseconds, implementation of a cycle-by-cycle control for PICSO based on this algorithm is feasible. In conclusion, the response time of reactive hyperemia is an important parameter which indicates the current pace of the heart in response to PICSO. This study has demonstrated a method to predict this response time using information obtained from the observable CSOP waveform. Accordingly, the result from this study should be useful for the optimization of PICSO cycle.

References

1. Aigner A, Mohl W, Timischl W (1984) Effects of PICSO on hemodynamic parameters. In: Mohl W, Wolner E, Glogar D (eds) The Coronary Sinus. Steinkopff Verlag, Darmstadt, pp 437–444

2. Ciuffo AA, Guerci AD, Halperin H, Bulkley G, Casale A, Weisfeldt ML (1984) Intermittent obstruction of the coronary sinus following coronary ligation in dogs reduces ischemic necrosis and increases myocardial perfusion. In: ibid (1), pp 454–464
3. Faxon DP, Jacobs AK, McSweeney SM, Coats WD, Kellett MA, Ryan TJ (1984) Coronary sinus assessment of left ventricular pressure in man. In: ibid (1), pp 424–429
4. Jacobs AK, Faxon DP, Apstein CS, Coats WD, Gottsman SB, Ryan TJ (1984) The hemodynamic consequences of coronary sinus occlusion. In: ibid (1), pp 430–436
5. Jacobs AK, Faxon DP, Mohl W, Coats WD, Gottsman SB, Ryan TJ (1984) The effect of pressure controlled intermittent coronary sinus occlusion during ischemia. In: ibid (1), pp 483–489
6. Kajiya F, Tsujioka K, Tomonaga G, Ogasawara Y, Tadaoka S, Goto M, Wada Y, Kagiyama M, Mito K (1984) Fluid dynamics in proximal and distal coronary artery measured by laser Doppler velocimeter. In: ibid (1) pp 73–78
7. Marcus M, Wright C, Doty D, Eastham C, Laughlin D, Krumm P, Fastenow C, Brody M (1981) Measurements of coronary velocity and reactive hyperemia in the coronary circulation of humans. Circ Res 49: 877–891
8. Mohl W, Aigner A, Moser M, Timischl W, Bauer R (1984) Changes in coronary artery flow as reaction to coronary sinus occlusion. In: ibid (1), pp 523–528
9. Mohl W, Glogar D, Kenner T, Klepetko W, Moritz A, Moser M, Muller M, Schuster J, Wolner E (1984) Enhancement of washout induced by pressure controlled intermittent coronary sinus occlusion (PICSO) in the canine and human heart. In: ibid (1), pp 537–548
10. Moser M, Mohl W, Gallasch E, Kenner T (1984) Optimization of pressure controlled intermittent coronary sinus occlusion intervals by density measurement. In: ibid (1), pp 529–536
11. Sabbah HN, Stein PD (1982) Effect of acute regional ischemia on pressure in the subepicardium and subendocardium. Am J Physiol 242: H240–H244

Authors' address:
Ying Sun, Ph.D.
Department of Electrical Engineering
University of Rhode Island
Kingston, RI 02881
U.S.A.

362

PICSO-Workshop

W. Mohl, P. Simon, Friedl Neumann, C. Punzengruber, W. Schreiner,
J. Schuster, C. Spiess, M. Müller, G. Tüchy, Astrid Cisar, R. Wenzel,
T. Czaky-Palawichini, P. Kemmetshofer, and Maria Fuchs

Whenever we are about to leave the trial stage and apply our experimental results in actual clinical settings we have to draw up a profit-loss account asking ourselves "which risks will the patient be exposed to and what does he stand to gain from the application of any such new technique?"

In the case of PICSO we were able to base our judgment on ample data from canine models in which PICSO was found to improve ischemic zone myocardial function and to reduce infarct size. Much of this evidence indicated that PICSO would produce the same beneficial effects in human settings and that we should go ahead with human trials. The problem is, however, that on the one hand we can never be absolutely certain that the human response will be identical to that of the animal while on the other hand we know that any new technique must be proven to be both 100% safe and efficient even *before* application in humans. This placed us in a dilemma and called for a trade-off, i.e. some modified version of the technique that allowed application and evaluation while at the same time imposing a minimum of risks on the patient.

In the case of PICSO it is our ultimate scientific target to apply it in settings of acute myocardial infarction or those of instable angina.

Neither of these cases lend themselves to first human trials since application in any such acute settings will definitely require an even greater amount of experience and routine to draw on. Furthermore, we are still short of measuring techniques refined enough to allow for a proper evaluation of the efficacy of the technique in acute settings.

In open heart surgery we are confronted with a totally different situation. Here a new technique such as PICSO is of hardly any risk to the patient since problems that might arise during application such as hemorrhages, arrhythmias or other negative influences on the myocardial performance can be dealt with promptly and without exposing the patient to additional risks. Moreover, since PICSO is applied when on extracorporeal circulation the method interferes little, if at all, with the operating procedure.

It is for this reason that we chose a surgical set of patients for our first human trials even though we knew that the multifactorial nature of open heart surgery would to some extent distort the effect of PICSO on myocardial function and make an evaluation difficult. From ethical considerations the safety of the patient was given priority over our ultimate scientific target. That PICSO is, in fact, a safe techniques was already established in 1984 when we first investigated its effect in humans (3).

The basic goal of this project was to determine the efficacy of PICSO as a means of protecting ischemic myocardium during coronary bypass grafting in 15 study patients vs. 15 controls. Evaluation of the study will have to take into account the multifactorial nature of open heart surgery (Fig. 1).

Our main objective was to determine the short and long term effects of PICSO when applied during the first hour of reperfusion.

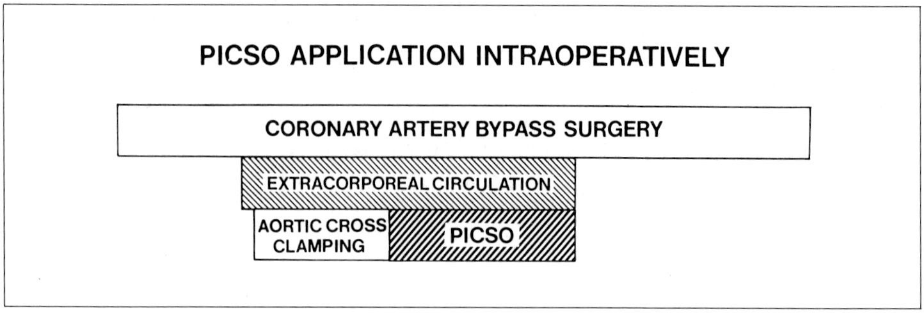

Fig. 1. Intraoperative application of PICSO, the catheter being inserted shortly after going on extracorporeal circulation. During aortic clamping the catheter is used for blood sampling without actually performing PICSO. PICSO is started shortly after aortic declamping and continued for 1 hour.

Patients selected for the human PICSO trial involved those admitted to the second surgical clinic for saphenous vein coronary bypass grafting. Inclusion criteria were male gender, an age of less than 70, two or three vessel diseases. Exclusion from the trial was indicated in patients with left main disease, valvular disease, unstable angina or myocardial infarction evolving as late as 30 days before surgery, and in patients with a significant coexisting medical disease.

All patients were randomized to ensure equal distribution of key parameters using a computer program to balance ejection fraction, cardiac index and revascularization score. This procedure of a balanced randomization allows us to have equal numbers of treatment and control patients with regard to the preoperatively selected parameters (1, 2) (Tables 1 and 2).

The technique of CS catheterization and PICSO intraoperatively

The CS catheter was inserted into the CS through a purse string suture in the free wall of the right atrium near the one stage venous cannula and positioned safely by manual control. This was done shortly before going on extracorporeal circulation to avoid possible air leakage. During aortic clamping the catheter was used for blood sampling without ac-

Table 1. Patient selection according to a balanced radomization, allowing for an equal number of control and treatment patients with regard to the preoperatively selected criteria.

	PICSO			Control		
	N	Mean	St. Dev.	N	Mean	St. Dev.
Age	15	55.867	9.680	15	55.467	7.472
Nr. infarcts	15	0.733	0.594	13	0.615	0.786
Nr. diseased vessels	14	3.000	0.392	15	2.733	0.594
Ejection fraction	15	45.467	15.137	15	50.133	13.495
Cardiac index	15	2.235	0.357	15	2.311	0.438

Table 2. Frequencies and mean values of randomization criteria for control group and treatment group.

Group	Criterium					
	Cardiac index (weight = 10)		Revascularization (weight = 5)		Ejection fraction (weight = 2)	
	2	2	0.85	0.85	45	45
Control						
freq.	5	10	6	9	7	8
mean ± s.e.m.	2.31 ± 0.11		0.93 ± 0.04		50.13 ± 3.48	
PICSO						
freq.	5	10	7	8	9	6
mean ± s.e.m.	2.23 ± 0.09		0.95 ± 0.08		45.47 ± 15.4	

tually performing PICSO. PICSO was started shortly after declamping of the aorta and continued for one hour in the treatment groups vs. reperfusion alone in controls.

Coronary sinus pressure dynamics

Processing of CSP data is a valuable tool for adjusting PICSO treatment, avoiding counterproductive cycles and analysing CSP dynamics for feedback control.

First the analog signals for CS pressure and the balloon inflation trigger were AD-converted. Subsequently, we did a peak detection of the CSP data, which allowed for a discrimination between systole and diastole. Then the time derivative dp/dt was calculated. As a result numerical values for the systolic and diastolic CSP were singled out to be passed on for further evaluation. The next and most important step was the mathematical modelling, i.e. representing the systolic and diastolic envelopes by a mathematical function characterized by only a few essential parameters. In our model we used a 3-parameter function to characterize the systolic and diastolic rise of CSP. The parameters were adjusted to fit the smooth curve as closely as possible (least squares fit), the shape of an entire envelope being reduced to as few as three numbers. Vice versa we reconstructed other features of the envelope curve, such as for instance the "plateau value" that can be reached towards the end of the CSP-rising phase, the "time" it takes for the CSP to get close to the plateau and the "slope" during the CSP rise.

It is important to point out that there is no a priori recipe for the selection of quantities to be calculated. As to the rising times we normally calculate the time necessary to reach 90% of the plateau levels. Another option would be to calculate 60 or 70% of the rising time.

This mathematical model places the responses of the CSP to the CS occlusion on a quantitative basis and allows diagnostic implications. Our model with a 90% rising time, for

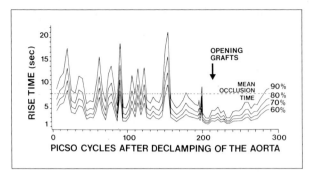

Fig. 2. Intraoperative time course of coronary sinus pressure (CSP) rise time. During the application of PICSO the systolic CSP envelope is fitted by a mathematical model for each single PICSO cycle. From the model parameters the derived quantity "rise time" is then calculated. According to definition the "rise time" is the time it takes for the CSP to reach a certain percentage (60%, 70%, 80%, 90%) of the extrapolated plateau which could eventually be reached after a prolonged occlusion. The plot of these quantities vs. time (i.e. vs. the number of PICSO cycles) allows a post hoc determination of whether actual occlusion time was adequate, rise times above the mean occlusion time indicating for example prematurely released occlusions. Conversely, after opening of the grafts occlusions are found to have been prolonged.

instance, found the systolic envelopes to take longer to get near the plateau than those of diastole.

What has been described so far refers to just one single PICSO cycle. Another interesting modality is to look at the changes of these quantities during surgery from the time of aortic declamping to the opening of the bypass grafts (Fig. 2).

For example, in a plot of the calculated plateau vs. the number of PICSO cycles after aortic declamping we noticed a very distinct rise of the plateau of the CSP due to an increased perfusion after opening of the bypass grafts. Conversely, shortly after aortic declamping we noticed a marked decline in the CSP plateau, most probably due to an overall decline in mean arterial pressure.

Likewise, it was interesting to look at the calculated rising times and their changes during application of PICSO. In addition to a rising time of 90% we also investigated those of 60 or 70%. What struck us most was the considerable increase in scatter with a 90% rising time as compared to other rising times investigated. One of our future goals will be to obtain estimates stable enough to be processed into a closed loop regulation to be set up in the future.

After the evaluation and interpretation of the data so far presented we then investigated the data to find out – post hoc – whether the timing of the PICSO cycles was adequate. We found it desirable to adjust the actual time of occlusion so as to be close to the level required for a 90% rising time. Subsequent plotting of the time of occlusion vs. the calculated 90% rising time allowed identification of prolonged or prematurely released occlusions. Evaluation of the model revealed the calculated rising times to scatter well around the mean value of the actual occlusion period during the first part of the operation while after opening of the bypass grafts all calculated rising times were distinctly below the actual occlusion time, indicating prolonged occlusions that had been poorly adjusted to the physiologic condition of the patient.

We assume these findings to clearly indicate the need for an automatic regulation mechanism of the occlusion/release pattern during the operation.

Biochemical remarks on reperfusion with PICSO

It is well established that cardiac metabolism is organized mainly to maintain the high intracellular concentration of high energy phosphates, which essentially govern the heart's contraction and relaxation pattern. At our last Symposium we reported on the dramatic decrease of myocardial HEPs during reperfusion following ischemic heart arrest.

Energy metabolism is also closely related to membrane function. Energy (ATP) is required for the maintenance of membrane-selective permeability and active processes of transport. Thus, the presence of abnormal amounts of ion or metabolites or proteins or enzymes in the extracellular space must be taken as evidence for alterations of membrane function due to disturbances in ATP production.

The purpose of this study was to evaluate the effect of PICSO on the ischemia-induced leakage of cytoplasmic constituents. Therefore a number of biochemical parameters were measured at fixed points of time, i.e. before bypass, 5 min after aortic declamping, and at 30 and 60 minutes of reperfusion, these time points corresponding to 5', 30' and 60' of PICSO in the treatment group.

The transport of most ions is achieved by an energy-dependent membrane pump, which ultimately establishes a transmembrane gradient. Early stage ischemic tissue injury considerably impairs the maintenance of the ionic gradients. Due to the cardioplegic solution used during open heart surgery, however, it is not possible to actually demonstrate the leakage of potassium ions. However, the behaviour of potassium clearly indicates that during reperfusion potassium blood levels return to normal within 10 minutes following declamping. There was no significant difference between the PICSO-treated group and controls.

Later stages at ischemic damage are reflected in a leakage of metabolites such as lactate or degradation products of ATP.

Lactate: As a result of myocardial ischemia anaerobic ATP production is enhanced, entailing an accumulation of lactate, which subsequently leaks from the cell. Highest lactate concentrations were observed immediately after going on extracorporeal circulation while 24 hours after aortic clamping blood lactate levels were found to have returned toward normal (Fig. 3).

Hypoxanthine/xanthine: Under conditions of ischemia ATP and ADP are degradated to AMP, large amounts of which are subsequently hydrolized irreversibly to adenosine, which in the process diffuses into the extracellular space and may be catabolized within endothelial cells and erythrocytes to hypoxanthine and xanthine. Even after 5 minutes of cardiac arrest a drastic release of hypoxanthine and xanthine into the coronary sinus was observed. Immediately after the initiation of reperfusion the contraction of purine bases in the coronary sinus decreased. Preliminary data indicate that during reperfusion with PICSO the degradation products of ATP are eliminated faster than with reperfusion alone.

Proteins and enzymes: Although cell membranes are almost impermeable to macromolecules there is evidence that proteins and enzymes are moved across membranes by exocytotic or pinocytotic processes. Increasing enzyme leakage during ischemia might be due to the impairment of membrane integrity based on reduced membrane biosynthesis and repair and the release and activation of lysosomal phospholipases, which may degrade membrane components, thus altering their stability. Furthermore high cytoplasmic calcium concentrations might increase the duration of slit opening.

367

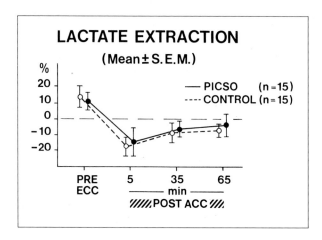

LACTATE EXTRACTION

(Mean ± S.E.M.)

— PICSO (n=15)
---- CONTROL (n=15)

PRE ECC 5 35 65
— min —
▨▨▨ POST ACC ▨▨▨

Fig. 3. % lactate extraction measured before going on extracorporeal circulation and at 5, 35, 65 minutes post ACC.

Although most enzymes used in clinical diagnosis are not tissue specific they are of importance owing to their prevalence in certain organs. Identification of CK and LDH isoenzymes has come to be of great importance in diagnosing myocardial ischemia. It is commonly accepted that irreversible damage is usually paralleled by significant enzyme release. The activities of LDH isoenzyme 1 give ample evidence of these mechanisms. There is a continuous rise in aHBDH activities during and after open heart surgery. Neither for arterial nor venous blood were significant differences observed between PICSO and control. However, it is evident that high levels of enzyme activities were measured several hours after the onset of ischemia because of later leakage from the cell and enzyme clearance via the slow flowing lymphatics.

From these data we conclude that differences in myocardial purine metabolism during reperfusion with or without PICSO are due to faster elimination of degradation products. However, the enhanced washout of purine bases during PICSO must be replaced because of the limited capacity of the de novo purine synthesis in the heart. This might be accomplished by simultaneous administration of purines and ribose.

Hemodynamics

Hemodynamic parameters were assessed intraoperatively at three time points: after the introduction of anesthesia (1), shortly before ECC (2) and 5–10 ' post ECC (3). The following parameters were measured: heart rate (HR), mean arterial pressure (MAP), central venous pressure (CVP), mean pulmonary arterial pressure (MPAP), pulmonary capillary wedge pressure (PCWP), cardiac output/index (CO/CI), stroke volume (SV), stroke volume index (SVI), left ventricular stroke work index (LVSWI) and systemic vascular resistance (SVR).

A significantly higher heart rate ($p < 0.05$) in controls after ECC with an equally high LVSWI and a slightly higher PCWP (n.s.) in controls suggested a more economical cardiac performance in the PICSO-treated group.

In addition to these parameters systolic coronary sinus occlusion pressure (CSOP) was measured at the onset of PICSO, before and after opening of the bypass grafts and prior to and following the end of ECC. While normally changes in systolic CSOP run parallel to changes in MAP, after opening of the bypass grafts a transient rise in systolic CSOP without concomitant variations in MAP was observed.

As to the bypass flows no significant differences were found between the treatment group and controls.

Intraoperative echocardiography

Myocardial function was assessed during coronary artery bypass surgery by means of 2D-echo.

Short axis cross sections at the level of mitral valve cordae tendineae and papillary muscle were measured at (1) baseline measurement prior to ECC, (2) 5–10' post ECC and (3) 20–30' post ECC.

We used either a commercially available echocardiograph (HP 77020A) with a phased array 5 MHz transducer or an ATL Mark 4 with a 5 MHz mechanical scanner.

Regional myocardial function was calculated for the cordae level cross section of the left ventricle. Wall motion analysis was done by outlining epicardial and endocardial interfaces during end-systolic and end-diastolic stop frames. Interfaces were then digitized into a computer (Kontron Cardio 200). Each short axis was subdivided into 8 equally segments using an internal referencing system.

End-diastolic endocardial areas, as a measure of pre- and afterload, did not differ significantly between PICSO and control. No significant changes were found for sectional myocardial areas, calculated as the difference between epicardial and endocardial, areas nor were there any significant differences between groups. For analysis of regional myocardial function segments were classified into 3 groups according to their %FAC at measurement (1): (A) – normocontractile, %FAC > 40%; (B) – intermediate, 20–40% FAC; (C) – hypocontractile, %FAC $\leqslant$ 20%.

Interestingly, in normocontractile and intermediate segments %FAC was found to significantly decrease from (1) to (2) while in the hypocontractile segments a significant increase in %FAC for both PICSO and control was found to occur.

At 30' after ECC (measurement 3) these changes tended to reverse. In the hypocontractile segments %FAC significantly exceeded baseline level in both PICSO and control. In the intermediate segments %FAC was slightly (n.s.) above baseline level. In the normal contractile segments controls significantly failed to reach baseline level ($p > 0.0004$) while in the treatment group %FAC in these segments was found to slightly exceed baseline level.

Thus, PICSO appears to have a positive effect on regional myocardial function during cardiac surgery.

Postoperative management of the PICSO and control groups

Hemodynamics via the Swan-Ganz catheter were measured 3, 6, 9 and 24 hours post aortic declamping. The 3 hour measurement was normally done within 30 minutes after admission of the patient in the ICU. Regular measurements of heart rate, mean arterial pressure and left atrial pressure as well as artificial respiration and biochemistry were done in two-hour intervals. Additionally, we recorded dosage and duration of drug medi-

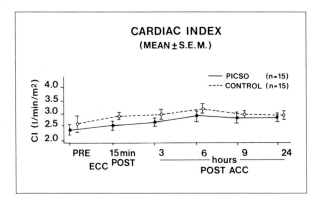

Fig. 4. Cardiac index remaining in a subnormal range between 2.5 and 31/min.

cation. 9 patients of each group were on low dose dopamine because of inadequate urine output. 4 patients of each group required dobutamine in mean dosages of 3.5 µg/kg/min over 11 hours in the PICSO group and 6.5 µg/kg/min over 17 hours in the control group to treat postoperative low cardiac output syndrome. 11 patients of each group received nitroglycerine in a mean dosage of 16 µg/min with a mean duration of 8 hours. Complications and interventions were also precisely documented.

In all the parameters measured we were unable to find any statistically significant differences between the two groups. Cardiac index remained in a subnormal range between 2.5 and 31/min (Fig. 4).

Left ventricular stroke work index, from our point of view one of the strongest parameters for defining the cardiovascular status of a patient since it includes measurements of both systolic and diastolic performance and contains the major variables that alter cardiac performance such as preload, afterload and heart rate, was in a range of 30 to 35 g.m/m² (normal value 45–60).

Systemic vascular resistance remained in a normal range between 1200 and 1400 after admission to ICU and decreased with a concomitant increase in body temperature (Fig. 5).

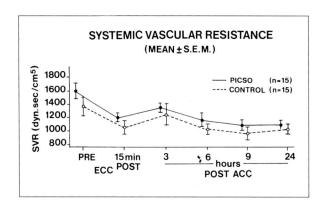

Fig. 5. Systemic vascular resistance remaining in a normal range between 1200 and 1400 after admission to the ICU and decreasing subsequently with a concomitant increase in body temperature.

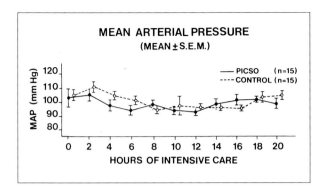

Fig. 6. Mean arterial pressure, recorded in two-hour intervals at the intensive care unit. Comparison between PICSO and control.

MAP, recorded in two-hour intervals, showed slightly elevated levels of 100 mm Hg at the beginning with a subsequent decrease toward the normal range of 80 when vasodilating therapy and rewarming initiated the drop in systemic vascular resistance (Fig. 6).

Heart rate was found to be lower in the PICSO group than in controls, this difference reaching almost statistical significance at the 4 and 6 hour measuring points.

The left atrial pressure as a measure of the left ventricular preload remained in the normal range of 10–12 mm Hg throughout the investigation period.

Table 3 shows some patient data with regard to artificial ventilation and weaning. Although both groups required IPPV between 14 and 15 hours, the control group needed longer continuous positive air way pressure. Also the duration of the stay at the ICU was longer in the control group.

As to complications in the course of the study one PICSO patient developed atrial flutter which was successfully treated with digitalis and quinidine. Life-threatening arrhythmias were observed in one case in the PICSO group and in two patients in the control group. One patient in the PICSO group developed ventricular fibrillation during his transfer from the OR to the ICU. He was rethoracotomized immediately but no pathological substrate was found and normal graft flows were measured. Hypokalemia appeared to have been responsible for this major complication. In the control group two patients developed mediastinitis. In both groups no perioperative myocardial infarction was detected.

Table 3. Comparison of duration of artificial respiration between PICSO and control.

	PICSO		Control	
	Mean	S.E.M.	Mean	S.E.M.
IPPV	14.9	3.8	13.6	3.3
CPAP	3.3	2.4	8.1	3.4
IPPV + CPAP	18.3	3.5	21.7	6.3
IC duration	35.4	5.4	49.8	9.5

371

Postoperative follow-up

A postoperative follow-up was performed in 15 treatment patients vs. 13 control patients, the period of follow-up being 7–17 weeks in 17 patients vs. 17–28 weeks in 11 patients (Table 4). As to the patients' self-assessment of their postoperative condition, in group I (7–17 weeks) 8 PICSO patients and 5 control patients said that they had considerably improved. The same holds true for 3 control patients and 2 PICSO patients whose condition had not improved falling within categories III and IV of NYHA grading. In a comparison of medication between PICSO and control groups it was interesting to note that the PICSO patients, who had taken more oral medication preoperatively than the control patients, managed with significantly less medication than the controls postoperatively, 3 PICSO patients needing no medication at all vs. only 1 patient out of the control group (Tables 5 and 6).

Table 4. Patients' self-assessment of their postoperative condition, 17 patients receiving 7–17 weeks of postoperative treatment vs. 11 patients receiving 17–18 weeks of postoperative treatment.

	7–17 weeks post op		17–28 weeks post op	
	PICSO	Control	PICSO	Control
State of health				
Much improved	8	5	2	3
Improved	0	2	2	0
Little improved	1	1	0	0
Not improved	0	0	2	2
	9	8	6	5

Table 5. Amount of preoperative medication in PICSO vs. control.

Preopoperatively	PICSO	Control
Cardiac stimulants	3	2
Cardioactive steroid glycosides	2	0
Diuretic agents	2	4
Vasodilators	18	13
Nitroglycerine	3	2
Alpha-adrenergic rec. blocking agents	0	0
Beta-adrenergic rec. blocking agents	3	3
Antiarrhythmic agents	2	1
Calcium channel blockers	12	13
Oral anticoagulants	1	0
Platelet aggregation reducing agents	0	0
Anti-anxiety drugs	0	1
Inhibition of xanthine oxidase	1	1
Clofibrate	0	2
	47	42

Table 6. Amount of preoperative medication in PICSO vs. control.

	PICSO	Control
No drugs	3	1
Cardiac stimulants	1	0
Cardioactive steroid glycosides	4	3
Diuretic agents	4	6
Vasodilators	3	3
Nitroglycerine (metered aerosol)	1	2
Alpha-adrenergic rec. blocking agents	0	1
Beta-adrenergic rec. blocking agents	3	2
Antiarrhythmic agents	0	1
Calcium channel blockers	2	4
Oral anticoagulants	2	1
Platelet aggregation reducing agents	4	1
Anti-anxiety drugs	1	2
Inhibition of xanthine oxidase	0	2
DHE, KCL, vit. B complex	3	0
Silymarin, euglycemic agent, clofibrate	0	3
Antibiotics	0	1
	31	33

Of the 28 patients investigated 25 went to a cardiological rehabilitation center postoperatively. Data on ergometrical checkups and ejection fraction measured by echocardiography as well as the clinical symptoms allowed for a comparison of pre- and postoperative classification according to NYHA standards (Figs. 7 and 8).

The data revealed that irrespective of the length of postoperative treatment the patients in grades III and IV either improved or stayed within the same category. No patient assigned to grade II preoperatively was assigned to groups II or IV postoperatively. In 2 control patients assigned to grades III and IV preoperatively no postoperative improvement was

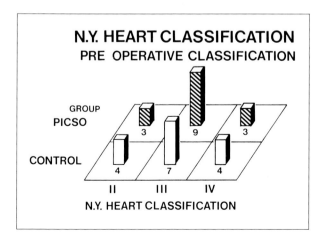

Fig. 7. NYHA classification preoperatively (PICSO vs. control).

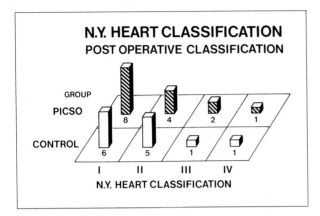

Fig. 8. NYHA classification postoperatively (PICSO vs. control).

found, the patient assigned to grade IV being subject to cerebral palsy with a subsequent speech disorder 1 month after treatment.

In the PICSO group 2 patients were assigned to grade III and 1 patient to grade IV. In the latter patient cardiac catheterization revealed stenosis of the coronary bypasses, while in the patient assigned to grade III myocardial function had not improved, the ejection fraction being 20% both pre- and postoperatively. No patient developed an acute myocardial infarction in the postoperative period investigated.

Discussion

Hugenholtz:
Could you give precise details of the randomization procedure, and which were your key parameters?

Mohl:
It was done as a balanced randomization, i.e. allocation of patients to categories of previously selected criteria so as to have equal numbers of treatment and control patients with regard to the various categories selected. This allows the detection of subtle changes, which is essential in intraoperative studies. Our key parameters were: 1) ejection fraction measured preoperatively during the angiographic procedure; 2) cardiac index after induction of anesthesia; 3) revascularization score.

Hugenholtz:
Have you considered measuring in addition to hypoxanthine adenosine and inosine? Adenosine is rapidly degraded but perhaps there is some information that might be gained in measuring all the nucleotides.

Müller:
As you told us adenosine is rapidly degraded to inosine and subsequently to hypoxanthine. And then, as reported by earlier studies from the U.S., adenosine excretion occurs within the first one or two minutes. It is thus technically impossible to take the blood samples at the patient's site and deproteinize the blood and start the analysis.

Remme:

I am surprised that you find such huge quantities of hypoxanthine that run into the 50 micromoles. I suppose you would have to pace to high heart rates to get those high levels of hypoxanthine. You said that there was a PICSO-induced improvement in metabolic function. I would say that actually it did not improve since there was a far greater difference in the PICSO group during the first measurements than in the controls.

Mohl:

Yes, but the high AV differences you are talking about were measured during global ischemia. Please note that PICSO had not yet started then. At that point we used our normal cardioplegia. Furthermore, nothing else was changed during the operation besides adding PICSO during the first hour of reperfusion.

Remme:

How are you going to interpret those metabolic graphs to support your hypothesis that PICSO is being used to initiate a washout phenomenon? You get a washout of hypoxanthine and lactate. Do you interpret this to be an improvement or as a sign of ongoing ischemia?

Mohl:

It is not possible to separate, first of all, the washout phenomenon on certain biochemical parameters and/or the effect of PICSO on the viability of the cell. Even more important is myocardial function and the protection of the structure. There is yet another problem; we did not measure the blood flow and therefore we could not establish an exact balance of these substances. There is also a mixture of ischemic and nonischemic blood and we know that there is a difference in the performance of certain myocardial areas, those with a good function being slightly depressed while some others improved. We admit that these are merely preliminary data, which one should not try to overinterpret.

Spotnitz:

You have a very ambitious study going here, but there is a number of potential problems on which I should like to comment. Firstly, I think that you need to reconsider the technique you are using to randomize the patient. First of all, on some of the subsequent hemodynamics and echo studies you are comparing courses of patients though you started out with different end-diastolic volumes, blood pressures etc. The cross-sectional areas of the left ventricular lumen seem to start out considerably apart.

My second problem is that most of the data in the literature would suggest what occurs when the proximal anastomoses are done does not have an impact on the postoperative course, and if those data are correct it is very unlikely that PICSO will have any effect after the patient leaves the operating room. So, if you wish to concentrate on PICSO in the ischemic period, when you are doing the proximal anastomoses, then you should look at wall motion abnormalities, the compliance changes, differences between the two groups. It is likely that this is the time when the differences will be seen, not later on.

Another point is the factors going on in the postoperative period that you have not mentioned. For example: What is the patient's temperature when leaving the operating room? What are the levels of circulating catecholamines which you should certainly measure if you are going to talk about segmental wall motion and different time periods. You said that several patients were on presser agents and nitroglycerine, but you did not say what criteria were being used to administer those agents because the agents themselves are affecting the other agents and nitroglycerine. Unless you are using a set protocol you will influence the hemodynamic results.

Because of the sensitive methods you are using, you might be able to detect an adverse effect of the technique you are using to do the operation. In other words, you are operating on patients with occluded coronaries and doing the distal anastomoses, and I would suggest that if you do demonstrate a problem there, it may be important to look at the other way of doing the operation, because no one has ever done as careful a study as you have done. You are not only evaluating PICSO, you are also evaluating cardiac surgery in general.

Mohl:

We were reluctant to look for changes in myocardial function during the period when the patient is on bypass because we thought that there was such a high variability. But now that you, being an expert in 2D-echo recommend it, I think we should go ahead with it.

The next thing is that there were no significant differences between treatment and control group. You were right to suspect that our groups started out differently because of the difference in global ischemia between baseline measurement and the onset of PICSO after declamping of the aorta. This is exactly the trade-off between safety of the patient and the ultimate scientific goal of our trial I was talking about earlier. Secondly, we also assume that the effects of PICSO are limited to the period of the operation itself without long-term effects. However, this might be different if you extent the treatment perioperatively. As to the different variables the surgeon is unable to control I – once again – have to say that bearing in mind both the safety of the patient and the research physician's target, this new technique, of necessity, can only be tested intraoperatively.

Weisel:

There is a group of patients who would probably benefit, namely those patients unresponsive to medical therapy who cannot get thrombolysis and require surgery, either today or tomorrow morning. The problem is trying to find out whether your PICSO treatment works or not. The recent data would suggest that if you do biopsies before the operation or just as you go on bypass there is a depression in glycogen and a decrease in the high-energy phosphates, which are lower after the operation in routine cases: this could be used as an end point to try to see if there is a benefit.

Mohl:
Yes, but where would you actually take the biopsies from?

Weisel:
We took biopsies from three different sites in the myocardium of sixty patients and were able to determine that you should do the biopsies where it is ischemic (determined from the angiogram and electrographic changes). You will find that most of the ischemia leading to unstable angina comes from LAD territory.

Faxon:
I think one of the questions a cardiologist and a non cardiac surgeon has during early

clinical trials is safety. Were there any complications from using coronary sinus catheters in the operating room and, if there were none, I think that is a valuable piece of information we should not overlook.

Mohl:

There were no complications apart from some problems in the early stage of the study, when we inserted the catheter when on bypass and produced an air lock. But otherwise there was no damage, hemorrhage or rupture in the coronary sinus. Blood loss was the same in both groups. There was no hemolysis or change in coagulation parameters. So I think we can definitely say that it is a safe procedure.

Meerbaum:

You said your heart is beating empty during PICSO; are your data relevant to the situation where the heart is filled?

Spotnitz:

Well, preload certainly affects what you see, and it also depends on exactly what technique you use. With no vent it is not true that the heart is completely unloaded. I think if your left atrial pressures are matched, it is perfectly valid to use the data, particularly if you use regional wall thickening rather than regional wall motion, which will solve some of these problems.

References

1. Dillon W, Goldstein M (1984) Multivariate Analysis. Methods and Applications. New York, pp 366–372
2. Draper N, Smith H (1981) Applied regression analysis, 2nd ed, New York, pp 307–310
3. Mohl W, Glogar D, Kenner Th, Klepetko A, Moritz M, Moser M, Müller M, Schuster J, Wolner E (1984) Enhancement of washout induced by intermittent coronary sinus occlusion (PICSO) in the canine and human heart. In: Mohl W, Glogar D, Wolner E (eds) The Coronary Sinus. Steinkopff Verlag, Darmstadt, pp 537–548

Authors' address:
Werner Mohl, M.D.,
2nd Surgical Clinic,
University of Vienna,
Spitalgasse 23,
1090 Vienna,
Austria

Summary statement – PICSO

D. P. Faxon

Department of Cardiology, University Hospital, Boston (U.S.A.)

The history of pressure controlled intermittent coronary sinus occlusion (PICSO) is relatively short, and the advances made in this area are attributable to the enormous efforts of those who are involved in the research. The accomplishments are remarkable as it has been only six years since its inception, and the first publication was only a few years ago.

The principle of PICSO is based upon intermittently occluding the coronary sinus, thus allowing the coronary sinus pressure to build to a plateau. Once the pressure reaches its maximal value, the balloon is released and the pressure returns to that of the right atrium. The cycle is then repeated. The increase in the pressure in the coronary sinus allows redistribution of blood to the ischemic zone and during release allows wash-out of toxic metabolites.

Dr. Mohl and others have also demonstrated that the pressure curve is a unique phenomenon containing important physiological information that is clinically useful in understanding coronary physiology. While the wave form is not fully understood, we do know that the rate of rise in this systolic and diastolic pressure and the time to the peak pressure are important.

As shown by Dr. Jacobs in experimental studies, there is an important relationship between coronary blood flow and the rate of change of the coronary sinus pressure during occlusion. Thus, the coronary sinus pressure might provide a direct measure of coronary blood flow in man. As reported by Dr. Mohl, analysis of the occluded pressure may give some clues as to the size of the area of risk of infarction, as well as infarct size. These measurements are very difficult for us to attain right now in the clinical setting and would be invaluable in monitoring the effectiveness of interventions aimed at reducing infarct size during acute myocardial infarction.

Additionally, in a study that Dr. Jacobs and I did in patients in the catheterization laboratory, the coronary sinus occlusion pressure contour was unique and the diastolic pressure very closely simulated that of the left ventricular diastolic pressure. This is not the case in animal models, particularly the dog and the pig model, where the diastolic pressure is significantly higher than the left ventricular pressure. This difference may be explained by differences in the venous drainage. In man, the measurement of coronary sinus diastolic pressure during occlusion is a very close approximation of left ventricular diastolic pressure and may provide a useful parameter in monitoring patients who are ill.

As reported in this symposium, not only is intermittent occlusion useful diagnostically, but also pressure controlled intermittent coronary sinus occlusion can significantly reduce infarct size during a permanent coronary occlusion. In addition, it has been shown to improve ventricular function as demonstrated by fractional shortening, and during reperfusion it can further reduce infarct size.

Thus, the technique may have usefulness in a variety of clinical settings such as during acute myocardial infarction. In acute myocardial infarction where no reperfusion occurs such as the patient who does not respond to thrombolysis, or has an unsuccessful angioplasty, PICSO would seem to perform a useful role in reducing infarct size. In addition, in successfully reperfused patients, PICSO may further reduce infarct size by reducing reperfusion injury. We do not yet have clinical experience in this area, but it seems likely that the technique may be a useful adjunct to current treatments of acute MI.

In addition, we have learned from Drs. Mohl, Lazar, and Roberts that PICSO may have an important application in coronary surgery. Dr. Lazar demonstrated impressive improvement in left ventricular function following 2 hours of coronary bypass and LAD occlusion when PICSO was used. Potential clinical applications are now being explored and early clinical studies by Dr. Mohl suggest benefit.

The issue of ischemia, however, is much less clear. The ability of PICSO and perhaps even synchronized retroperfusion to reduce brief ischemia has not been shown in experimental studies. In a study by Dr. Jacobs, no significant difference in segment thickening or shortening in a canine model of brief coronary ischemia was noted with PICSO. However, in a study by Capone et al., the mean lactate consumption, a measure of myocardial metabolism during ischemia, was significantly less with PICSO. In this study, brief ischemia was created by an increase in myocardial demand, rather than purely a reduction in supply. Thus, PICSO may have some application in chronic myocardial ischemia, where the demand rather than supply is the primary problem.

A number of questions about PICSO remain unanswered, most importantly its mechanism of action. The elegant study by Dr. Mohl and Dr. Kenner using blood density measurements suggests that PICSO works by wash-out of edema fluid and toxic metabolites. Confirmation of the mechanism is necessary so we can understand how this technique works and where its limitations and greatest applications might be. In addition, the potential to administer antiarrhythmic agents or other drugs into the infarct area is an important area for future research. The potential applications of all coronary sinus techniques are numerous and include acute myocardial infarction, unstable angina, cardiac surgery, malignant tachyarrhythmias, PTCA, and cardiac transplantation. As we proceed now, into early clinical studies, we need to look very carefully at each of these possible applications and design appropriate clinical trials to determine the effectiveness of these techniques.

Author's address:
David P. Faxon, M. D.
Department of Cardiology
University Hospital
75 East Newton Street
Boston, MA 02118
U.S.A.

Coronary sinus interventions and interventional therapy

Pros and cons of coronary sinus interventions versus conventional therapy

D. P. Faxon, and P. G. Hugenholtz*

Department of Cardiology, University Hospital Boston (U.S.A.), and Akademisch Ziekenhuis, Thoraxcentrum, Rotterdam (The Netherlands)

Faxon:

Over the last few days we have heard presented an enormous amount of experimental data. As Dr. Harken pointed out so nicely, we are now on the threshold of clinical studies. So let me briefly outline what clinical and experimental evidence exists that coronary sinus techniques will, in fact, be useful in the treatment of patients, and which settings will be most likely to benefit.

Cardiac surgery

We heard very compelling evidence of potential benefits of coronary sinus interventions in cardiac surgery. At the last meeting two years ago, we heard that retrograde cardioplegia had great advantages over antegrade cardioplegia. In particular, retrograde cardioplegia resulted in better cooling and provided an unobstructive route to the ischemic myocardium. The potential disadvantage of requiring a longer time to institute therapy, as mentioned by Dr. Menasché is not the case if one cannulates in a proper way using current equipment. We are therefore in need of randomized clinical trials and a good registry to demonstrate conclusively if retrograde cardioplegia is superior to antegrade. The same holds true for the role of PICSO or SRP since both might have a role in the treatment of patients in the postoperative period. This again is an area in need of clinical investigation. However, as pointed out by Dr. Weisel more refined tools will be needed to determine the efficacy of these techniques in cardiac surgery where end points are difficult to determine and measure. The experimental studies of Drs. Roberts and Lazar at our institution, do suggest that PICSO in the immediate postoperative situation has potential to improve ventricular function in animal models. Early clinical studies by Dr. Mohl and colleagues also suggest clinical benefit in the reperfusion period.

Acute myocardial infarction

Thrombolysis and angioplasty are increasingly being used in the treatment of patients with acute myocardial infarction. This is based upon the very convincing evidence from recent clinical trials. In particular, the recent GISSI trial clearly suggests that thrombolysis benefits patients with acute myocardial infarction by significantly reducing short term mortality. Thrombolysis does have some limitations and drawbacks: First of all, it takes some time for the thrombolytic agent to work (about 40 minutes in most studies). Moreover, in most of the reported studies, the patency rate is 60%–70%. In fact, in the recent TIMI trial, the incidence of vessel patency within 90 minutes after giving an intravenous thrombolytic agent, rtPA or streptokinase, was rather dismal. Streptokinase and rt-PA had patency rates of 30% and 60% respectively. Thus, a very large percentage of patients (40% to be optimistic) will not have arterial reperfusion with thrombolysis. While angioplasty may result in a higher reperfusion rate, angioplasty takes more time to institute and is a more complicated and costly procedure. It is also a procedure that can not be done in a community hospital.

Another problem of all reperfusion techniques is that they can result in reperfusion injury. Studies on synchronized retroperfusion and Dr. Jacob's studies with PICSO, provide evidence that these approaches can reduce reperfusion injury even in settings of successful thrombolysis or successful angioplasty. These studies suggest that in the settings of acute myocardial infarction there is, in fact, an adjunct role for these techniques to further reduce myocardial damage with or without successful reperfusion.

Unstable angina

As compared to acute myocardial infarction, unstable angina is much more controversial. In general, patients can be very successfully treated by medical therapy. The administration of triple drug therapy (beta blockers, calcium antagonists, and nitrates including intravenous nitroglycerine), is a very potent means of reducing episodes of ischemia, stabilizing the patient, and allowing a revascularization procedure if necessary. There are subsets of patients in which this therapy fails to control symptoms. In this subgroup of patients with unstable angina, coronary sinus interventions might have an important role to play, particularly since there is evidence from experimental studies to indicate a benefit. The preliminary clinical studies of Dr. Gore also support this notion and give us some glimmer of hope that high-risk patients with unstable angina may benefit from these techniques. In our own hospital, the unstable patient who is refractory to medical therapy comprises about 17% of our unstable population. Most of the complications occur in these patients since they constitute a high-risk group. The end points of acute myocardial infarction or death could be measured and meaningful comparisons made between conventional therapy and coronary sinus interventions. Thus, early clinical studies with coronary sinus interventions should be directed toward the patient with unstable angina who has a high risk of myocardial infarction or death.

Angioplasty

Another potential area of application of coronary sinus technique is during angioplasty. My own bias about the use of coronary sinus intervention techniques in angioplasty is that they will not prove to be very useful as angioplasty is already quite safe and effective. A successful angioplasty occurs in more than 90% of patients and balloon inflations of 30 to 90 seconds can easily be done without harming the patient. Whether more prolonged inflations of the balloon are necessary in order to reduce the incidence of restenosis is currently unknown and unless this becomes evident, the use of coronary sinus intervention during a routine angioplasty would probably not be likely to improve the current success of the technique. This would not be the case if complications occur during angioplasty. In patients who need to go to the operating room emergently, particularly in the presence of multivessel disease or incomplete revascularization, the application of a coronary sinus interventions could help stabilize the patient and reduce myocardial damage until the patient is on cardiopulmonary bypass. Thus in summary, coronary sinus intervention appears promising and may have an important role to play, during cardiac surgery, acute myocardial infarction, unstable angina, and during a failed angioplasty when emergency surgery is needed.

Hugenholtz:

Thank you, Dr. Faxon. In a large measure, I would agree with you. I was pleased that you showed a systematic discussion of all the areas that we might focus on for our pro and con attitude. And I again want to repeat that I am not against anything you said, because it *does* make sense. But I would like to be a bit more precise about a number of these points. I think the first issue we have to address is that for yet another technique in the area of cardiac protection to be promoted, we have to realize that resistance from various quarters is increasing. When we are talking about a complex procedure in a complex area, obviously costing a major investment in time, energy, and money, I think it would be best to actually figure out where any of these techniques will be most likely to succeed rather than say that these are *all* areas we might look at. Not that I think that I should become still more conservative, but everybody in this room knows how it is having to divide up the Schilling or the Dollar in even smaller pieces. So, on which target you will put your bets is really the question I want to address.

Unstable angina

I honestly believe that if we could teach doctors to properly use the current pharmacological triple therapy, intravenous nitroglycerine and a combination of beta-blockers plus calcium antagonists in right amounts at the right time with a certain progression in terms of dosing, at least 40–45%, if not more than half of the current problems with unstable angina could be cooled off by the optimal use of this currently available and cheap pharmacological therapy. And as to the problem cases which you said comprise some 17%, data that has been acquired in our institution over the past two years in some 140 patients who were therapy-resistant for 24–36 hours, indicating that this figure is somewhat higher at 30%. These patients are showing persistent signs of ischemia and one definitely wants to do something about it. In this subset, PTCA has been a major breakthrough and I think it can solve nearly all of this problem. In our 140 therapy-resistant patients, we have had one late death and a 5% incidence of myocardial infarction. And with the years, I am sure, reperfusion will do away with any other complications related to this particular subset of patients. Therefore unstable angina is not an area I would put my bets on, just yet. This leaves us with patients where the PTCA failed in the first place, or where complications occurred, or where a surgical intervention was necessary, or the procedure

385

was longer than desired. And here I agree that surgeons, even when being quick, cannot avoid the infarction. And it is for this group that I would primarily like to investigate this technique. It is this group that, as Dr. Weisel pointed out, you would previously have put on a balloon pump before entering the operating room. Now let us put the retrograde support system in *before* you get into a problem. This particular subset of patients comprises some 5% of the population we would see.

So there remains a small group of 5%, not 17% where I would think active support by mechanical retroperfusion would be appropriate and in these cases, I would give preference to PICSO.

Myocardial infarction

I think you are underestimating slightly the efficacy of thrombolysis, since you did not mention that the GISSI trial done in Italy involved some 13,000 patients. This trial clearly shows that when intravenous streptokinase is given within the first 3 hours the acute death rate is halved. To be specific, it dropped from 14 or 15% to something like 7%. This is a myocardial mortality reduction of major proportions. Admittedly, they have not proven whether this is achieved through spontaneous patency of a vessel or the dissolution of the plug, but the mortality figure is compelling. Likewise there is data from the Netherlands which appears to be even stronger. It shows that if you apply within the first few hours, a strategy which is one step further than GISSI, i.e., to begin with half a million units of streptokinase at the hospital door which gives you a patency rate within the first few hours of only 40%, but then proceed with intracoronary streptokinase, a mortality figure of a few per cent in a first year follow-up can be achieved. Provided the job is completed with properly executed PTCA, it may be even lower. In other words, although it is not yet the ideal solution and a complex procedure since it requires intravenous plus intracoronary streptokinase and PTCA, for me it is *the* proper physiological approach for the restoration of antegrade flow. It *is* the dominant numero uno appropriate strategy. Such early intravenous use of a lytic agent gains a critical amount of time allowing to proceed with subsequent steps. I would say that a properly structured, stepped approach with the best lytic agent, intravenously first, followed when needed (and I think this is required in only half the cases) by an intracoronary manipulation, can achieve patency rates of about 85% or even higher. And that, I think, is a tremendous figure. Yet, among these patients, if you are late but still in time, I can see that further support in terms of the technique you have discussed may have a major role to play. I would rate this group, however, as less likely to succeed, since these are usually patients with necrosed tissue in whom it will be difficult to prove how much you can preserve cardiac tissue.

Cardiac surgery

I must compliment the Vienna group on having made a very careful study in this area. However, I also think that some of the points raised during the discussion are valid and deserve reconsideration. What is it really that you are after in cardiac surgery? What is the hypothesis that you are trying to test? As to the measurements, these again show how difficult this area is for all of us doctors, because whether we are talking about unstable

angina or an ischemic state in cardiac surgery, we just do not have the right tools to measure ischemia. Yes, there is the echo technique, but there is only so much you can get out
of it. You can try to do biopsies but the fact that you have ATP in the cell does not mean
that the cell is going to contract. So I have to repeat that cardiac surgery to me would
seem to be the area least worthy of being tested, because of the difficulty in providing the
point in having the right hypothesis. Most exciting in the list and figuring even above unstable angina is what Harken and others discussed this morning, that is the matter of *malignant arrhythmias*. When you wish to deliver a high concentration of a given drug, and
that goes for the dismutase, and other O_3 scavengers, again I think the whole reperfusion
area is of great promise.

So in summary, we do not disagree on major points. I would, however, put the likeli-
hoods for this specific technique to succeed in a slightly different order. I would put on
top the local delivery of drugs for a specific situation, testing a specific hypothesis and
delivering the drug where it has to be delivered. Then I would take the setting of unstable
angina involving totally therapy resistant cases because there again you have something
specific. And in the third place I would put acute infarction. Fourth, surgery, because it is
a very difficult area to be tested.

Faxon:

As you mentioned, the GISSI trial only examined mortality as an end point. We do not
know the mechanisms of the improvement in mortality rate. Likewise the WIST trial reported by Kennedy showed a significant reduction in mortality rate but no improvement
in ventricular function.

Hugenholtz:

That point has been taken care of by the Dutch Interuniversity Trial, a randomized
investigation into the effects of streptokinase given early, because not only do we have
data on the ventricular function over a course of months with data on mortality, but we
also have the data on infarct size and on the angiography subsequently. And within that
trial, not only was the short-term mortality cut in half but this striking reduction persisted for a full year or even longer, because we now have longer follow-ups. That highly significant difference in survival was explained by the fact that those who survived had a
much higher ejection fraction (53 vs. 46% in controls), something that Kennedy could not
prove because he did not test for it in a systematic fashion. Furthermore, we proved that
the earlier you commenced the intervention, the better the outcome with still lower mortality and entirely normal ventricular function. And, furthermore, we proved with careful
regional wall motion analysis, that this was due to an improvement in the affected segments. It was not a general rheological afterload reduction that improved the ejection
fraction. It was because function in the ischemic segments was restored. And the overall
results were best in that group which received first early intravenous, then the IC streptokinase and then the PTCA procedures. Therefore mortality is just part of the puzzle. You
need to prove that the reduction in mortality and the improved survival is related to improved function, which in turn relates to the fact that infarct size was smaller. And in-

deed, in the cases we have studied was on average infarct size, limited by one third in comparison to controls.

Faxon:

Well, it is still a fact that patients have myocardial infarction despite all of this therapy. The principle still remains that the smaller the infarct size, the better the patient is going to do, and the data you presented support this. So, it makes logical sense that if I could further reduce the infarct size even with thrombolysis, angioplasty, surgery, or whatever it will be, it will be better for the patient. For this reason, I think these coronary sinus techniques have the possibility of being additive and therefore important new treatment modalities in acute myocardial infarction.

Hugenholtz:

Allright, but then they have to be applied quickly because I have to become convinced that the only thing that really matters is time. Stanley Sarnoff has paraphrased: ,,Time is money" into ,,Time is muscle". And so if the technique requires time, and any technique cost-time, I would go for the one that gives me the quickest results. And that is still an intravenous injection at the earliest moment by the most alert physician who is nearest to the patient. And here is the great hope for rt-PA, since it attacks the clot directly. The very next step would be, of course, to look whether there are residual signs of ischemia. Then clearly we would not have done enough and then I would go to the arterial site first. I would not put something through the coronary sinus as a first approach. And then, if I still had time, I would support the notirn that you do it through the coronary sinus pump.

Faxon:

That is perhaps one area. But I think the difference is that a right-sided venous catheter in the coronary sinus is a relatively simple technique that a community hospital physician can do. It does not involve a coronary cathezerization laboratory and is not time consuming nor costly. It is a technique that can be done right after the paramedics gives the rt-PA. Somebody can insert the coronary sinus catheter and then move the patient to the appropriate place to do a cardiac catheterization or angioplasty if needed at that particular point. Even in a situation where you do angioplasty or intracroronary streptokinase, there is still the additional benefit of these techniques in reducing reperfusion injury, so why not, when you insert your arterial catheter, also put in a venous catheter? Why not give the patient the greatest possible benefit?

Hugenholtz:

What we need is proof for that, but I am willing to go along with your basic idea. However, I am not so convinced that a doctor in a regional hospital will insert a right-sided catheter in the coronary sinus as a first line of defense. I would concur with you that this is an area of investigation. I think I would very much like to investigate a patient who has had the best intravenous lytic therapy and in whom signs of ischemia recur whilst being far away from a catheterization laboratory. There we should try this technique. That to me would be a very good area of investigation.

Authors' addresses:

David P. Faxon, M.D.
Department of Cardiology
University Hospital
75 East Newton Street
Boston, MA 02118
U.S.A.

P. G. Hugenholtz, Prof.
Akademisch Ziekenhuis
Thoraxcentrum
Molewaterplein 40
3015 DG Rotterdam
Niederlande

The transfemoral catheterization of the coronary sinus in the clinical practice

B. Heublein[1], G. Linß[1], N. Franz[1], P. Romaniuk[2], D. Modersohn[1], and D. Strangfeld[3]

Humboldt-University, Medical Division (Charité) Berlin (G.D.R.)

Summary: The transfemoral route is favoured in complex diagnostic and therapeutic strategy in acute or chronic coronary heart disease. Transfemoral catheterization of the coronary sinus (CS) and the great cardiac vein (GCV) with a pre-shaped normal 7F catheter is – according to experiences over a number of months – successful in about 90%. Variably shaped CS valves and the long and power consuming catheter route with unfavourable curves are responsible for the lower success rate using balloon catheters for temporary occlusion. The completeness, duration and localization of balloon blocking depends on the CS morphology, size and the stability of the deflated balloon. Mostly only the GCV and the anterior interventricular vein are superselectively blockable. The junction near the orifice of the CS caused retrograde filling of the posterior interventricular vein along superficial connections and the intramural venous network. These are important factors for the effect of drug retroinfusion.

Heparinization induced partly distinct differences in concentrations of important pressure-regulating substances in central venous blood. Both the localizations of the catheter for standardized blood sampling and the actual conditions of anticoagulation seem to be important for comparable data.

Introduction

Manipulations of the coronary sinus (CS) in attempts to protect ischemic myocardium and for validation of biochemical changes in man are at present problematical. In the clinic special conditions are taken into consideration for catheterization and blood recruitment. Normally CS intervention techniques are (potentially) one part of a more complex diagnostic or therapeutic regime in patients with acute or chronic ischemic heart disease, like myocardial protection during PTCA, in unstable angina or acute myocardial infarction. Such conditions are, among others:

– with the aim of retroperfusion, retroinfusion or retroocclusion;
   I) high success rate for catheter placement in a relatively short time,
  II) feasibility under high fibrinolytic activity induced by thrombolytic therapy,
 III) stabile localization of the balloon for temporary occlusion in different CS and great cardiac vein (GCV) morphology, size and curvature,
  IV) to produce a temporary total occlusion for retrograde drug administration as an important precondition of drug action.

– for biochemical studies with coronary venous blood;
   I) localization and stability of the catheter for blood sampling,
  II) stability of measurements under different level of heparin.

---

[1] Clinic of Internal Medicine
[2] Institute of Cardiovascular Diagnostic
[3] Clinic of Nuclear Medicine

This study was performed in order to evaluate
- the feasibility of transfemoral catheterization of CS and GCV by normal and balloon-carrying catheter,
- the influence of CS morphology on the stability of balloon localization and completeness of temporary occlusion,
- heparinization and contrast ventriculography and their influence on concentrations of important pressure-regulating substances in right atrial or GCV sampled blood.

Methods

Great cardiac vein catheterization

In 40 patients with angiographically proven coronary artery disease (n = 28) and without significant coronary obstructions (n = 12) transfemoral catheterization of the GCV was performed by means of 7F-PE-catheters, shaped in our own laboratory. In addition, in 10 patients with significant coronary artery obstructions the catheterization and temporary occlusion of CS or GCV was performed by a balloon catheter (Mansfield Sci. Inc.) to show the coronary venous vasculature and filling characteristics retrogradely, to test the completeness of the occlusion and the balloon stability.

Biochemical data

In 18 patients blood sampling in the right atrium or GCV was performed to estimate the concentrations of epinephrine, norepinephrine, dopamin-beta-hydroxylase (DBH), callicrein and angiotensin before treatment (a), 5 min after heparinization (100 Iu/kg) (b) and 3 min after left ventriculography (Visotrast, 40 ml, flow 12) (c).

Results

Success rate in catheterization of great cardiac vein

According to a typical learning curve for some months in 36 of the last 40 patients (90%) catheterization of the GCV by a 7F catheter (without balloon) was successful. The catheterization of the GCV via the Vv. femoralis by a balloon catheter using the analog curved guide-wire technique was found to be much more difficult. Only in 7 (of 10) patients could we attain the GCV.

Coronary sinus occlusion

A stable (about 20 s) occlusion by inflated balloon was obtained in 3 patients. In all other cases the occlusion was incomplete, due to displacement of the balloon during the inflation or extensive shunting along the posterior interventricular vein, mostly in the distal part of the CS.

392

Biochemical data

Table 1 shows some results according to the time of sampling. Additionally the deviations obtained were significantly different in the subgroups (DBH in patients with a history of infarct and with coronary artery disease, epinephrine in patients without a history of infarction, callicrein in patients with increased left ventricular wall volume).

Discussion

Catheterization and occlusion

It is well known that transfemoral catheterization of the GCV is much more difficult than the way via the v. cava superior. But the physicians are well trained and the management in case of complications is easier, especially in haemorrhage due to thrombolysis considering the relatively thick catheter sheath. Thus, the relatively high success rate with a specially formed catheter and guide-wire is encouraging. Using this method the blood sampling without any influence from the so-called reflux phenomenon is reliable and the additional placement of other interesting devices through an ultra-thin teflon sheath is possible, such as a micromanometer for registration of real pressure and, perhaps, also the flow. Figure 1 shows an example of the catheter shape employed after rotation and placement in the GCV. On the other hand, the placement of a balloon catheter in this way needs more skill, sometimes additional procedures and therefore more time. In particular the passage of the balloon at different CS valves (1), whose shapes are not known, both at the point of entrance and in more remote places (for example at the junction of the GCV into the CS) is sometimes very difficult, considering the long and power-

Table 1. Concentrations of some vasoactive substances in blood sampled in the right atrium just after catheterization without heparinization (a), 5 min after heparinization sampled in the GCV (b) and 3 min after left ventriculography sampled at the same place in the GCV (c).

Parameter	Number of patients	Sampling				
		a	b	t-value (a/b)	c	t-value (b/c)
Epinephrine	17	1.77 ±0.92	1.55 ±0.62	1.10	1.80 ± 1.27	−1.04
Norepinephrine	17	3.92 ±1.76	3.88 ±1.32	1.35	3.89 ±2.47	−1.23
DBH	18	43 ±69	32 ±45	0.47	36 ±64	−0.15
Callicrein	16	15.9 ±2.4	14.5 ±2.2	2.29*	13.8 ±3.8	0.66
Angiotensin	13	1.6 ±1.3	2.0 ±1.7	0.39	1.8 ±1.6	1.45

* $p < 0.5$.

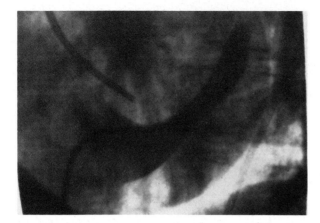

Fig. 1. Coronary sinus and great cardiac vein after contrasting. Tip of the catheter is placed in the GCV, LAD projection; micromanometer in the left ventricle; transfemoral catheterization.

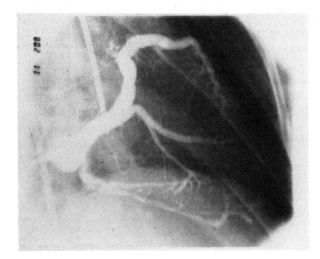

Fig. 2. Retrograde filling of the coronary venous vasculature after total and stable occlusion (20 s) of the coronary sinus; (30° RAO projection, 6 ml visotrast). Showing CS and in the continuity the GCV and (from top to the bottom) the anterior interventricular vein, posterior left ventricular veins and the posterior interventricular vein. The balloon is inflated just behind the CS orifice.

consuming method and unfavourable curves (Fig. 1). These preliminary results – the low success rate and the long X-ray exposure time – must be considered in any therapeutic CS intervention, especially in urgent situations like myocardial infarction.

An important question for CS interventions, especially in CS infusion, is the stable localization and total occlusion temporarily after inflation of the balloon (Fig. 2). In this patient the retroinfused drug should reach the capillary bed retrogradely. The stability and completeness in such situations is also demonstrable by retrograde Xe^{133} injection and registration of plateau and washout-curve after deflation of the balloon. However, such a stable and total occlusion by inflated balloon was only obtained in 3 patients. Often during the inflation or deflation we could notice a distinct displacement of the balloon in the direction of the CS orifice or out in the right atrium. We could avoid this in most cases with a higher placement of the balloon (Fig. 3). But than we retroinfuse a superselected region of ventricular wall! With this position of the balloon the posterior interventricular

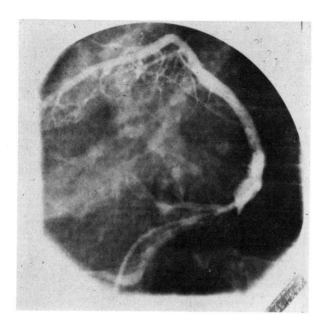

Fig. 3. Retrograde filling of great cardiac vein and anterior interventricular vein (above) and visualization of posterior interventricular vein (bottom); (60 ° LAD, 20 s occlusion time with high balloon position, 6 ml visotrast).

veins can be filled along superficial connections and the intramural venous network. But the blood flow overcomes the pressure gradient and the direct route via the posterior interventricular vein into the CS has the lowest resistance. Thus, drug retroinfusion in the venous capillary bed in this region cannot be expected. The localization and the completeness of the ballooning seem to be very important for drug reaction, the duration of effect and the efficiency.

The reasons for the described displacement during inflation or collapse of the balloon could be the increased pressure behind the balloon and the conical shape of the CS in connection with failing resistance caused by the catheter curvature in the right atrium – v. cava inferior (Fig. 1). We need more experience under clearly defined clinical conditions and some modifications of the catheter and the technique (including twistable catheter material, preshaped, low profile balloon with improved wall surface resistance under deflation, and a soft tip) to render the intervention safe, quick and effective.

Biochemical data

Table 1 shows the great variation of blood concentrations sampled under strictly standardized conditions. The partly distinct differences after heparinization are unexpected. These differences caused by heparinization are obviously more important than the results due to contrast ventriculography. The reasons for these results and the partly significant changing in defined subgroups of patients are unknown at this time. But in any case we have to keep in view that both the localization of the catheter for standardized blood sampling (2) and the actual condition during this procedure are important for comparable data.

References

1. Tschabitscher M (1984) Anatomy of Coronary Veins. In: Mohl W, Wolner E, Glogar D (eds) The Coronary Sinus. Steinkopff Verlag, Darmstadt, pp 8–25
2. Steingart RM, Scheuer J (1982) Assessment of Myocardial Ischemia and Infarction. In: Hurst JW (ed) The Heart arteries and veins. McGraw-Hill Book Company, New York, pp 357–378

Authors' address:
Prof. B. Heublein, M.D.
Clinic of Internal Medicine
Humboldt-University, Medical Division (Charité)
Schumannstraße 20/21
1040 Berlin
G.D.R.

Evaluation of coronary sinus interventions by two-dimensional echocardiography

G. Maurer

Division of Cardiology, Department of Medicine, Cedars-Sinai Medical Center and UCLA School of Medicine, Los Angeles (U.S.A.)

Summary: In canine models of experimental occlusion of the left anterior descending coronary artery (LAD), 2-dimensional echocardiography (2DE) has demonstrated significant improvement of left ventricular (LV) ejection fraction after instituting synchronized diastolic retroperfusion (SRP). Regional function analysis demonstrated improved contractility in previously dysfunctioning segments, suggesting a beneficial effect of SRP on ischemic myocardium. 2DE has also been used to study modifications of the SRP methodology and could demonstrate the superiority of hypothermic over normothermic SRP for salvage of ischemic myocardium as well as its utility for prevention of reperfusion injury.

Similarly, initial studies suggest that pressure controlled intermittent coronary sinus occlusion (PICSO) led to improvements of both global and regional LV function for up to 3 hours following LAD occlusion.

Contrast 2DE has demonstrated the ability of retrograde coronary venous injectates to penetrate into myocardial regions rendered ischemic by LAD occlusion. Penetration of echo-contrast into the region supplied by the circumflex coronary artery was less successful, presumably because of veno-venous shunts which prevented an adequate build-up of intravascular pressure in this particular area. The noninvasive nature of 2DE and its ability to study beat to beat changes suggest its utility for future clinical assessment of coronary sinus interventions.

Introduction

Echocardiography has gained widespread clinical acceptance as a versatile noninvasive imaging modality. In addition to its early applications, such as evaluating pericardial effusions and valvular heart disease, it is being used increasingly in the setting of ischemic heart disease because of its ability to evaluate ventricular function. A number of parameters of left ventricular function can be determined by 2-dimensional echocardiography (2DE). Both end-diastolic (EDV) and end-systolic volumes (ESV) and therefore ejection fraction can be measured by various methods in both humans (2, 16) and dogs (18), yielding good correlation with angiography. 2DE is also capable of giving detailed information about regional systolic function (6) and offers reliable measurements of wall thickness and myocardial mass (8, 15, 17), as well as of systolic wall thickening (4), which is a highly specific indicator for myocardial viability. The use of contrast injections into coronary arteries or the aortic root permits assessment of myocardial blood flow in experimental animals: both successful delineation the underperfused zone (1), as well as estimation of the magnitude of regional myocardial blood flow (10) have been demonstrated. Because of the ability of 2DE to observe beat to beat changes and to perform serial noninvasive studies, it has been applied in a number of studies to evaluate the effects of coronary sinus interventions on ventricular function, as well as to study the mechanisms of coronary sinus interventions.

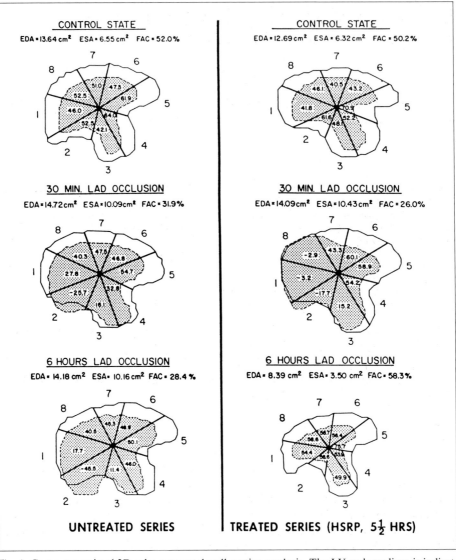

Fig. 1. Computer-assisted 2D echo segmental wall motion analysis. The LV endocardium is indicated in end-diastole (continuous line) and in end-systole (dashed line). Each cross-sectional area was subdivided into 8 equally distributed segments, and segmental areas automatically calculated by the computer. FAC was calculated for the entire cross-section as well as for individual segments (1 through 8), according to the formula: FAC = (EDA − ESA)/EDA × 100. Untreated (top left) and HSRP treated dogs (top right) during preocclusion control state, showing normal FAC for the overall section and its sub-segments; 30 minutes after LAD coronary occlusion and prior to treatment, segmental wall motion abnormalities developed in the anteroseptal region in both series, coupled with increased global section ESA and reduced FAC. Marked improvement in wall motion is seen in the dog treated with HSRP (bottom right panel) during maintained LAD occlusion from 30 minutes to 6 hours; also note the significant reduction in chamber size, in contrast with the untreated dog (bottom left panel) which exhibited further functional deterioration in corresponding LV regions (Segments 1, 2, and 3),

EDA: end-diastolic area; ESA: end-systolic area; FAC: fractional area change; HSRP: hypothermic synchronized retroperfusion; LAD: left anterior descending coronary artery. Reproduced from Haendchen et al. in (7), p. 399.

Retroperfusion

Synchronized coronary venous retroperfusion initiated 30 minutes after occlusion of the left anterior descending coronary artery, has been shown to alter global and regional left ventricular function (12, 19), as compared to untreated controls. As illustrated in Figure 1, a number of changes occur with SRP.

For reasons that are currently not well understood, EDV generally decreases after institution of SRP, not only compared to the untreated control group, but also compared to initial EDV prior to coronary occlusion. The decrease in ESV is even greater, resulting in an ejection fraction that is significantly higher than in the untreated group, but is slightly diminished compared to the baseline state.

This increase in ejection fraction is directly due to an improvement of regional wall motion in the segments rendered ischemic by coronary occlusion, as evidenced by improved fractional area change. In addition, return of systolic wall thickening has been reported even in some instances when systolic thinning had initially been seen after LAD occlusion.

Similar findings have been obtained by other means of experimentally measuring regional myocardial contractility, such as implanted ultrasonic crystals (3).

These observations suggest a direct beneficial effect of SRP on canine ischemic myocardium in the setting of LAD occlusion.

SRP may also play a role in the prevention of reperfusion injury that is caused by restoration of arterial blood flow, as shown in another dog study (5), where the proximal LAD was occluded for 3 hours and then reperfused for 7 days. SRP was applied from 30 minutes up to 3 hours of the occlusion period. After 7 days ejection fraction was higher in the treated group ($55 \pm 5\%$, as compared to $43 \pm 7\%$ for controls), as was fractional area change (at mid-papillary level $40 \pm 17\%$ vs. $11 \pm 20\%$ for controls) and systolic wall thickening (at mid-papillary level $25 \pm 24\%$ vs. $-2 \pm 17\%$ for controls). Because SRP apparently delays the evolution of myocardial necrosis, its application may be beneficial in the setting of acute infarction before achieving surgical or nonsurgical reperfusion.

2DE has also been utilized to study the effectiveness of different modes of SRP in relation to each other. Thus hypothermic SRP was shown to be superior to SRP with warm blood (7), as manifested by greater improvement of global and ischemic regional left ventricular function, although both modalities resulted in improved function compared to untreated controls.

Pressure-controlled intermittent coronary sinus occlusion

Fewer echocardiographic data are available regarding the effects of pressure-controlled intermittent coronary sinus occlusion (PICSO) on ventricular function. One study (14) applied PICSO for 2.5 hours between 30 minutes and 3 hours of proximal LAD occlusion. Fractional area change in all severely ischemic segments was $-4.0 \pm 4.7\%$ at 30 minutes after occlusion, and increased to $7.0 \pm 3.3\%$ with 150 minutes of treatment. At the most extensively involved low papillary muscle level, regional ischemic fractional area change was increased from -0.4 ± 0.1 to $14.4 \pm 4\%$, whereas a further deterioration was noted in untreated dogs with coronary occlusion.

Assessment of distribution of retrograde injections

In addition to retrograde infusion of blood by SRP, attempts are being made to utilize the coronary venous system as an alternate route for delivery of pharmacological interventions. Initial results with retrograde infusion of cardioplegic solution (13) and procainamide (9) appear promising and suggest that this route may have advantages over application via the arterial pathway.

The ability of coronary venous injections to actually reach myocardial regions rendered ischemic by LAD occlusion could be demonstrated by contrast echocardiography (11). Sonicated Renografin-76 was injected retrogradely via a balloon catheter which was wedged inside the great cardiac vein to prevent backflow of the injectate to the coronary sinus. Retrograde injections after LAD occlusion in 7 dogs resulted in transmural myocardial opacification which occupied $42.8 \pm 8.6\%$ of the LV cross-sectional circumference. Opacification always included the entire ischemic zone ($30 \pm 6.3\%$ of the of myocardial circumference, as determined by left main coronary artery contrast injections) and extended into adjacent nonischemic myocardium. Extensive shunting to the right atrium, right ventricle and left ventricle via the Thebesian circulation was seen. Attempts to penetrate into myocardium subserved by the circumflex coronary artery have so far been unsuccessful, presumably because large veno-venous shunts, which prevented the necessary build-up of intravascular pressure in this particular area.

Coronary venous contrast 2DE may help define regions of myocardium that are accessible to retrograde interventions and could therefore potentially serve as an early indicator for the success of such interventions in individual patients.

Assessment by Doppler echocardiography

So far, little has been done to evaluate coronary sinus interventions by Doppler echocardiography. This method could be utilized to study the instantaneous effects of these interventions on left ventricular stroke volume, as evidenced by changes in aortic flow velocity curves. Mitral inflow patterns can provide information about changes in left ventricular diastolic compliance. In addition, Doppler can provide information about the effects of interventions on valvular regurgitation.

Using the newest technology, Doppler color flow mapping, we have been able to directly visualize coronary sinus flow (Figure 2), and may ultimately be able to perform quantitative assessment.

Conclusion

2DE provides assessment of effects of coronary sinus interventions on global and regional LV function and offers information about penetration and regional distribution of retrograde injectates. The noninvasive nature of 2DE and its ability to study beat to beat changes suggest its utility for future clinical assessment of coronary sinus interventions.

400

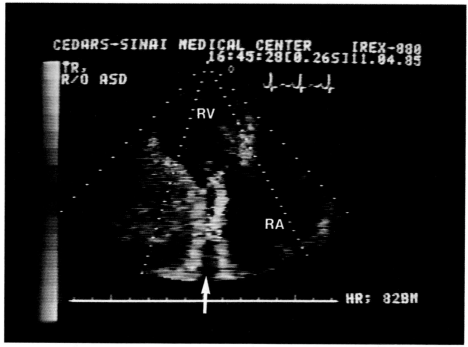

Fig. 2. Visualization of human coronary sinus flow by color Doppler echocardiography. This technology allows for nonivasive imaging of intracardiac blood flow, displayed superimposed on the 2D echocardiogram. Flow toward the transducer is shown as red (or orange), flow away from the transducer as blue. The color intensity corresponds to flow velocity. In this systolic frame the coronary sinus (arrow) is seen entering the right atrium. Coronary sinus flow is seen as an orange jet, which appears directed toward the closed tricuspid valve. RA: right atrium; RV: right ventricular outflow tract.

Acknowledgements

The author would like to thank Drs. Roberto Haendchen and Eliot Corday for supplying Figure 1.

References

1. Armstrong WF, Mueller TM, Kinney E, Tickner EG, Dillon JC, Feigenbaum H (1982) Assessment of myocardial perfusion abnormalities with contrast-enhanced two-dimensional echocardiography. Circulation 66: 166–174
2. Carr KW, Engler RL, Forsythe JR, Johnson AD, Gosink B (1979) Measurement of left ventricular ejection fraction by mechanical cross-sectional echocardiography. Circulation 59: 1196–1205
3. Farcot JC, Berdeaux A, Giudicelli JF, Vilaine JP, Bourdarias JP (1983) Diastolic synchronized retroperfusion versus reperfusion: effects on regional left ventricular function and myocardial blood flow during acute coronary occlusion in dogs. Am J Cardiol 51: 1414–1421
4. Fenely MP, Hickie JB (1984) Validity of echocardiographic determination of left ventricular systolic wall thickening. Circulation 70: 226–232

401

5. Haendchen RV, Corday E, Meerbaum S, Povzhitkov M, Rit J, Fishbein MC (1983) Prevention of ischemic injury and early reperfusion derangements by hypothermic retroperfusion. J Am Coll Cardiol 1: 1067–1080
6. Haendchen RV, Wyatt HL, Maurer G, Zwehl W, Bear M, Meerbaum S, Corday E (1983) Quantitation of regional cardiac function bt two-dimensional echocardiography. I. Patterns of contraction of the normal left ventricle. Circulation 67: 1234–1245
7. Haendchen RV, Fishbein MC, Meerbaum S, Corday E (1984) Superiority of hypothermic vs. normothermic synchronized coronary venous retroperfusion for protection of acutely ischemic myocardium. In: Mohl W, Wolner E, Glogar D (eds) The Coronary Sinus. Steinkopff Verlag, Darmstadt, pp 392–402
8. Helak JW, Reichek N (1984) Quantitation of left ventricular mass and volume by two-dimensional echocardiography. In vitro anatomic validation. Circulation 63: 1398–1407
9. Karagueuzian H, Ohta M, Drury JK, Fishbein MC, Meerbaum S, Corday E, Mandel WJ, Peter T (1986) Coronary venous retroinfusion of Procainamide: a new approach for the management of spontaneous and inducible sustained ventricular tachycardia during myocardial infarction. J Am Coll Cardiol 7: 551–563
10. Maurer G, Ong K, Haendchen R, Torres M, Tei C, Wood F, Meerbaum S, Shah P, Corday E (1984) Myocardial contrast two-dimensional echocardiography: comparison of contrast disappearance rates in normal and underperfused myocardium. Circulation 69: 418–429
11. Maurer G, Punzengruber C, Haendchen RV, Torres MAR, Heublein B, Meerbaum S, Corday E (1984) Retrograde coronary venous contrast echocardiography: assessment of shunting and delineation of regional myocardium in the normal and ischemic canine heart. J Am Coll Cardiol 4: 577–586
12. Meerbaum S, Haendchen RV, Corday E, Povzhitkov M, Fishbein MC, Rit JY, Lang TW, Uchiyama T, Aosaki N, Broffman J (1982) Hypothermic coronary venous phased retroperfusion: a closed chest treatment of acute regional myocardial ischemia. Circulation 65: 1435–1445
13. Menasche P, Kural S, Fauchet M, Lavergne A, Commin P, Bercot M, Touchot B, Georgiopoulos G, Piwnica A (1982) Retrograde coronary sinus perfusion: As a safe alternative for ensuring cardioplegic delivery in aortic valve surgery. Ann Thorac Surg 34: 647–659
14. Mohl W, Punzengruber C, Moser M, Kenner T, Heimisch W, Haendchen R, Meerbaum S, Maurer G, Corday E (1985) Effects of pressure-controlled intermittent coronary sinus occlusion on regional ischemic function. J Am Coll Cardiol 5: 939–947
15. Reichek N, Helak J, Plappert TA, St. John Sutton MG, Weber KT (1983) Anatomic validation of left ventricular mass estimates from clinical two-dimensional echocardiography: Initial results. Circulation 67: 348–352
16. Schiller NB, Acquatella H, Ports TA, Drew D, Goerke J, Ringertz H, Silverman NH, Brundage B, Botwinick EH, Boswell R, Carlsson E, Parmley WW (1979) Left ventricular volume from paired biplane two-dimensional echocardiography. Circulation 60: 547–555
17. Wyatt HL, Heng MK, Meerbaum S, Hestenes JD, Cobo JM, Davidson RM, Corday E (1979) Cross-sectional echocardiography. I. Analysis of mathematic models for quantifying the mass of the left ventricle in dogs. Circulation 60: 1104–1113
18. Wyatt HL, Meerbaum S, Heng MK, Gueret P, Corday E (1980) Cross-sectional echocardiography. III. Analysis of mathematic models for quantifying volume of symmetric and asymmetric left ventricles. Am Heart J 100: 821–829
19. Yamazaki S, Drury JK, Meerbaum S, Corday E (1985) Synchronized coronay venous retroperfusion: Prompt improvement of left ventricular function in experimental myocardial ischemia. J Am Coll Cardiol 5: 655–663

Author's address:
Gerald Maurer, M.D.
Division of Cardiology
Cedars-Sinai Medical Center
8700 Beverly Boulevard
Los Angeles, CA 90048
U.S.A.

Concluding remarks on coronary sinus interventions in cardiology

Thomas J. Ryan

Boston University Medical Center, Boston, MA (U.S.A.)

Following this 2nd International Symposium on Myocardial Protection via the Coronary Sinus it seems abundantly clear that the cardiologist of today has long neglected a true understanding of the physiology of the venous circulation of the heart. From these proceedings it seems equally clear that the retrograde interventions utilizing synchronized diastolic retroperfusion with arterial blood, pressure controlled intermittent coronary sinus occlusion and retroinfusion of pharmacologic agents hold brilliant promise for protecting the ischemic myocardium.

Since he now plays a central role in revascularizing the myocardium either by the use of thrombolytic agents in the setting of acute infarction or performing balloon angioplasty in both the acute and chronic setting, it is imperative that today's cardiologist not only expand his awareness of reperfusion injury but also devise new means of protecting ischemic myocardium during his nonoperative procedures.

We have absorbed the brilliant studies relating to the complex reflexes originating in the venous system presented at these meetings and we have had lucid presentations of the measurable benefit of SRP and PICSO in the experimental animal. The clinical and experimental data relating to retroinfusion of cardioplegia shows continued promise. It seems both timely and attractively simple for the cardiologist to return his focus to the readily accessible right side of the heart and exploit the access provided by the coronary sinus and great cardiac veins to that fragile territory we all know so well, the metabolizing myocardium.

Author's address:
Thomas J. Ryan, M.D.
Boston University Medical Center
Boston, MA 02118
U.S.A.

Coronary sinus interventions during cardiac surgery

H. L. Lazar and A. J. Roberts,
Department of Cardiothoracic Surgery, University Hospital, Boston, MA
(U.S.A.)

In recent years, coronary sinus interventions during cardiac surgery have included techniques directed toward retrograde infusion of cardioplegic solutions. Retrograde cardioplegic infusion may provide more uniform cardioplegic delivery than the antegrade method especially in the presence of multiple coronary artery stenoses. The retrograde technique avoids trauma to the coronary arteries and results in minimal interference with the performance of surgery. The limitations of this technique include the potential for inadequate preservation of the right ventricle because of the lack of venous communications to the coronary sinus, the potential for coronary venous injuries and a higher incidence of supraventricular arrhythmias, heart block, and other conduction abnormalities in the perioperative period. Another limitation is the necessity for an extra suture line in the right atrium to insert the catheter. These potential limitations have limited the use of coronary sinus retroperfusion in clinical practice at this time.

Pressure-controlled intermittent coronary sinus occlusion (PICSO) has emerged as another potential coronary sinus intervention during cardiac surgery. PICSO has been shown to significantly reduce both infarct size and myocardium at risk following periods of coronary artery occlusion in experimental animals. Possible mechanisms to explain the improvements seen with PICSO include retroperfusion of the ischemic zone and enhanced washout of toxic metabolites formed during ischemia. The effects of PICSO following a period of global ischemia on cardiopulmonary bypass (CPB) are presently undefined. Dr. Werner Mohl of Vienna has successfully performed PICSO in patients on cardiopulmonary bypass following periods of ischemic cardioplegic arrest without complications. His results are preliminary but seem to suggest some improvement in the PICSO group. His favorable findings and the improvements seen with PICSO following regional ischemia prompted us to undertake an experimental study to determine whether PICSO could reverse reperfusion damage following a period of ischemic arrest on CPB.

We placed fourteen pigs on CPB and subjected them to 2 hours of ischemic arrest with multidose, potassium, crystalloid cardioplegia supplemented with topical and systemic ($28\,°C$) hypothermia. During arrest, the mid left anterior descending coronary artery (LAD) was occluded with a snare which was released immediately following aortic unclamping. Seven pigs underwent PICSO for 60 minutes following aortic unclamping; while seven others served as controls. The PICSO group had the best recovery of ejection (33 ± 6 vs. $50 \pm 2\%$ $p < 0.01$), the highest stroke work index (0.61 ± 0.05 vs. 0.87 ± 0.07 g-m/kg $p < 0.01$) and higher pH values in the area beyond the LAD occlusion (6.67 ± 0.05 vs. 6.99 ± 0.06 $p < 0.01$) when final measurements were made after 60 minutes of reperfusion. Our data along with Dr. Mohl's preliminary clinical results suggest that PICSO may play an important role in reversing reperfusion injury following cardioplegic arrest during cardiac surgery. Its ability to reduce infarct size following coronary occlusion and its beneficial effects following cardioplegic arrest may make PICSO an important intervention in patients with acute coronary ischemia. Further studies are underway in our laboratory to determine the effects of PICSO during cardioplegic arrest and to further define its potential role during cardiac surgery. For example, during hypothermic potassium cardioplegic arrest, PICSO may improve cardioplegic distribution toward ischemic areas. Consequently, regional pH may be preserved at a higher level and myocardial hypothermia at a lower temperature. These changes may also be associated with improved left ventricular performance following reperfusion. Proof of these relationships awaits further experiments employing PICSO-supported antegrade cardioplegic delivery.

Authors' address:
Harald L. Lazar, M.D.
Department of Cardiothoracic Surgery
University Hospital
Boston, MA 02118
U.S.A.

Concluding remarks on interventions perioperatively

A. S. Wechsler

Division of General and Thoracic Surgery, Duke University Medical Center, Durham, N.C. (U.S.A.)

My task is to summarize some of the perioperative concepts of CSI and problems that might lend themselves to these approaches. If everything were ideal in the setting of cardiac surgery, there would be little need to apply adjunctive measures to the currently available techniques mentioned by Dr. Roberts. However, as identified by Dr. Weisel (see this volume pp 169–174), there exists a strong metabolic deficit in the early moments following even carefully planned and highly elective surgery. These very moments might be particularly likely to benefit from CSI. I assume that an intervention during this time, using a technology – perhaps less invasive than those primarily designed to unload the myocardium but yet likely to enhance metabolic performance of the myocardium by modifying regional flow factors – might be a potential application holding great promise in the delivery of rapid metabolic recovery following operation. I assume that this could either take the form of PICSO or that of regional synchronized retroperfusion to deliver, not antiarrhythmics, as has been done by the group in Los Angeles, but precursors of high energy metabolism, which, owing to their profound systemic effects, have been very difficult to deliver directly into the arterial system. Probably, such an approach would, in fact, permit delivery of very high concentrations to regions of the myocardium from which these substances have been depleted. Likewise this might allow for a more rapid regeneration of high energy phosphate stores.

The area, however, where I see these techniques most applicable, is an area which I perceive from my own practice within the United States as evolving rapidly. At present, 60% of the cardiac surgical practice at our institution and at many others is related to treatment of conditions requiring urgent or emergency revascularization procedures. As a consequence of the highly aggressive approach to coronary artery disease and myocardial infarction taken by the cardiologist it is clearly accepted now that early revascularization of acutely occluded vessels provides myocardial salvage. The six hour magical time that has been placed on it I regard as highly arbitrary, and in human beings as compared to animal models, not yet adequately established by testing. These "six hours" are based on currently available technology. But as the technology for improving regional perfusion improves, the time-span permissible for revascularization, be it chemical or medical interventional, such as PCTA (percutaneous transluminal angioplasty) or by surgery, is clearly going to be extended.

A typical practice in a very contemporary community would be for an acute myocardial infarction patient, seen by his family physician, to receive a large intravenous dose of streptokinase, to be given emergency transport to a hospital prepared to receive such patients, to have visualization of this coronary bed and to have interventional opening of that vessel. (Even though this is controversial we know that only 60% of lesions are generally opened with streptokinase, the rate being perhaps slightly higher with specific plasminogen activator.) Many patients, of course, are not candidates for interventional opening of the vessel, and others have severe vessel disease which cannot be treated in that manner. However, in our setting all such patients would, in fact, be subjected to an emergency operation. If some means of interim support providing improvement of perfusion of the myocardium could be routinely provided, one could imagine that these patients would come to the operating room with far greater potential for myocardial salvage since it is extremely difficult for the cardiac surgeon to do anything better than that with which he is presented. In operational settings with regions of extremely poor highy-energy phosphate stores to start with for example, it is predictable, and almost guaranteed, that these regions of myocardium will tend to have poor function and metabolism also in the immediate and perhaps subsequent perioperative time.

If I were to paint an even broader scenario with a glimpse of the future I could also conceive that the technology of coronary sinus catheter implantation would become so routine and so easy that in concert with the administration of a thrombolytic agent such catheters could well be inserted by intensivists at community hospitals, and used during transport of patients to major surgical centers where further interventional therapy would be used. It is precisely in this setting that a device such as PICSO, which requires no arterial intervention and hence does not interfere in any way with obstructed arteries, and which allows very easy and rapid insertion and does not require infusion of any substance, could be employed as an efficient and potent interim measure. Given such an approach it will be entirely unpredictable to which point the time of revascularization with minimalization of cardiac injury might yet be extended, which I think is the gold standard for which we are all striving.

The one setting in which I could imagine an appropriate clinical study to begin is the setting of coronary arteries – whether in acutely ill patients or patients electively undergoing angioplasty – which occlude acutely and cannot be opened in the interventional laboratory. In our experience this cluster of patients virtually always does well with surgery. However, every patient seen in that setting develops full progression of his acute myocardial infarction on his electrocardiogram and a significant enzyme release, which, in my mind, provides an ideal opportunity for an intervention to be performed.

Comment by Prof. Tom Ryan

Certainly, in the United States the scenario Dr. Wechsler just pictured is increasingly occurring, and thrombolytic therapy and early reperfusion of the acutely occluded coronary artery are well established in the community today. I think just the fact that PICSO as applied has been shown to reduce infarct size in acute settings is a reason to go forward immediately with that study. The most recent data from the United States report 90,000 PTCAs performed in 1985; 63,000 were performed in 1984. We are now established as interventionalists, and I think that the time for the potential of these coronary sinus interventions has certainly come even though we do not yet have a definite answer to what the future will actually hold for them.

Author's address:
Professor A. S. Wechsler
Department of General and Thoracic Surgery
Duke University Medical Center
P.O. Box 3174
Durham, N.C. 27710
U.S.A.

408

Summary statement

A. J. Roberts

University Hospital, Boston (U.S.A.)

There is an increasing interest in coronary sinus interventions related to cardiac surgery. This has become obvious since the first international symposium on coronary sinus interventions some two years ago. At the present meeting, there is abundant evidence that coronary sinus research is thriving. This observation is supported by the many clinical trials with retroperfusion during cardiac surgery occurring in Europe. In addition, the first clinical trial with pressure controlled intermittent coronary sinus occlusion (PICSO) has been recorded from the second surgical clinic at the University of Vienna. In the United States of America, there has been abundant research activity related to coronary sinus interventions. Furthermore, we have been presented with the results of a USA survey showing as many as 25% of surgeons are willing to try coronary venous bypass grafting in certain selected cases undergoing myocardial revascularization.

In terms of retroperfusion via the coronary sinus during cardiac surgery, there are several apparent advantages to this technique during valvular surgery. For example, this route of retrograde delivery of cardioplegia leaves an uncluttered field for the surgical team. In addition, the retrograde method should decrease the incidence of iatrogenic coronary ostial lesions related to direct cannulization procedures. In operations for coronary artery diseases, in theory, many of the limitations of heterogeneous myocardial protection, offered by the delivery of aortic root cardioplegia, can be overcome by the retrograde delivery technique.

It appears that myocardial cooling, maintenance of myocardial high-energy phosphate stores and fatty acid metabolism as well as myocardial functional recovery are preserved by the retrograde perfusion technique at least as well as by the conventional antegrade method. However, the reports that we have heard at this meeting describing vascular endothelial injury and myocardial edema as well as occasional gross disruption of the coronary sinus related to coronary sinus cannulation are alarming. What remains to be seen is whether changes in catheter design, further clinical experience with catheter insertion and better understanding of pressure-volume relationships in the coronary sinus during cardioplegic arrest will allow the surgeon to decrease the occurrence of such complications. However, it is noteworthy that the addition of pulsatile cardioplegic delivery by the coronary sinus appears to offer some physiologic advantage compared to continuous or intermittent non-pulsatile delivery modes. Consequently, it would appear appropriate for surgeons to have familiarity with a retrograde cardioplegic delivery technique as part of the surgical armamentarium for achieving myocardial protection. For example, certain cases of valvular heart disease or more extensive, diffuse, coronary artery disease might lend themselves to preferential advantage with retrograde cardioplegic techniques as compared to antegrade measures. Furthermore, the combined usage of both antegrade and retrograde cardioplegic delivery modalities might give additional myocardial protection during and following global myocardial ischemia. Certainly, the time to complete diastolic arrest after aortic cross-clamping is less with antegrade cardioplegia and cardioplegic delivery distal to proximal coronary artery improved by retrograde infusion.

Furthermore, certain "high-risk" patients like those with evolving myocardial necrosis might be a sub-group of patients which could be expected to have a greater chance of benefit by retroperfusion modalities.

Such patients might be treated preoperatively by synchronized retroperfusion in a coronary care unit and, later, during the operative procedure by retrograde cardioplegic delivery during aortic cross-clamping utilizing the same catheter positioned preoperatively. In this fashion, the patient might potentially benefit from pre-operative clinical stabilization and additive intra-operative myocardial protection with minimal interference with the conduct of surgery.

In terms of right atrial cardioplegia, the group from the Hôpital Broussais in Paris has suggested benefit using this atrial delivery technique in comparison to the direct coronary sinus cannulation method. However, the overt distension of the right heart chambers during the right atrial infusions is a concern. We have heard during this meeting that such distension or other characteristics associated with right atrial cardioplegic infusions may be associated with some subsequent functional myocardial damage or metabolic derangements. Although the right atrial delivery technique appears easier to employ than direct coronary sinus cannulation methods, further studies are necessary to insure that early and late results following the right atrial technique are comparable to other more conventional cardioplegic methods.

The use of PICSO during the reperfusion period immediately following global myocardial ischemia continues to be intriguing. Although the precise mechanism associated with the beneficial results of PICSO therapy during and following myocardial ischemia remain to be defined, increasing experimental evidence suggest beneficial defects of PICSO treatment. The initial clinical application of PICSO during cardiac surgery has been to minimize reperfusion injury. Dr. Werner Mohl has reported at this meeting that the initial clinical studies in Vienna, employing PICSO during a 1 hour period following global myocardial ischemia during uncomplicated coronary bypass graft surgery, have been completed. His results show that the technique is relatively safe and that the patient's clinical course is uncomplicated. In addition, there is a suggestion that regional changes in left ventricular wall motion are better preserved when PICSO is added to the reperfusion period. My associate, Dr. Harold Lazar, has applied PICSO during reperfusion in a coronary occlusion model in the experimental laboratory. Two-dimensional echocardiography was employed to assess left ventricular performance. We chose a two hour period of global myocardial ischemia with a temporary left anterior descending coronary artery occlusion during this time. Myocardial ischemic injury was minimized by the application of a multidose hypothermic, hyperkalemic cardioplegic method during aortic cross-clamping. Topical hypothermia and mild systemic hypothermia were also employed. After the aortic cross-clamp was released in these experiments, the LAD occlusion was removed and half of the group was treated by PICSO therapy during 60 minutes of reperfusion. The other half of the entire group did not receive PICSO during reperfusion. We found that left ventricular compliance was similar between PICSO and control groups, but left ventricular performance curves and ejection fraction measurements were better after PICSO mediated reperfusion. In addition, regional measurements of myocardial pH were better maintained in the PICSO group as compared to control animals. Preliminary work by Dr. Lazar also suggests that in this experimental swine model, PICSO treatment during antegrade, crystalloid, potassium, cardioplegia may be better than antegrade cardioplegia alone. Presumably, better cardioplegic distribution occurs related to a PICSO effect. Nevertheless, further work is necessary before this relationship is confirmed.

In summary, the experimental and clinical observations provided at this meeting offer a strong basis for the potential value of further clinical and experimental efforts. Newer, and more sensitive, techniques described at this meeting for assessing hemodynamic, metabolic and structural changes involving the myocardium during the perioperative period have been reported. These methods undoubtedly will allow a greater discrimination of the potential benefits from the various myocardial protective techniques presented during this symposium. Nevertheless, it is doubtful that many of the "low-risk" patients undergoing cardiac surgery will show clear-cut benefit from coronary sinus interventions. The reason for this bias is that the current level of myocardial protection during open heart surgery, although imperfect, is sufficiently well defined to allow for adequate myocardial protection at a low operative risk for most patients. However, "high-risk" patients, such as those with active, evolving, myocardial necrosis might potentially benefit from one or more of the various coronary sinus related interventions. In my opinion, it would be justified to proceed with clinical trials in patients with acute myocardial ischemia or otherwise "high-risk" preoperative conditions. I would suggest that the close coordination between the interventional cardiologist and cardiac surgeon could lead to the successful application of coronary sinus interventions to promote myocardial salvage in groups of patients who are at a relatively high risk of evolving myocardial damage perioperatively.

Author's address:
A. J. Roberts, M.D.
University Hospital
75 East Newton Street
Boston, Mass. 02118
U.S.A.

411

Author Index

The Coronary Sinus

Proceedings of the 1ˢᵗ International Symposium on Myocardial Protection Via the Coronary Sinus Vienna, February 27-29, 1984

W. MOHL / E. WOLNER / D. GLOGAR (eds.)

1984. 560 pages, extensively illustrated with figures and tables.
Cloth DM 140,–; US $ 63.00
ISBN 3-7985-0634-4 (Steinkopff)
ISBN 0-387-91250-9 (Springer-Verlag New York)

Contents: 1. Anatomy and Pathophysiology of Venous System. 2. Interventions Using the Coronary Sinus Route: Intraoperative Protection Via the Coronary Sinus − Basic Physiology on Retroperfusion and Coronary Sinus Occlusion − Intermittent Coronary Sinus Occlusion Modalities − Synchronized Retroperfusion Modalities.

This book is the first to deal with the coronary sinus as an alternative access route, as part of the heart-vein system, to the diseased heart muscle.

Not only are the scientific fundamentals from biophysics, biochemistry, computer science and anatomy discussed, the latest perspectives in coronary venous anatomy and physiology, as well as technical aspects of measurements and pump systems are also dealt with. The principal aim of the book is to describe the types of interventions currently being developed which have been proved valid to protect ischemic myocardium. The papers give an account of the results from the latest experimental and clinical research. The book also focuses on techniques such as retrograde coronary sinus perfusion and coronary sinus occlusion. Of special importance are the papers on intermittent occlusion and synchronized retroperfusion modalities.

These proceedings address basic scientists in microcirculation, cardiologists, cardiac surgeons, pathologists, physiologists, anatomists, and students, for whom retroperfusion techniques via the coronary sinus may have great clinical potential.

Distribution in US and Canada through Springer-Verlag, 175 Fifth Avenue, New York, NY 10010; for other countries through your bookseller or directly from Dr. Dietrich Steinkopff Verlag, P. O. Box 11 1008, 6100 Darmstadt/West Germany.

Steinkopff Verlag Darmstadt
Springer-Verlag New York